Hartman's Nursing Assistant Care
The Basics

Hartman Publishing, Inc.
with Jetta Fuzy, RN, MS

FOURTH EDITION

hartmanonline.com

Hartman

ii

Credits

Managing Editor
Susan Alvare Hedman

Designer
Kirsten Browne

Cover Illustrator
Jo Tronc

Production
Thad Castillo

Photography
Matt Pence, Pat Berrett, Art Clifton, and Dick Ruddy

Proofreaders
Kristin Calderon, Kristin Cartwright, Melanie Futrell, and Eliza Martin

Sales/Marketing
Deborah Rinker, Kendra Robertson, Erika Walker, and Belinda Midyette

Customer Service
Fran Desmond, Thomas Noble, Angela Storey, Eliza Martin, and Col Foley

Warehouse Coordinator
Chris Midyette

Copyright Information

Notice to Readers

Though the guidelines and procedures contained in this text are based on consultations with healthcare professionals, they should not be considered absolute recommendations. The instructor and readers should follow employer, local, state, and federal guidelines concerning healthcare practices. These guidelines change, and it is the reader's responsibility to be aware of these changes and of the policies and procedures of his or her healthcare facility.

The publisher, authors, editors, and reviewers cannot accept any responsibility for errors or omissions or for any consequences from application of the information in this book and make no warranty, express or implied, with respect to the contents of the book. The publisher does not warrant or guarantee any of the products described herein or perform any analysis in connection with any of the product information contained herein.

Special Thanks

A heartfelt thank you goes to our insightful and wonderful reviewers, listed in alphabetical order:

Theresa J. DeBon, RN, BS
Tulsa, OK

Ruth Hardke, RN
Stow, OH

Charles Illian, RN, BSN, Infection Preventionist
Orlando, FL

Marie Johnston, RN
Harrisburg, PA

Sally Lyle, RN, BSN
Rock Hill, SC

Wendy Pickard-Tanios, RN, BS, ONC
Round Rock, TX

Christine A. Smith, RN, MSN
Poquoson, VA

We are very appreciative of the many sources who shared their informative photos with us:

- Briggs Corporation
- Detecto
- Dreamstime
- Exergen Corporation
- Harrisburg Area Community College
- Dr. James Heilman
- Hollister Incorporated
- Invacare Corporation
- Medline Industries
- National Pressure Ulcer Advisory Panel
- North Coast Medical, Inc.
- Nova Medical Products
- RG Medical Diagnostics of Wixom, MI
- Starkey Hearing Technologies
- Vancare, Inc.
- Welch Allyn

Gender Usage

This textbook utilizes the pronouns *he*, *his*, *she*, and *her* interchangeably to denote healthcare team members and residents.

Please email corrections and suggestions to editor@hartmanonline.com.

Contents

Procedure	Page

Procedures

Procedure	Page

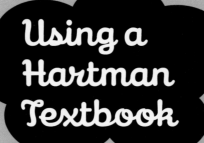

Using a Hartman Textbook

Understanding how this book is organized and what its special features are will help you make the most of this resource!

We have assigned each chapter its own colored tab. Each colored tab contains the chapter number and title, and it is on the side of every page.

1. List examples of legal and ethical behavior

Everything in this book, the student workbook, and the instructor's teaching material is organized around learning objectives. A learning objective is a very specific piece of knowledge or a very specific skill. After reading the text, if you can do what the learning objective says, you know you have mastered the material.

bloodborne pathogens

Bold key terms are located throughout the text, followed by their definitions. They are also listed in the glossary at the back of this book.

Making an occupied bed

All care procedures are highlighted by the same black bar for easy recognition.

Guidelines: Preventing Falls

Guidelines and Observing and Reporting lists are colored green for easy reference.

Residents' Rights
Abuse and Alzheimer's Disease
...ase may b

These boxes teach important information on how to support and promote Residents' Rights.

Beginning and ending steps in care procedures

For most care procedures, these steps should be performed. Understanding why they are important will help you remember to perform each step every time care is provided.

Beginning Steps

Identify yourself by name. Identify the resident by name.

A resident's room is his home. Residents have a right to privacy. Before any procedure, knock and wait for permission to enter the resident's room. Upon entering his room, identify yourself and state your title. Residents have the right to know who is providing their care. Identify and greet the resident. This shows courtesy and respect. It also establishes correct identification. This prevents care from being performed on the wrong person.

Wash your hands.

Handwashing provides for infection prevention. Nothing fights infection in facilities like performing consistent, proper hand hygiene. Handwashing may need to be done more than once during a procedure. Practice Standard Precautions with every resident.

Explain procedure to resident. Speak clearly, slowly, and directly. Maintain face-to-face contact whenever possible.

Residents have a right to know exactly what care you will provide. It promotes understanding, cooperation, and independence. Residents are able to do more for themselves if they know what needs to happen.

Provide for the resident's privacy with a curtain, screen, or door.

Doing this maintains residents' right to privacy and dignity. Providing for privacy in a facility is not simply a courtesy; it is a legal right.

Adjust the bed to a safe level, usually waist high. Lock the bed wheels.

Locking the bed wheels is an important safety measure. It ensures that the bed will not move as you are performing care. Raising the bed helps you to remember to use proper body mechanics. This prevents injury to you and to residents.

Ending Steps

Return bed to lowest position. Remove privacy measures.	Lowering the bed provides for residents' safety. Remove extra privacy measures added during the procedure. This includes anything you may have draped over and around residents, as well as privacy screens.
Place call light within resident's reach.	A call light allows residents to communicate with staff as necessary. It must always be left within the resident's reach. You must respond to call lights promptly.
Wash your hands.	Handwashing is the most important thing you can do to prevent the spread of infection.
Report any changes in resident to the nurse. Document procedure using facility guidelines.	You will often be the person who spends the most time with a resident, so you are in the best position to note any changes in a resident's condition. Every time you provide care, observe the resident's physical and mental capabilities, as well as the condition of his or her body. For example, a change in a resident's ability to dress himself may signal a greater problem. After you have finished giving care, document the care using facility guidelines. Do not record care before it is given. If you do not document the care you gave, legally it did not happen.

In addition to the beginning and ending steps listed above, remember to follow infection prevention guidelines. Even if a procedure in this book does not tell you to wear gloves or other PPE, there may be times when it is appropriate.

A few procedures in this book mention positioning side rails on beds, but most references to side rails have been omitted. This is due to the decline in their use because of risk of injury. Follow your facility's policies regarding side rails.

1
The Nursing Assistant in Long-Term Care

1. Compare long-term care to other healthcare settings

Welcome to the world of health care. Health care happens in many places. Nursing assistants work in many of these settings. In each setting similar tasks will be performed. However, each setting is also unique.

This textbook will focus on long-term care. **Long-term care** (**LTC**) is given in long-term care facilities (LTCFs) for persons who need 24-hour skilled care. **Skilled care** is medically necessary care given by a skilled nurse or therapist; it is available 24 hours a day. It is ordered by a doctor and involves a treatment plan. This type of care is given to people who need a high level of care for ongoing conditions. The term *nursing homes* was once widely used to refer to these facilities. Now they are often known as *long-term care facilities, skilled nursing facilities, rehabilitation centers,* or *extended care facilities.*

People who live in long-term care facilities may be disabled. They are often elderly, but younger adults sometimes require long-term care, too. They may arrive from hospitals or other healthcare settings. Their **length of stay** (the number of days a person stays in a care facility) may be short, such as a few days or months, or longer than six months. Some of these people will have a **terminal illness**. This means that the illness will eventually cause death. Other people may recover and return to their homes or to other care facilities or situations.

Most people who live in long-term care facilities have **chronic** conditions. This means the conditions last a long period of time, even a lifetime. Chronic conditions include physical disabilities, heart disease, and dementia. (Chapters 4 and 5 have more information about these disorders and diseases.) People who live in these facilities are usually referred to as *residents* because the facility is where they reside or live. These places are their homes for the duration of their stay.

People who need long-term care will have different **diagnoses**, or medical conditions determined by a doctor. The stages of illnesses or diseases affect how sick people are and how much care they will need. The jobs of nursing assistants will also vary. This is due to the fact that each person has different symptoms, abilities, and needs.

Other healthcare settings include the following:

Home health care is provided in a person's home (Fig. 1-1). This type of care is also generally given to people who are older and are chronically ill but who are able to and wish to remain at home. Home care may also be needed when a person is weak after a recent hospital stay. Home care includes many of the services offered in other settings.

Fig. 1-1. Home care is performed in a person's home.

Assisted living facilities are residences for people who need some help with daily care, such as showers, meals, and dressing. Help with medications may also be given. People who live in these facilities do not need 24-hour skilled care. Assisted living facilities allow more independent living in a home-like environment. An assisted living facility may be attached to a long-term care facility, or it may stand alone.

Adult day services are for people who need some help and supervision during certain hours, but who do not live in the facility where care is provided. Generally, adult day services are for people who are not seriously ill or disabled. Adult day services can also provide a break for spouses, family members, and friends.

Acute care is 24-hour skilled care given in hospitals and ambulatory surgical centers. It is for people who require short-term, immediate care for illnesses or injuries (Fig. 1-2). People are also admitted for short stays for surgery.

Fig. 1-2. Acute care is performed in hospitals for illnesses or injuries that require immediate care.

Subacute care is care given in a hospital or in a long-term care facility. It is used for people who need less care than for an acute (sudden onset, short-term) illness, but more care than for a chronic (long-term) illness. Treatment usually ends when the condition has stabilized or after the set time for treatment has been completed. The cost is usually less than a hospital but more than long-term care.

Outpatient care is usually given for less than 24 hours. It is for people who have had treatments or surgery and need short-term skilled care.

Rehabilitation is care given by specialists. Physical, occupational, and speech therapists restore or improve function after an illness or injury. Chapter 9 has information about rehabilitation.

Hospice care is given in facilities or homes for people who have about six months or less to live. Hospice workers give physical and emotional care and comfort. They also support families. Information about hospice care can be found in Chapter 3.

2. Describe a typical long-term care facility

Long-term care facilities (LTCFs) are businesses that provide skilled nursing care 24 hours a day. These facilities may offer assisted living housing, dementia care, or subacute care. Some facilities offer specialized care. Others care for all types of residents. The typical long-term care facility offers personal care for all residents and focused care for residents with special needs. Personal care includes bathing, skin, nail and hair care, and assistance with walking, eating, dressing, transferring, and toileting. All of these daily personal care tasks are called **activities of daily living**, or **ADLs**. Other common services offered at these facilities include the following:

- Physical, occupational, and speech therapy

- Wound care

- Care of different types of tubes, such as catheters (thin tubes inserted into the body to drain fluids or inject fluids)

- Nutrition therapy

- Management of chronic diseases, such as Alzheimer's disease, AIDS, diabetes, chronic obstructive pulmonary disease (COPD), cancer, and congestive heart failure (CHF)

When specialized care is offered at long-term care facilities, the employees must have special training. Residents with similar needs may be placed in units together. Non-profit companies or for-profit companies can own long-term care facilities.

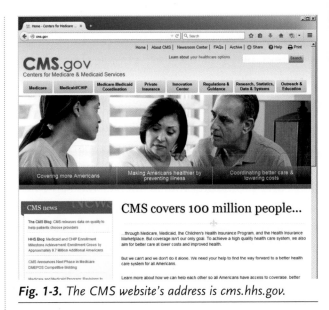

Fig. 1-3. The CMS website's address is cms.hhs.gov.

Residents' Rights

Culture Change and Person-Directed Care
Some long-term care facilities are adopting newer models of care. These models promote meaningful environments with individualized approaches to care. **Culture change** is a term given to the process of transforming services for elders so that they are based on the values and practices of the person receiving care. Culture change involves respecting both elders and those working with them. Core values are promoting choice, dignity, respect, self-determination, and purposeful living. To honor culture change, care settings may need to change their organization practices, physical environments, and relationships. **Person-directed care** emphasizes the individuality of the person who needs care, and seeks to build community by recognizing and developing each person's capabilities. Promoting dignity and providing caring environments is key. The Pioneer Network's website, pioneernetwork.net, and the Eden Alternative's website, edenalt.org, have more information.

3. Explain Medicare and Medicaid

The Centers for Medicare & Medicaid Services (CMS) is a federal agency within the U.S. Department of Health and Human Services (Fig. 1-3). CMS runs two national healthcare programs—Medicare and Medicaid. They both help pay for health care and health insurance for millions of Americans. CMS has many other responsibilities as well.

Medicare is a federal health insurance program that was established in 1965 for people aged 65 or older. It also covers people of any age with permanent kidney failure or certain disabilities. Medicare has four parts. Part A helps pay for care in a hospital or skilled nursing facility or for care from a home health agency or hospice. Part B helps pay for doctor services and other medical services and equipment. Part C allows private health insurance companies to provide Medicare benefits. Part D helps pay for medications prescribed for treatment. Medicare will only pay for care it determines to be medically necessary.

Medicaid is a medical assistance program for low-income people, as well as for people with disabilities. It is funded by both the federal government and each state. Eligibility and coverage varies from state to state and is determined by income and special circumstances. People must qualify for this program.

Medicare and Medicaid pay long-term care facilities a fixed amount for services. This amount is based on the resident's needs upon admission and throughout his stay at the facility.

4. Describe the nursing assistant's role

Nursing assistants can have many different titles. *Nurse aide, certified nurse aide, patient care technician*, and *certified nursing assistant* are some examples. The title given varies by state requirements. This textbook will use the term *nursing assistant*.

Nursing assistants (NAs) perform assigned nursing tasks, such as taking a resident's temperature. Nursing assistants also provide personal care, such as bathing residents and helping with hair care. Promoting independence and self-care are other very important tasks that nursing assistants do. Other nursing assistant duties include the following:

- Helping residents with toileting needs

- Assisting residents to move around safely

- Keeping residents' living areas neat and clean

- Assisting with meals (Fig. 1-4)

- Caring for supplies and equipment

- Helping residents dress

- Making beds

- Giving backrubs

- Helping residents with mouth care

Fig. 1-4. *Helping residents eat and drink is an important part of an NA's job.*

Nursing assistants are not allowed to insert or remove tubes, change sterile dressings, or give tube feedings. Nursing assistants are not allowed to give medications; nurses are responsible for giving medications.

Nursing assistants spend more time with residents than other care team members. They act as the "eyes and ears" of the team. Observing changes in a resident's condition and reporting them is a very important duty of the NA. Residents' care can be revised or updated as conditions change. Another duty of the NA is noting important information about the resident (Fig. 1-5). This is called **charting**, or documenting.

Fig. 1-5. *Observing carefully and reporting accurately are some of the most important duties an NA will have.*

Nursing assistants are part of a team of health professionals. The team includes doctors, nurses, social workers, therapists, dietitians, and specialists. The resident and resident's family are part of the team. Everyone, including the resident, works closely together to meet goals. Goals include helping residents to recover from illnesses and to do as much as possible for themselves.

Residents' Rights

Responsibility for Residents

All residents are the responsibility of each nursing assistant. An NA will receive assignments to perform tasks, care, and other duties for specific residents. If he sees a resident who needs help, even if the resident is not on his assignment sheet, the NA should provide the needed care.

5. Describe the care team and the chain of command

Residents will have different needs and problems. Healthcare professionals with a wide range of education and experience will help care for them. This group is known as the *care team*. Members of the care team include the following:

Nursing Assistant (NA) or Certified Nursing Assistant (CNA): The nursing assistant (NA) performs assigned tasks, such as taking vital signs. The NA also provides or assists with personal care, such as bathing residents and helping with toileting. Nursing assistants must have at least 75 hours of training, and in many states, training exceeds 100 hours.

Registered Nurse (RN): In long-term care, a registered nurse coordinates, manages, and provides skilled nursing care. This includes giving special treatments and medications as prescribed by a doctor. An RN also assigns tasks and supervises daily care of residents by nursing assistants. A registered nurse is a licensed professional who has graduated from a two- to four-year nursing program. RNs have diplomas or college degrees. They have passed a licensing examination. Registered nurses may have additional academic degrees or education in specialty areas.

Licensed Practical Nurse (LPN) or Licensed Vocational Nurse (LVN): A licensed practical nurse or licensed vocational nurse gives medications and treatments. LPNs may also supervise nursing assistants' daily care of residents. An LPN/LVN is a licensed professional who has completed one to two years of education and has passed a licensing examination.

Physician or Doctor (MD [medical doctor] or DO [doctor of osteopathy]): A doctor's job is to diagnose disease or disability and prescribe treatment (Fig. 1-6). Doctors have graduated from four-year medical schools, which they attended after receiving bachelor's degrees. Many doctors also attend specialized training programs after medical school.

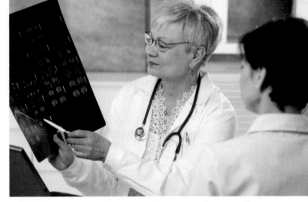

Fig. 1-6. *Doctors diagnose disease and prescribe treatment.*

Physical Therapist (PT or DPT): A physical therapist evaluates a person and develops a treatment plan. Goals are to increase movement, improve circulation, promote healing, reduce pain, prevent disability, and regain or maintain mobility (Fig. 1-7). A PT gives therapy in the form of heat, cold, massage, ultrasound, electrical stimulation, and exercise to muscles, bones, and joints. Physical therapist education programs are mostly offered at the doctoral degree level (doctor of physical therapy, or DPT). Entrance into these programs usually requires an undergraduate degree. Doctoral degree programs usually last three years. PTs have to pass national and state licensure exams before they can practice.

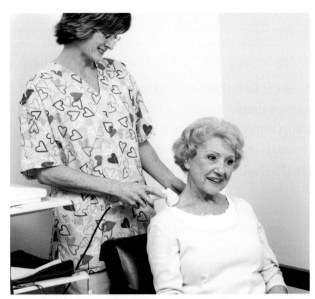

Fig. 1-7. *A physical therapist will help reduce pain and restore specific abilities.*

Occupational Therapist (OT): An occupational therapist helps residents learn to adapt to disabilities. An OT may help train residents to perform activities of daily living (ADLs). This often involves the use of equipment called **assistive** or **adaptive devices**. The OT evaluates the resident's needs and plans a treatment program. Occupational therapists are required to have a minimum of a master's degree. OTs have to pass a national certification examination, and most must be licensed within their state.

Speech-Language Pathologist (SLP): A speech-language pathologist, or speech therapist, identifies communication disorders, addresses factors involved in recovery, and develops a plan of care to meet recovery goals. An SLP teaches exercises to help the resident improve or overcome speech problems. An SLP also evaluates a person's ability to swallow food and drink. Speech-language pathologists are required to have a master's degree in speech-language pathology. Most states require that SLPs be licensed or certified to work.

Registered Dietitian (RDT): A registered dietitian creates diets for residents with special needs. Special diets can improve health and help manage illness. RDTs may supervise the preparation and service of food and educate others about healthy eating habits. Registered dietitians have completed a bachelor's degree. They may also have completed a postgraduate degree. Most states require that RDTs be licensed or certified.

Medical Social Worker (MSW): A medical social worker determines residents' needs and helps get them support services, such as counseling or financial assistance. He or she may help residents obtain clothing and personal items if the family is not involved or does not visit often. A medical social worker may book appointments and transportation. Generally, MSWs hold a master's degree in social work.

Activities Director: The activities director plans activities for residents to help them socialize and stay active. These activities are meant to improve and maintain residents' well-being and to prevent further complications from illness or disability. An activities director may have a bachelor's degree, associate's degree, or qualifying work experience. An activities director may be called a *recreational therapist* depending upon education and experience.

Resident and Resident's Family: The resident is an important member of the care team. The resident has the right to make decisions about his or her own care. The resident helps plan care and makes choices. The resident's family may also be involved in these decisions. The family is a great source of information. They know the resident's personal preferences, history, diet, rituals, and routines.

Residents' Rights

Resident as Member of Care Team
All members of the care team should focus on the resident. The team revolves around the resident and his or her condition, treatment, and progress. Without the resident, there is no care team.

A nursing assistant carries out instructions given to her by a nurse. The nurse is acting on the instructions of a doctor or other member of the care team. This is called the **chain of command**. It describes the line of authority and helps to make sure that residents get proper health care. The chain of command also protects employees and employers from liability. **Liability** is a legal term. It means that someone can be held responsible for harming someone else. For example, imagine that something an NA does for a resident harms that resident. However, what the NA did was in the care plan and was done according to policy and procedure. In that case she may not be liable, or responsible, for hurting the resident. However, if an NA does something not in the care plan that harms a resident, she could be held responsible. That is why it is important for the team to follow instructions in the care plan and for the facility to have a chain of command (Fig. 1-8).

Administrator: manages non-medical aspects of the facility, administers finances, and coordinates policy in consultation with medical professionals

Medical Director (MD): reviews and consults on medical aspects of care, coordinating with attending physicians and nursing staff and encouraging quality care

Director of Nursing (DON): manages the nursing staff at a facility

Assistant Director of Nursing (ADON): assists the DON with management of nursing staff

Staff Development Coordinator: directs the training of employees at a facility

Minimum Data Set (MDS) Coordinator/Resident Assessment Coordinator: manages the assessment of resident needs and delivery of required care in a long-term care facility (usually a specially trained nurse)

Nursing Supervisor: supervises and supports nursing staff of entire facility or multiple nursing units, assisting with resident care as needed

Charge Nurse: supervises and supports nursing staff of a particular unit and treats a limited number of residents

Staff Nurses (RNs, LPNs/LVNs): provide nursing care as prescribed by a physician

Nursing Assistants (NAs, CNAs): perform assigned nursing tasks, assist with routine personal care, and observe and report any changes in residents' conditions and abilities

Other Services

Physical Therapist (PT): administers therapy to increase movement, promote healing, reduce pain, and prevent disability

Occupational Therapist (OT): helps residents learn to adapt to disabilities and trains them to perform ADLs

Speech-Language Pathologist (SLP): identifies communication disorders and swallowing problems and develops a plan of care

Fig. 1-8. The chain of command describes the line of authority and helps ensure that the resident receives proper care.

Nursing assistants must understand what they can and cannot do. This is so that they do not harm residents or involve themselves or their employer in a lawsuit. States certify that nursing assistants are qualified to work. However, nursing assistants are not licensed healthcare providers. Everything they do in their job is assigned by a licensed healthcare professional. They work under the authority of another person's license. That is why these professionals will show great interest in what NAs do and how they do it.

Every state grants the right to practice various jobs in health care through licensure. Examples include a license to practice nursing, medicine, or physical therapy. Each member of the care team works within his or her scope of practice. A **scope of practice** defines the tasks that healthcare providers are allowed to do and how to do them correctly. Laws and regulations on what NAs can and cannot do vary from state to state. It is important that NAs know which tasks are outside their scope of practice and not perform them.

The resident **care plan** is individualized for each resident. It is developed to help achieve the goals of care. A nurse creates the care plan. The resident is also involved in the planning. The care plan lists the tasks that the care team, including NAs, must perform. It states how often these tasks should be performed and how they should be carried out.

The care plan is a guide to help the resident be as healthy as possible. It is critical that NAs make observations and report them to the nurse. Even simple observations can be very important. The information that NAs collect and the changes they observe help determine how care plans may need to change. NAs spend so much time with residents; they are likely to have valuable information that will help in care planning.

6. Define policies, procedures, and professionalism

All facilities have manuals outlining their policies and procedures. A **policy** is a course of action that should be taken every time a certain situation occurs. For example, a very basic policy is that healthcare information must remain confidential. A **procedure** is a method, or way, of doing something. For example, a facility will have a procedure for reporting information about residents. The procedure explains what form to complete, when and how often to fill it out, and to whom it is given. New employees will be told where to find a list of policies and procedures that all staff are expected to follow. Common policies at long-term care facilities include the following:

- All resident information must remain confidential. This is not only a facility rule, it is also the law. More information on confidentiality, including the Health Insurance Portability and Accountability Act (HIPAA) can be found later in the chapter.

- The plan of care must always be followed. **Tasks not listed in the care plan or approved by the nurse should not be performed.**

- Nursing assistants should not do tasks that are not included in the job description.

- Nursing assistants must report important events or changes in residents to a nurse.

- Personal problems must not be discussed with the resident or the resident's family.

- Nursing assistants should not take money or gifts from residents or their families.

- Nursing assistants must be on time for work and must be dependable.

Employers will have policies and procedures for every resident care situation. Written procedures may seem long and complicated, but each step is important. NAs must become familiar with and follow their facility's policies and procedures.

Professional means having to do with work or a job. The opposite of professional is **personal**. It refers to life outside a job, such as family, friends, and home life. **Professionalism** is behaving properly when on the job. It includes dressing appropriately and speaking well. It also includes being on time, completing tasks, and reporting to the nurse. For an NA, professionalism means following the care plan, making careful observations, and reporting accurately. Following policies and procedures is an

important part of professionalism. Residents, coworkers, and supervisors respect employees who behave in a professional way. Professionalism helps people keep their jobs. It may also help them earn promotions and raises.

A professional relationship with residents includes the following:

- Keeping a positive attitude

- Doing only the assigned tasks that are in the care plan and that the NA is trained to do

- Keeping all residents' information confidential

- Being polite and cheerful at all times (Fig. 1-9)

- Not discussing personal problems

- Not using personal cell phones in residents' rooms or in any resident care area

- Not using profanity, even if a resident does

- Listening to the resident

- Calling a resident *Mr., Mrs., Ms.,* or *Miss,* and his or her last name, or by the name he or she prefers. Terms such as *sweetie, honey, dearie,* etc., are disrespectful and should not be used.

- Never giving or accepting gifts

- Always explaining care before providing it

- Following practices, such as handwashing, to protect care providers and residents

Fig. 1-9. Nursing assistants are expected to be polite and cheerful.

A professional relationship with employers includes the following:

- Completing tasks efficiently

- Always following all policies and procedures

- Always documenting and reporting carefully and correctly

- Reporting problems with residents or tasks

- Reporting anything that keeps an NA from completing duties

- Asking questions when the NA does not know or understand something

- Taking directions or criticism without getting upset

- Being clean and neatly dressed and groomed

- Always being on time

- Telling his employer if the NA cannot report for work

- Following the chain of command

- Participating in education programs

- Being a positive role model for the facility

Nursing assistants must be

- **Compassionate:** Being **compassionate** is being caring, concerned, empathetic, and understanding. Demonstrating **empathy** means identifying with the feelings of others. People who are compassionate understand others' problems. They care about them. Compassionate people are also sympathetic. Showing **sympathy** means sharing in the feelings and difficulties of others.

- **Honest:** An honest person tells the truth and can be trusted. Residents need to feel that they can trust those who care for them. The care team depends on honesty in planning care. Employers count on truthful records of care and observations.

- **Tactful:** Being **tactful** means showing sensitivity and having a sense of what is appropriate when dealing with others.

- **Conscientious:** People who are **conscientious** try to do their best. They are guided by a sense of right and wrong. They are alert, observant, accurate, and responsible. Giving conscientious care means making accurate observations and reports, following the care plan, and taking responsibility for actions (Fig. 1-10).

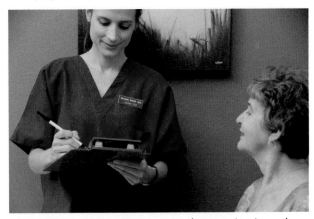

Fig. 1-10. *Nursing assistants must be conscientious about documenting observations.*

- **Dependable:** NAs must be able to make and keep commitments. They must be at work on time. They must skillfully do tasks, avoid too many absences, and help their peers when needed.

- **Patient:** People who are patient do not lose their temper easily. They do not act irritated or complain when things are hard. Residents are often elderly and may be sick or in pain. They may take a long time to do things. They may become upset. Nursing assistants must be patient. They must not rush residents or act annoyed.

- **Respectful:** Being respectful means valuing other people's individuality. This includes their age, religion, culture, feelings, practices, and beliefs. People who are respectful treat others politely and kindly.

- **Unprejudiced:** NAs work with people from many different backgrounds. They must give each resident the same quality care regardless of age, gender, sexual orientation, religion, race, ethnicity, or condition.

- **Tolerant**: Being tolerant means respecting others' beliefs and practices and not judging them. NAs may not like or agree with things that residents or their families do or have done. However, their job is to care for each resident as assigned, not to judge him or her. NAs should put aside their opinions. They should see each resident as an individual who needs their care.

7. List examples of legal and ethical behavior and explain Residents' Rights

Ethics and laws guide behavior. **Ethics** are the knowledge of right and wrong. An ethical person has a sense of duty toward others. He tries to do what is right. **Laws** are rules set by the government to help people live peacefully together and to ensure order and safety. Ethics and laws are very important in health care. They protect people receiving care and guide those giving care. NAs and all care team members should be guided by a code of ethics. They must know the laws that apply to their jobs.

Guidelines: Legal and Ethical Behavior

G   Be honest at all times.

G   Protect residents' privacy and confidentiality. Do not discuss their cases except with other members of the care team.

G   Keep staff information confidential.

G   Report abuse or suspected abuse of residents. Assist residents in reporting abuse if they wish to make a complaint of abuse.

G   Follow the care plan and assignments. If you make a mistake, report it promptly.

G   Do not perform any tasks outside your scope of practice.

G   Report all resident observations and incidents to the nurse.

G   Document accurately and promptly.

G   Follow rules on safety and infection prevention (see Chapter 2).

G   Do not accept gifts or tips (Fig. 1-11).

Fig. 1-11. *Nursing assistants should not accept money or gifts because it is unprofessional and may lead to conflict.*

G   Do not get personally or sexually involved with residents or their family members or friends.

Due to reports of poor care and abuse in long-term care facilities, the U.S. government passed the **Omnibus Budget Reconciliation Act** (**OBRA**) in 1987. It has been updated several times. OBRA requires that the Nurse Aide Training and Competency Evaluation Program (NATCEP) set minimum standards for nursing assistant training. NAs must complete at least 75 hours of training that covers topics like communication, preventing infections, safety and emergency procedures, and how to promote residents' independence and legal rights. Training must also include specific nursing skills, such as how to take vital signs. NAs must also know how to respond to mental health and social services needs, rehabilitative needs, and how to care for residents who are cognitively impaired.

OBRA requires that NAs pass a competency evaluation (testing program) before they can be employed. They must attend regular in-service education (a minimum of 12 hours per year) to keep their skills updated.

OBRA also requires that states keep a current list of nursing assistants in a state registry. In addition, OBRA identifies standards that instructors must meet in order to train nursing assistants. OBRA sets guidelines for minimum staff requirements. It specifies the minimum services that long-term care facilities must provide.

The resident assessment requirements are another important part of OBRA. OBRA requires that complete assessments be done on every resident. The assessment forms are the same for every facility.

OBRA made major changes in the survey process. Surveys are inspections that help make sure that long-term care facilities follow state and federal regulations. Surveys are done periodically by the state agency that licenses facilities. They may be done more often if a facility has been cited for problems. To **cite** means to find a problem through a survey. Inspections may be done less often if the facility has a good record. Inspection teams include a variety of trained healthcare professionals. The results from surveys are available to the public and posted in the facility.

OBRA also identifies important rights for residents in long-term care facilities. **Residents' Rights** relate to how residents must be treated while living in a facility. They are an ethical code of conduct for healthcare workers. Facilities give residents a list of these rights and review each right with them. NAs should be familiar with these legal rights. Residents' Rights are very detailed and include the following:

Quality of life: Residents have the right to the best care available. Dignity, choice, and independence are important parts of quality of life.

Services and activities to maintain a high level of wellness: Residents must receive the correct care. Facilities must develop care plans for residents, and their care should keep them as healthy as possible. Residents' health should not decline as a direct result of the facility's care.

The right to be fully informed about rights and services: Residents must be told what services

are available. They must be told what the fee is for each service. Residents must be given a written copy of their legal rights, along with the facility's rules. Legal rights must be explained in a language they can understand. Residents must be given contact information for state agencies relating to quality of care, such as the ombudsmen program. When requested, survey results must be shared with residents. Residents have the right to be notified in advance of any change of room or roommate. They have the right to communicate with someone who speaks their language. They have the right to assistance for any sensory impairment, such as blindness.

The right to participate in their own care: Residents have the right to participate in planning their treatment, care, and discharge. Residents have the right to refuse medication, treatment, care, and restraints. They have the right to be told of changes in their condition. They have the right to review their medical record. Informed consent is a concept that is part of participating in one's own care. A person has the legal and ethical right to direct what happens to his or her body. Doctors also have an ethical duty to involve the person in his or her health care. **Informed consent** is the process in which a person, with the help of a doctor, makes informed decisions about his or her health care.

The right to make independent choices: Residents can make choices about their doctors, care, and treatments. They can make personal decisions, such as what to wear and how to spend their time. They can join in community activities, both inside and outside the care facility. They have the right to a reasonable accommodation of their needs and preferences.

The right to privacy and confidentiality: Residents have a right to privacy when care is given. Their medical, personal, and financial information cannot be shared with anyone but the care team. Residents have the right to private, unrestricted communication with anyone (Fig. 1-12).

Fig. 1-12. Residents have the right to private communication with anyone; they have the right to send and receive mail that is unopened.

The right to dignity, respect, and freedom: Residents must be respected and treated with dignity by caregivers. They cannot be abused, mistreated, or neglected in any way.

The right to security of possessions: Residents' personal possessions must be safe at all times. They cannot be taken or used by anyone without a resident's permission. Residents have the right to manage their own finances or to choose someone else to do it for them. Residents can ask that the facility handle their money. If the care facility handles residents' financial affairs, residents must have access to their accounts and financial records. They must receive quarterly statements, among other things.

Residents have the right to file a complaint with the state survey and certification agency for abuse, neglect, or misappropriation of their property if the facility is handling their financial affairs. They also have the right to be free from charge for services covered by Medicaid or Medicare.

Rights during transfers and discharges: Location changes must be made safely and with the resident's knowledge and consent. Residents have the right to stay in a facility unless a transfer or discharge is needed. They also have the right to appeal a transfer or discharge.

The right to complain: Residents have the right to make complaints without fear of punishment.

Facilities must work quickly to try to resolve complaints.

The right to visits: Residents have the right to have visits from doctors, family, friends, clergy members, ombudsmen, legal representatives, or any other person.

Rights with social services: The facility must provide residents with access to social services. This includes counseling, assistance in solving problems with others, and help contacting legal and financial professionals.

Guidelines: Protecting Residents' Rights

G   Never abuse a resident physically, emotionally, verbally, or sexually. Watch for and immediately report any signs of abuse or neglect.

G   Call the resident by the name he or she prefers.

G   Involve residents in planning. Allow residents to make as many choices as possible about when, where, and how care is performed.

G   Always explain a procedure to a resident before performing it.

G   Do not unnecessarily expose a resident while giving care.

G   Respect a resident's refusal of care. Residents have a legal right to refuse treatment and care. However, report the refusal to the nurse immediately.

G   Tell the nurse if a resident has questions, concerns, or complaints about treatment or the goals of care.

G   Be truthful when documenting care.

G   Do not talk or gossip about residents. Keep all resident information confidential.

G   Knock and ask for permission before entering a resident's room (Fig. 1-13).

G   Do not accept gifts or money from residents.

G   Do not open a resident's mail or look through his belongings.

Fig. 1-13. To respect privacy, NAs should always knock before entering residents' rooms, even if the door is open.

G Respect residents' personal possessions. Handle them gently and carefully.

G Report observations about a resident's condition or care.

G Help resolve disputes by reporting them to the nurse.

Residents' Rights

Maintaining Boundaries

In professional relationships, boundaries must be set. Boundaries are the limits to or within relationships. Nursing assistants are guided by ethics and laws that set limits for their relationships with residents. These boundaries help support a healthy resident-staff relationship. Working closely with residents on a regular basis may make it more difficult to honor the boundaries of professional relationships. Residents may feel that NAs are their friends. If a staff member and resident become personally involved with each other, it becomes more difficult to enforce rules. The resident may expect the NA to break the rules because she thinks they are friends. Emotional attachments to residents are unprofessional and may weaken an NA's judgment. NAs should be friendly, warm, and caring with residents. But they should behave professionally and stay within the limits of set boundaries. Facility rules and the care plan's instructions should be followed. They are in place for everyone's protection.

A very important part of protecting residents' rights is preventing abuse and neglect. **Abuse** is purposeful mistreatment that causes physical, mental, or emotional pain or injury to someone. **Neglect** is the failure to provide needed care that results in physical, mental, or emotional

harm to a person. There are many forms of abuse, including the following:

- **Physical abuse** is any treatment, intentional or not, that causes harm to a person's body. This includes slapping, bruising, cutting, burning, physically restraining, pushing, shoving, or even rough handling.

- **Psychological abuse** is emotional harm caused by threatening, scaring, humiliating, intimidating, isolating, or insulting a person, or treating him or her as a child. It also includes verbal abuse. **Verbal abuse** is the use of spoken or written words, pictures, or gestures that threaten, embarrass, or insult a person.

- **Sexual abuse** is the forcing of a person to perform or participate in sexual acts against his or her will. This includes unwanted touching and exposing oneself to a person. It also includes the sharing of pornographic material.

- **Financial abuse** is the improper or illegal use of a person's money, possessions, property, or other assets.

- **Assault** is a threat to harm a person, resulting in the person feeling fearful that he or she will be harmed. Telling a resident that she will be slapped if she does not stop yelling is an example of assault.

- **Battery** is the intentional touching of a person without his or her consent. An example is an NA hitting or pushing a resident. This is also considered physical abuse. Forcing a resident to eat a meal is another example of battery.

- **Domestic violence** is abuse by spouses, intimate partners, or family members. It can be physical, sexual, or emotional. The victim can be a woman or man of any age or a child.

- **False imprisonment** is unlawful restraint that affects a person's freedom of movement.

Both the threat of being physically restrained and actually being physically restrained are types of false imprisonment. Not allowing a resident to leave the facility is also considered false imprisonment.

- **Involuntary seclusion** is the separation of a person from others against the person's will. An example is an NA confining a resident to his room.

- **Workplace violence** is abuse of staff by other staff members, residents, or visitors. It can be verbal, physical, or sexual. This includes improper touching and discussion about sexual subjects.

- **Sexual harassment** is any unwelcome sexual advance or behavior that creates an intimidating, hostile, or offensive working environment. Requests for sexual favors, unwanted touching, and other acts of a sexual nature are examples of sexual harassment.

- **Substance abuse** is the use of legal or illegal drugs, cigarettes, or alcohol in a way that harms oneself or others. For the NA, substance abuse can lead to unsafe practices that result in negligence, malpractice, neglect, and abuse. It can also lead to the loss of the NA's certification.

Neglect can be put into two categories: active neglect and passive neglect. **Active neglect** is the purposeful failure to provide needed care, resulting in harm to a person. **Passive neglect** is the unintentional failure to provide needed care, resulting in physical, mental, or emotional harm to a person. The caregiver may not know how to properly care for the resident, or may not understand the resident's needs.

Negligence means actions, or the failure to act or provide the proper care for a resident, resulting in unintended injury. An example of negligence is an NA forgetting to lock a resident's wheelchair before transferring her. The resident falls and is injured. **Malpractice** occurs when a

person is injured due to professional misconduct through negligence, carelessness, or lack of skill.

Nursing assistants must never abuse residents in any way. They must also try to protect residents from others who abuse them. If an NA ever sees or suspects that another caregiver, family member, or resident is abusing a resident, she must report this immediately to the nurse in charge. **Reporting abuse is not an option—it is the law.**

Observing and Reporting: Abuse and Neglect

The following injuries are considered suspicious and should be reported:

- O/R Poisoning or traumatic injury
- O/R Teeth marks
- O/R Belt buckle or strap marks
- O/R Bruises, contusions, and welts
- O/R Scars
- O/R Fractures, dislocation
- O/R Burns of unusual shape and in unusual locations, cigarette burns
- O/R Scalding burns
- O/R Scratches or puncture wounds
- O/R Scalp tenderness or patches of missing hair
- O/R Swelling in the face, broken teeth, nasal discharge
- O/R Bruises, bleeding, or discharge from the vaginal area

These signs could indicate abuse:

- O/R Yelling obscenities
- O/R Fear, apprehension, fear of being alone
- O/R Poor self-control
- O/R Constant pain
- O/R Threatening to hurt others
- O/R Withdrawal or apathy (Fig. 1-14)

Fig. 1-14. *Withdrawing from others is an important change to report.*

°/ʀ Alcohol or drug abuse

°/ʀ Agitation or anxiety, signs of stress

°/ʀ Low self-esteem

°/ʀ Mood changes, confusion, disorientation

°/ʀ Private conversations not allowed, or the family member/caregiver is present during all conversations

°/ʀ Reports of questionable care by the resident or his family

These signs could indicate neglect:

°/ʀ Pressure ulcers

°/ʀ Unclean body

°/ʀ Body lice

°/ʀ Unanswered call lights

°/ʀ Soiled bedding or incontinence briefs not being changed

°/ʀ Poorly-fitting clothing

°/ʀ Unmet needs relating to hearing aids, eyeglasses, etc.

°/ʀ Weight loss, poor appetite

°/ʀ Uneaten food

°/ʀ Dehydration

°/ʀ Fresh water or beverages not being offered regularly

°/ʀ Reports of not receiving prescribed medication by the resident or his family

Nursing assistants are in an excellent position to observe and report abuse or neglect. NAs have an ethical and legal responsibility to observe for signs of abuse and to report suspected cases to the proper person. NAs must follow the chain of command when reporting abuse. If action is not taken, the NA should keep reporting up the chain of command until action is taken. If no action is taken at the facility level, she can call the state abuse hotline, which is an anonymous call. If a life-or-death situation is witnessed, the NA should remove the resident to a safe place if possible. The NA should get help immediately or have someone go for help. The resident should not be left alone.

If abuse is suspected or observed, the NA should give the nurse as much information as possible. If residents want to make a complaint of abuse, NAs must help them in every way. This includes telling them of the process and their rights. NAs must never retaliate against (punish) residents complaining of abuse. If an NA sees someone being cruel or abusive to a resident who made a complaint, she must report it.

An ombudsman can assist residents, too. An **ombudsman** is assigned by law as the legal advocate for residents (ltcombudsman.org). The Older Americans Act (OAA) is a federal law that requires all states to have an ombudsman program. An ombudsman visits facilities and listens to residents. He or she decides what action to take if there are problems. Ombudsmen can help resolve conflicts and settle disputes concerning residents' health, safety, welfare, and rights. The ombudsman will gather information and try to resolve the problem on the resident's behalf and may suggest ways to solve the problem. Ombudsmen provide an ongoing presence in long-term care facilities. They monitor care and conditions (Fig. 1-15).

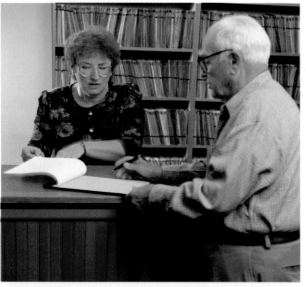

Fig. 1-15. *An ombudsman is a legal advocate for residents. He or she may work with other agencies to resolve complaints.*

Residents' Rights

Residents' Council

A Residents' Council is a group of residents who meet regularly to discuss issues related to the care facility. This council gives residents a voice in facility operations. Topics of discussion may include facility policies, decisions regarding activities, concerns, and problems. The Residents' Council offers residents a chance to provide suggestions on improving the quality of care. Council executives are elected by residents. Family members are invited to attend meetings with or on behalf of residents. Staff may participate in this process when invited by council members.

To respect **confidentiality** means to keep private things private. Nursing assistants will learn confidential (private) information about residents. They may learn about a resident's health, finances, and relationships. Ethically and legally, they must protect this information. NAs should not share information about residents with anyone other than the care team.

Congress passed the **Health Insurance Portability and Accountability Act (HIPAA)** (hhs.gov/hipaa) in 1996. It has been further de-

fined and revised since then. One reason this law was passed is to help keep health information private and secure. All healthcare organizations must take special steps to protect health information. Their employees can be fined and/ or imprisoned if they do not follow rules to protect patient privacy.

Under HIPAA, a person's health information must be kept private. It is called **protected health information (PHI)**. Examples of PHI include name, address, telephone number, social security number, email address, and medical record number. Only those who must have information for care or to process records should know a person's private health information. They must protect the information. It must not become known or used by anyone else. It must be kept confidential.

HIPAA applies to all healthcare providers, including doctors, nurses, nursing assistants, and any other care team members. NAs cannot give out any information about a resident to anyone who is not directly involved in the resident's care unless the resident gives official consent or unless the law requires it. For example, if a neighbor asks an NA how a resident is doing, she should reply, "I'm sorry, but I cannot share that information. It's confidential." That is the correct response to anyone who does not have a legal reason to know about the resident.

Guidelines: Protecting Privacy

G   Make sure you are in a private area when you listen to or read your messages.

G   Know with whom you are speaking on the phone. If you are not sure, get a name and number. Call back after you find out it is all right to do so.

G   Do not talk about residents in public (Fig. 1-16). Public areas include elevators, grocery stores, lounges, waiting rooms, parking garages, schools, restaurants, etc.

Fig. 1-16. *NAs should not discuss any information about residents in public places.*

G   Use confidential rooms for reports to other care team members.

G   If you see a resident's family member or a former resident in public, be careful with your greeting. He or she may not want others to know about the family member or that he or she has been a resident.

G   Do not bring family or friends to the facility to meet residents.

G   Make sure nobody can see health or personal information on your computer screen while you are working. Log out and/or exit the web browser when finished with computer work.

G   Do not give confidential information in emails. You do not know who has access to your messages.

G   Do not take photos of residents. Do not share resident information or photos on social networking sites, such as Facebook, Twitter, Instagram, or Pinterest.

G   Make sure fax numbers are correct before faxing information. Use a cover sheet with a confidentiality statement.

G   Do not leave documents where others may see them.

G   Store, file, or shred documents according to facility policy. If you find documents with a resident's information, give them to the nurse.

All healthcare workers must follow HIPAA regulations no matter where they are or what they are doing. There are serious penalties for violating these rules, including

•   Fines ranging from $100 to $1.5 million

•   Prison sentences of up to ten years

Maintaining confidentiality is a legal and ethical obligation. It is part of respecting residents and their rights. Discussing a resident's care or personal affairs with anyone other than members of the care team violates the law.

8. Explain legal aspects of the resident's medical record

The resident's medical record or chart is a legal document. What is documented in the chart is considered in court to be what actually happened. In general, if something does not appear in a resident's chart, it did not legally happen. Failing to document care could cause very serious legal problems for NAs and their employers. It could also harm residents. NAs must remember that if it was not documented, it was not done. Careful charting is important for these reasons:

•   It is the only way to guarantee clear and complete communication among all the members of the care team.

•   Documentation is a legal record of every resident's treatment. Medical charts can be used in court as legal evidence.

•   Documentation helps protect nursing assistants and their employers from liability by proving what they did when caring for residents.

•   Documentation gives an up-to-date record of the status and care of each resident.

Guidelines: Careful Documentation

G   Document care immediately after it is given. This makes details easier to remember. **Do not record any care before it has been done.**

G   Think about what you want to say before documenting. Be as brief and as clear as possible.

G   Use facts, not opinions.

G   Use black ink when documenting by hand. Write as neatly as you can.

G   If you make a mistake, draw one line through it. Write the correct information. Put your initials and the date (Fig. 1-17). Do not erase what you have written. Do not use correction fluid. Documentation done on a computer is time-stamped; it can only be changed by entering another notation.

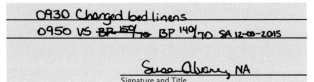

Fig. 1-17. One example of how to correct a mistake.

G   Sign your full name and title (for example, Sara Martinez, CNA). Write the correct date.

G   Document as specified in the care plan. Some facilities have a check-off sheet for documenting care. It is also called an ADL (activities of daily living) or flow sheet.

G   Documentation may need to be done using the 24-hour clock, or military time (Fig. 1-18). Regular time uses the numbers 1 to 12 to show each of the 24 hours in a day. In military time, the hours are numbered from 00 to 23 or 24. Midnight is expressed as 0000 (although it can also be written as 2400), 1:00 a.m. is 0100, 1:00 p.m. is 1300, and so on.

To change regular hours between 1:00 p.m. to 11:59 p.m. to military time, add 12 to the regular time. For example, to change 4:00 p.m. to military time, add 4 + 12. The time is expressed as 1600 (sixteen hundred) hours. To change from military time to regular time, subtract 12. For example, to change 2200 hours to standard time, subtract 12 from 22. The answer is 10:00 p.m.

Both regular and military time list minutes and seconds the same way. The minutes and seconds do not change when converting from regular to military time. For example, to change 4:22 p.m. to military time, add 4 + 12. The minutes do not change. The time is expressed as 1622 (sixteen twenty-two) hours.

Midnight can be expressed two different ways in military time. It can be written as 0000, and it can also be written as 2400. This follows the rule of adding 12 to the regular time. Follow facility policy on how to express midnight.

Fig. 1-18. Divisions in the 24-hour clock.

G   At some facilities, computers are used to document information. Computers record and store information. It can be retrieved when it is needed. This is faster and more accurate than writing information by hand. If your facility uses computers for documentation, you will be trained to use them. HIPAA privacy guidelines apply to computer use. Make sure nobody can see private and protected health information on your computer screen. Confidential information should not be shared with anyone except the care team.

9. Explain the Minimum Data Set (MDS)

A resident assessment system was developed by the federal government in 1990 and is revised periodically. It is called the **Minimum Data Set (MDS)**. The MDS is a detailed form with guidelines for assessing residents. It also lists what to do if resident problems are identified. Staff must complete the MDS for each resident within 14 days of admission and again each year. In addition, each resident's MDS must be reviewed every three months. A new MDS must be done when there is any major change in the resident's condition. NAs contribute to the MDS by reporting changes in residents promptly and documenting accurately. Doing this means a new MDS can be completed when needed.

10. Discuss incident reports

An **incident** is an accident, problem, or unexpected event during the course of care. It is something that is not part of the normal routine. A mistake in care, such as feeding a resident from the wrong meal tray, is an incident. A resident falling or being injured is another type of incident. Accusations made by residents against staff and employee injuries are other types of incidents. State and federal guidelines require that incidents be recorded in an incident report. An incident report (also called an occurrence or event report) is a report that documents the incident and the response to it. The information in an incident report is confidential. Incident reports should be done when any of the following occurs:

- A resident falls (all falls must be reported, even if the resident says he or she is fine)

- An NA or a resident breaks or damages something

- An NA makes a mistake in care

- A resident or a family member makes a request that is out of the NA's scope of practice

- A resident or a family member makes sexual advances or remarks

- Anything happens that makes an NA feel uncomfortable, threatened, or unsafe

- An NA gets injured on the job

- An NA is exposed to blood or body fluids

Reporting and documenting incidents is done to protect everyone involved. This includes the resident, the employer, and the nursing assistant. NAs must report any incident, including job-related injuries, immediately to the charge nurse. When documenting incidents, NAs should complete the report as soon as possible and give it to the charge nurse. This is important so that details are not forgotten.

If a resident falls and the NA did not see it, he should not write, "Mr. G fell." Instead he should write, "Found Mr. G on the floor," or, "Mr. G states that he fell." NAs should write brief and accurate descriptions of the events as they happened. They should not place blame or liability within the report. Incident reports help demonstrate areas where changes can be made to avoid repeating the same incident.

***

Guidelines: Incident Reporting

G   Tell what happened. State the time and the mental and physical condition of the person.

G   Tell how the person tolerated the incident (his reaction).

G   State the facts; do not give opinions.

G   Do not write anything in the incident report on the medical record.

G   Describe the action taken to give care.

2

Foundations of Resident Care

1. Understand the importance of verbal and written communications

Effective communication is a critical part of a nursing assistant's job. Nursing assistants must communicate with supervisors, the care team, residents, and family members. A resident's health depends on how well NAs communicate observations and concerns to the nurse.

Communication is the process of exchanging information with others. It is a process of sending and receiving messages. People communicate with signs and symbols, such as words, drawings, and pictures. They also communicate through their behavior.

Verbal communication uses spoken or written words. Oral reports are an example of verbal communication. **Nonverbal communication** is communicating without using words. An example is a person shrugging his shoulders. Nonverbal communication also includes how a person says something. Body language is another form of nonverbal communication. Movements, facial expressions, and posture can express different attitudes or emotions (Fig. 2-1).

Residents' Rights

Different Languages
When caring for residents, NAs should speak in a language that residents can understand or find an interpreter (someone who speaks the resident's language). Picture cards or gestures can help with communication. NAs should not use a different language when speaking with staff in front of residents.

Fig. 2-1. *Body language sends messages just as words do. Which of these people seems more interested in their conversation—the person on the right who is looking down with her arms crossed or the person on the left who is sitting up straight and smiling?*

Nursing assistants must make brief, accurate oral and written reports to residents and staff. Careful observations are used to make these reports and are important to the health and well-being of all residents. Signs and symptoms that should be reported will be discussed throughout this textbook. Some observations will need to be reported immediately to the nurse. Deciding what to report immediately involves critical thinking. Anything that endangers residents should be reported immediately, including the following:

- Falls

- Chest pain

- Severe headache

- Trouble breathing

- Abnormal pulse, respiration, or blood pressure

- Change in mental status
- Sudden weakness or loss of mobility
- High fever
- Loss of consciousness
- Change in level of consciousness
- Bleeding
- Change in resident's condition
- Bruises, abrasions, or other signs of possible abuse

When making reports about residents, NAs must remember that all resident information is confidential. Information should only be shared with the care team.

When residents report symptoms, events, or feelings, the NA should have them repeat what they have said. He should ask for more information. The NA should ask open-ended questions that need more than a "yes" or "no" answer. For example, an NA should not ask, "Did you sleep well last night?" Instead, he should ask, "Can you tell me about your night and how you slept?" This will encourage the resident to offer facts and details.

Proper Communication

When communicating with residents, the NA should remember to use these tips:

- Always greet the resident by his or her preferred name.
- Identify himself.
- Focus on the topic to be discussed.
- Face the resident while speaking and avoid talking into space.
- Talk with the resident, not other staff members, while giving care.
- Listen and respond when the resident speaks.
- Praise the resident and smile often.
- Encourage the resident to interact with him and others.

- Be courteous.
- Tell the resident when he is leaving the room.

Residents' Rights

Names

NAs should call residents by the names residents prefer. NAs should not refer to residents by their first names unless a resident has asked them to do so. Terms such as *sweetie*, *honey*, or *dearie* are disrespectful and should not be used.

When making any report, the right information must be collected before documenting it. Facts, not opinions, are most useful to the nurse and the care team. Two kinds of factual information are needed in reporting. **Objective information** is based on what a person sees, hears, touches, or smells. Objective information is collected by using the senses. It is also called *signs*. **Subjective information** is something a person cannot or did not observe. It is based on something that the resident reported that may or may not be true. It is also called *symptoms*. An example of objective information is, "Mr. Hartman is holding his head and rubbing his temples." A subjective report of the same situation might be, "Mr. Hartman says he has a headache." The nurse needs factual information in order to make decisions about care and treatment. Both objective and subjective reports are valuable.

In any report, what is observed (signs) and what the resident reports (symptoms) need to be clearly noted. "Ms. Scott reports pain in left shoulder" is an example of clear reporting. NAs are not expected to make diagnoses based on signs and symptoms they observe. Their observations, however, can alert staff to possible problems. In order to report accurately, NAs must observe residents accurately. To observe accurately, NAs need to use as many senses as possible to gather information (Fig. 2-2).

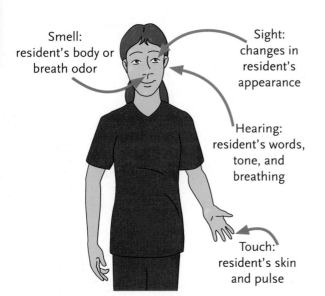

Fig. 2-2. *Reporting observations means using more than one sense.*

Sight. The NA should look for changes in the resident's appearance. These include rashes, redness, paleness, swelling, discharge, weakness, sunken eyes, and posture or gait (walking) changes.

Hearing. The NA should listen to what the resident says about his condition, family, or needs. Is the resident speaking clearly and making sense? Does he show emotions, such as anger, frustration, or sadness? Is his breathing normal? Does he wheeze, gasp, or cough? Is the area quiet enough for him to rest as needed?

Touch. Does the resident's skin feel hot or cool, moist or dry? Is the pulse rate regular?

Smell. Are there any odors coming from the resident's body? Odors could suggest poor bathing, infections, or incontinence. **Incontinence** is the inability to control the bladder or bowels. Breath odor could suggest use of alcohol or tobacco, indigestion, or poor mouth care.

For oral reports, the NA should write notes so that important details are not forgotten. Following an oral report, the NA must document when, why, about what, and to whom an oral report was given.

Sometimes the nurse or another member of the care team will give an NA a brief oral report on one of her residents. The NA should listen carefully and take notes (Fig. 2-3). She should ask about anything she does not understand. At the end of the report, the NA can restate what she has been told to make sure she understands.

Fig. 2-3. *Taking notes helps nursing assistants remember facts and report accurately.*

NAs will learn medical terms for specific conditions during their training. Medical terms are made up of roots, prefixes, and suffixes. A root is a part of a word that contains its basic meaning. The prefix is the word part that comes before the root to help form a new word. The suffix is the word part added to the end of a root that helps form a new word. Prefixes and suffixes are called *affixes* because they are attached, or affixed, to a root. Here are some examples:

- The root *derm* or *derma* means skin. The suffix *itis* means inflammation. Dermatitis is an inflammation of the skin.

- The prefix *brady* means slow. The root *cardia* means heart. Bradycardia is slow heartbeat or pulse.

- The suffix *pathy* means disease. The root *neuro* means of the nerve or nervous system. Neuropathy is a nerve disease or disease of the nervous system.

When speaking with residents and their families, NAs should use simple, non-medical terms. Medical terms may not be understood. But when speaking with the care team, using medical terms will help NAs give more complete information.

Abbreviations are another way to help the care team communicate more efficiently with each other. For example, the abbreviation *prn* means *as necessary*. NAs should learn the standard medical abbreviations their facility uses. They can use them to report information briefly and accurately. NAs may need to know these abbreviations to read assignments or care plans. A brief list of abbreviations is located at the end of this textbook. There may be other terms in use at a facility, so NAs should follow facility policy.

Telephone Communication

Nursing assistants may be asked to answer the telephone at their facility. Here are guidelines they should follow:

Guidelines: Answering the Facility Telephone

G   Always identify your facility's name, your name, and your position. Be friendly and professional.

G   If you need to find the person the caller wishes to speak with, place the caller on hold after asking if it is okay to do so.

G   If the caller has to leave a message, write it down and repeat it to make sure you have the correct message. Ask for proper spellings of names. Do not ask for more information than the person needs to return the call; a name, short message, and phone number is enough. Do not give out any information about staff or residents.

G   Thank the person for calling; say goodbye.

Call Lights

Long-term care facilities are required to have call systems, often called *call lights*, so that residents can call for help whenever they need it. They are in resident rooms and bathrooms. Some have strings for residents to pull, and others have buttons to push. The signal is usually both a light outside the room and a sound and can be heard in the nurses' station. This is the primary way a resident can call for help. NAs must always respond immediately when they see the light or hear the sound. They should do so even if the resident who needs help is not on their assignment sheet. All residents are the responsibility of each NA. NAs should respond to call lights in a courteous and respectful manner. They must check each time before leaving a room to make sure that the call light is within the resident's reach and that the resident knows how to use it.

---

2. Describe barriers to communication

Communication can be blocked or disrupted in many ways (Fig. 2-4). These are some barriers and ways for nursing assistants to avoid them:

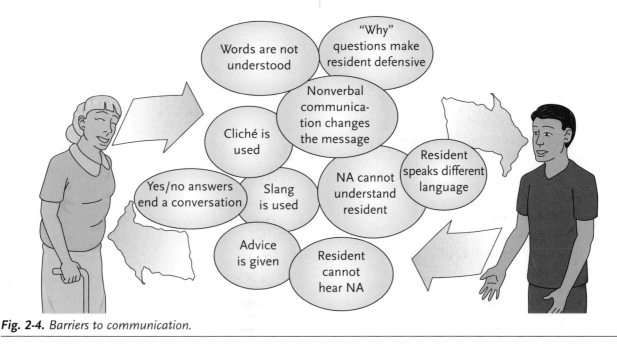

Fig. 2-4. Barriers to communication.

Resident does not hear NA, does not hear correctly, or does not understand. The NA should face the resident. He should speak slowly and clearly. He should not shout, whisper, or mumble. The NA should speak in a low voice, using a pleasant tone. If the resident wears a hearing aid, he should check that it is on and is working.

Resident is difficult to understand. The NA should be patient and take time to listen. He can ask the resident to repeat or explain the message. He should then state the message in his own words to make sure he has understood.

NA, resident, or others use words that are not understood. An NA should not use medical terms with residents or their families. He should use simple, everyday words and ask what a word means if he is not sure.

NA uses slang or profanity. The NA should avoid using slang words. They are unprofessional and may not be understood. He should not use profanity, even if the resident does.

NA uses clichés. Clichés are phrases that are used over and over again and do not really mean anything. For example, "Everything will be fine" is a cliché. Instead of using a cliché, the NA should listen to what a resident is really saying. He should respond with a meaningful message.

NA responds with "Why?" The NA should avoid asking "Why?" when a resident makes a statement. "Why" questions make people feel defensive.

NA gives advice. The NA should not offer his opinion or give advice. Giving medical advice is not within an NA's scope of practice. It could be dangerous.

NA asks questions that only require yes/no answers. The NA should ask open-ended questions that need more than a "yes" or "no" answer. Yes and no answers end conversation. For example, if an NA wants to know what a resident likes to eat, he should not ask, "Do you like vegetables?" Instead, he should ask, "Which vegetables do you like best?"

Resident speaks a different language. If a resident speaks a different language than the NA does, the NA should speak slowly and clearly. He should keep his messages short and simple and he should limit distractions. He should be alert for words the resident understands, as well as signs that the resident is only pretending to understand. He may need to use pictures or gestures to communicate. The NA can ask the resident's family or other staff members who speak the resident's language for help. He should be patient and calm.

NA or resident uses nonverbal communication. Nonverbal communication can change a message. The NA should be aware of his body language and gestures. He can look for nonverbal messages from residents and clarify them. For example, "Mr. Feldman, you say you're feeling fine but you seem to be in pain. Can I help?"

Defense mechanisms may be considered barriers to communication. **Defense mechanisms** are unconscious behaviors used to release tension or cope with stress. They help to block uncomfortable or threatening feelings. These are some common defense mechanisms:

- **Denial**: Completely rejecting the thought or feeling—"I'm not upset with you!"

- **Projection**: Seeing feelings in others that are really one's own—"My teacher hates me."

- **Displacement**: Transferring a strong negative feeling to a safer situation—for example, an unhappy employee cannot yell at his boss for fear of losing his job. He later yells at his wife.

- **Rationalization**: Making excuses to justify a situation—for example, after stealing something, saying, "Everybody does it."

- **Repression**: Blocking painful thoughts or feelings from the mind—for example, forgetting sexual abuse.

- **Regression**: Going back to an old, usually immature behavior—for example, throwing a temper tantrum as an adult.

Culture can affect communication. A **culture** is a system of learned behaviors, practiced by a group of people, that is considered to be the tradition of that group and is passed on from one generation to the next. Each culture may have different knowledge, behaviors, beliefs, values, attitudes, religions, and customs. When an NA communicates with residents from different cultures, she should ask herself these questions:

- What information do I need to communicate to this person?

- Does this person speak English as a first or second language?

- Do I speak this person's language, or do I need an interpreter?

- Does this person have any cultural practices about touch or gestures I should adapt to?

Learning each resident's behavior and preferences can be a challenge. However, it is an important part of communication. It is especially vital in a multicultural society (a society made up of many cultures), such as the United States. NAs should be aware of all the messages they send and receive. Listening and observing carefully will help NAs better understand residents' needs and feelings.

3. List guidelines for communicating with residents with special needs

Due to illness or impairments, some residents will need special techniques to aid communication. An **impairment** is a loss of function or ability; it can be a partial or complete loss. Special techniques for different conditions are listed below. Information on communicating with residents who have Alzheimer's disease is in Chapter 5.

Hearing Impairment

There are many different kinds of hearing loss. People who have impaired hearing or are deaf may have lost their hearing gradually, or they may have been born with the impairment. People who are hearing impaired may use a hearing aid, read lips, or use sign language. People with impaired hearing also closely observe the facial expressions and body language of others to add to their knowledge of what is being said. Hearing loss may affect how well residents can express their needs.

Guidelines: Hearing Impairment

G   If the person has a hearing aid, make sure he or she is wearing it and that it is turned on. There are many types of hearing aids (Fig. 2-5). Follow manufacturer's directions for cleaning. In general, the hearing aid needs to be cleaned daily. Wipe it with special cleaning solution or alcohol, using a soft cloth. Do not put the hearing aid in water. Handle it carefully; do not drop it. Always store it inside its case when it is not being worn. Turn it off when it is not in use. Remove it before bathing, showering, or shampooing hair. Some hearing aids need to be recharged nightly. Some have rechargable batteries. Follow the care plan's instructions.

Fig. 2-5. *The top photo shows an older type of hearing aid. The bottom photo shows a different type of hearing aid that is worn inside the ear. (BOTTOM PHOTO COURTESY OF STARKEY HEARING TECHNOLOGIES, STARKEY.COM)*

G Reduce or remove noise, such as TVs, radios, and loud speech. Close doors if needed.

G Get residents' attention before speaking. Do not startle them by approaching from behind. Walk in front or touch them lightly on the arm to let them know you are near.

G Speak clearly, slowly, and in good lighting. Directly face the person (Fig. 2-6). The light should be on your face, not on the resident's. Ask if she can hear what you are saying.

Fig. 2-6. *When communicating with a resident who has a hearing impairment, the nursing assistant should speak face-to-face in good light.*

G Do not shout. Do not mouth the words in an exaggerated way.

G Keep the pitch of your voice low.

G Residents may read lips, so do not chew gum or eat while speaking. Keep your hands away from your face while talking.

G If the resident hears better out of one ear, try to speak and stand on that side.

G Use short sentences and simple words. Avoid sudden topic changes.

G Repeat what you have said using different words when needed. Some hearing-impaired people want you to repeat exactly what you said. This is because they miss only a few words.

G Use picture cards or a notepad as needed.

G Hearing-impaired residents may hear less when they are tired or ill. This is true of everyone. Be patient and empathetic.

G Some hearing-impaired residents have speech problems and may be difficult to understand. Do not pretend you understand if you do not. Ask the resident to repeat what was said. Observe the lips, facial expressions, and body language. Then tell the resident what you think you heard. You can also request that the resident write down words.

G Hearing decline can be a normal aspect of aging. Be understanding and supportive.

Vision Impairment

Vision impairment can affect people of all ages. It can exist at birth or develop gradually. It can occur in one eye or in both. It can also be the result of injury, illness, or aging. Some vision impairment causes people to wear corrective lenses, such as contact lenses or eyeglasses. Some people need to wear eyeglasses all the time. Others only need them to read or for activities that require seeing distant objects, such as driving.

Guidelines: Vision Impairment

G If the resident has eyeglasses, make sure they are clean and that he or she wears them. Clean glass lenses with water and soft tissue. Clean plastic lenses with cleaning fluid and a lens cloth. Make sure that eyeglasses are in good condition and fit well. Report to the nurse if they do not.

G Contact lenses are made of many types of plastic. Some can be worn and disposed of daily; others are worn for longer periods. If the resident is able, it is best to leave contact lens care to him or her.

G Knock on the door and identify yourself as soon as you enter the room. Do not touch the resident until you have said your name. Explain why you are there and what you would like to do. Let the resident know when you are leaving the room.

G Make sure there is proper lighting in the room. Face the resident when speaking.

G When you enter a new room with the resident, orient him or her to where things are. Describe the things you see around you. Try not to use words such as "see," "look," and "watch."

G Always tell the resident what you are doing while caring for him. Give specific directions, such as, "on your right" or, "in front of you." Talk directly to the resident whom you are assisting. Do not talk to other residents or staff members.

G Use the face of an imaginary clock as a guide to explain the position of objects that are in front of the resident. For example, "There is a sofa at 7 o'clock" (Fig. 2-7).

Fig. 2-7. Using the face of an imaginary clock to explain the position of objects can be helpful.

G Do not move personal items or furniture. Put everything back where you found it.

G Tell the resident where the call light is. Make sure it is within the resident's reach.

G Leave doors completely open or completely closed, never partly open.

G If the resident needs guidance in getting around, walk slightly ahead. Let the resident touch or grasp your arm lightly.

G Encourage the use of the other senses, such as hearing, touch, and smell. Encourage the resident to feel and touch things, such as clothing, furniture, or items in the room.

G Use large clocks, clocks that chime, and radios to help keep track of time.

G Large-print books, audiobooks, digital books, and Braille books are available. Learning to read Braille, however, takes a long time and requires training.

G If the resident has a guide dog, do not play with, distract, or feed it.

Mental Illness

Mental health is the normal functioning of emotional and intellectual abilities. A person who is mentally healthy is able to

- Get along with others (Fig. 2-8)

- Adapt to change

- Care for self and others

- Give and accept love

- Deal with situations that cause anxiety, disappointment, and frustration

- Take responsibility for decisions, feelings, and actions

- Control and fulfill desires and impulses appropriately

Fig. 2-8. The ability to interact well with other people is a characteristic of mental health.

While it involves the emotions and mental functions, **mental illness** is a disorder. It produces signs and symptoms and affects the body's ability to function. It responds to proper treatment and care. Mental illness disrupts a person's ability to function at a normal level in the family, home, or community. It often causes inappropriate behavior. Some signs and symptoms of mental illness are confusion, disorientation, agitation, and anxiety.

People who are mentally ill cannot simply choose to be well. People who are mentally healthy are usually able to control their emotions and actions. People who are mentally ill may not have this control.

Different types of mental illness will affect how well residents communicate. Nursing assistants should treat each resident as an individual. They should tailor their approach to the situation.

Guidelines: Communication and Mental Illness

G   Do not talk to adults as if they were children.

G   Use simple, clear statements and a normal tone of voice.

G   Be sure that what you say and how you say it show respect and concern.

G   Sit or stand at a normal distance from the resident. Be aware of your body language.

G   Be honest and direct, as you would with any resident.

G   Avoid arguments.

G   Maintain eye contact and listen carefully (Fig. 2-9).

Fig. 2-9. Nursing assistants should maintain eye contact and sit a normal distance when communicating with residents who are mentally ill.

Learning Objective 9 in Chapter 3 has more information on mental illness.

Combative Behavior

Residents may display **combative**, meaning violent or hostile, behavior. Such behavior may include hitting, pushing, kicking, or verbal attacks. It may be the result of disease affecting the brain. It may also be due to frustration. Or it may just be part of someone's personality. In general, combative behavior is not a reaction to the caregiver and should not be taken personally. NAs should always report and document combative behavior. Even if they are not upset by the behavior, the care team needs to be aware of it.

Guidelines: Combative Behavior

G   Block physical blows or step out of the way, but never hit back (Fig. 2-10). No matter how much a resident hurts you, or how angry or afraid you are, never hit or threaten a resident.

Fig. 2-10. When dealing with combative residents, nursing assistants should step out of the way, but never hit back.

G   Allow the resident time to calm down before the next interaction.

G   Ensure the resident is safe and give him or her space. When possible, stand at least an arm's length away.

G   Remain calm. Lower the tone of your voice.

G   Be flexible and patient.

G   Stay neutral. Do not respond to verbal attacks. Do not argue or accuse the resident of wrongdoing. If you must respond, say something like, "I understand that you're angry and frustrated. How can I make things better?"

G Do not use gestures that could frighten or startle the resident.

G Be reassuring and supportive.

G Consider what provoked the resident. Sometimes something as simple as a change in caregiver or routine can be very upsetting to a resident. Get help to take the resident to a quieter place if needed.

G Report inappropriate behavior to the nurse.

Anger

Anger is a natural emotion that has many causes. These include disease, fear, pain, loneliness, and loss of independence. Anger may also just be a part of someone's personality. Some people get angry more easily than others.

People express anger in different ways. Some may shout, yell, threaten, throw things, or pace. Others express their anger by withdrawing, being silent, or sulking. Angry behavior should always be reported to the nurse.

Guidelines: Angry Behavior

G Stay calm. Do not argue or respond to verbal attacks.

G Empathize with the resident. Try to understand what he or she is feeling.

G Try to find out what caused the resident's anger. Using silence may help the resident explain. Listen attentively as the resident speaks.

G Treat the resident with dignity and respect. Explain what you are going to do and when you will do it.

G Answer call lights promptly.

G Stay at a safe distance if the resident becomes combative.

Inappropriate Behavior

Inappropriate behavior from a resident includes trying to establish a personal, rather than a professional, relationship. Examples include asking personal questions, requesting visits on personal time, asking for or doing favors, giving tips or gifts, and lending or borrowing money.

Inappropriate behavior also includes making sexual advances and comments to staff or other residents. Sexual advances include any sexual words, comments, or behavior that makes the person to whom the advances are directed feel uncomfortable.

Inappropriate behavior may include residents removing their clothes or touching themselves in public. Illness, dementia, confusion, and medication may cause this behavior. If an NA encounters a resident in any embarrassing situation, she should remain professional. She should not overreact, as that may actually reinforce the behavior. Trying to distract the resident may help. If it does not, the resident should be taken to a private area. The nurse should be notified.

Confused residents may have problems that mimic inappropriate sexual behavior. They may have an uncomfortable rash, clothes that are too tight, too hot, or too scratchy, or they may need to go to the bathroom. NAs need to observe for these problems. When residents act inappropriately, NAs should report the behavior, even if they think it was harmless.

Residents' Rights

Communicating with Residents

Nursing assistants' interactions with residents are important. Residents' physical and psychological health can depend a great deal on how NAs communicate. This is especially true for residents who are cognitively impaired, lonely, helpless, or bored. NAs should be comforting and kind with residents. They should listen if residents want to talk. Just the presence of a caring person can reassure residents that they are not alone.

4. Identify ways to promote safety and handle non-medical emergencies

Safety

All staff members, including nursing assistants, are responsible for safety in a facility. It is very important to try to prevent accidents *before* they occur. Prevention is the key to safety. As NAs work, they should watch for safety hazards. They should report unsafe conditions to the supervisor promptly. Before leaving a resident's room, an NA should do a final check and ask himself:

• Is the call light within the resident's reach?

• Is the room tidy? Are the resident's items in their proper places?

• Is the furniture in the same place as I found it? Is the bed in its lowest position?

• Does the resident have a clear walkway around the room and into the bathroom?

Principles of Body Mechanics

Back strain or injury is a serious problem for nursing assistants. Using proper body mechanics is an important step in preventing back strain and injury. **Body mechanics** is the way the parts of the body work together when a person moves. Using proper body mechanics helps save energy and prevent injury.

Alignment. When standing, sitting, or lying down, the body should be in alignment and should have good posture. This means that the two sides of the body are mirror images of each other, with body parts lined up naturally. **Posture** is the way a person holds and positions his body. A person can maintain correct body alignment when lifting or carrying an object by keeping it close to his body (Fig. 2-11). His feet and body should be pointed in the direction he is moving. He should avoid twisting at the waist.

Base of support. The base of support is the foundation that supports an object. The feet are the body's base of support. The wider the support,

the more stable a person will be. Standing with legs apart allows for a greater base of support. This is more stable than standing with feet together.

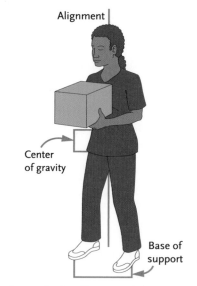

Fig. 2-11. Proper body alignment is important when standing and when sitting.

Center of gravity. The center of gravity in the body is the point where the most weight is concentrated. This point will depend on the position of the body. When a person stands, weight is centered in the pelvis. A low center of gravity gives a more stable base of support. Bending the knees when lifting an object lowers the pelvis and, therefore, lowers a person's center of gravity. This gives the person more stability. It makes him less likely to fall or strain the working muscles.

Guidelines: Using Proper Body Mechanics

G   Assess the situation first. Clear the path. Remove any obstacles.

G   Use both arms and hands to lift, push, or carry objects.

G   When lifting a heavy object from the floor, spread your feet shoulder-width apart. Bend your knees. Use the strong, large muscles in your thighs, upper arms, and shoulders to lift the object. Raise your body and the object together (Fig. 2-12).

Back muscles must lift the object and half of the body

Legs and thighs do the lifting

Fig. 2-12. In this illustration, which person is lifting correctly?

G Hold objects close to you when you are lifting or carrying them. This keeps the object closer to your center of gravity and base of support.

G Push or slide objects rather than lifting them.

G Avoid bending and reaching as much as possible. Move or position furniture so that you do not have to bend or reach.

G If you are making a bed, adjust the height to a safe working level, usually waist high. Avoid bending at the waist.

G When a task requires bending, use a good stance. Bend your knees to lower yourself, rather than bending from the waist. This uses the big muscles in your legs and thighs rather than the smaller muscles in your back.

G Do not twist when you are lifting or moving an object. Instead, turn your whole body. Pivot your feet instead of twisting at the waist. Your feet should point toward what you are lifting or moving.

G Get help when possible for lifting or helping residents.

G Talk to residents before moving them. Let them know what you will do so they can help if possible. Agree on a signal, such as counting to three. Lift or move on three so that everyone moves together.

G To help a resident sit up, stand up, or walk, place your feet 12 inches, or shoulder-width, apart. Put one foot in front of the other, and

bend your knees. Your upper body should stay upright and in alignment. Do this whenever you have to support a resident's weight.

G Never try to catch a falling resident. If the resident falls, assist her to the floor. If you try to reverse a fall in progress, you could injure yourself and/or the resident.

G Report to the nurse any task that you cannot safely do. Never try to lift an object or a resident that you feel you cannot handle.

Accident Prevention

Falls

A fall is any sudden, uncontrollable descent from a higher to a lower level, with or without injury resulting. Falls make up most of the accidents that occur in care facilities. They can be caused by an unsafe environment, loss of abilities, diseases, and medications. Problems resulting from falls range from minor bruises to fractures and life-threatening injuries. A **fracture** is a broken bone. Falls are particularly common among the elderly. Older people are often more seriously injured by falls because their bones are more fragile. NAs should be especially alert to the risk of falls. All falls must be reported to the supervisor.

These factors increase the risk of falls:

* Clutter

* Throw rugs

* Exposed electrical cords

* Slippery or wet floors

* Uneven floors or stairs

* Poor lighting

* Call lights that are out of reach or not promptly answered

Personal conditions that increase the risk of falls include medications, loss of vision, gait (walking) or balance problems, weakness, paralysis, and disorientation. **Disorientation** means confusion about person, place, or time.

Guidelines: Preventing Falls

G Clear all walkways of clutter, trash, throw rugs, and cords.

G Use rugs with a non-slip backing.

G Have residents wear non-skid, sturdy shoes. Make sure shoelaces are tied.

G Residents should avoid wearing clothing that is too long or drags on the floor.

G Keep items that are used often close to residents, including call lights.

G Answer call lights right away.

G Immediately clean up spills on the floor.

G Report loose hand rails immediately.

G If used, check placement of body or bed alarms and see if they are working.

G Mark uneven flooring or stairs with tape of a contrasting color to indicate a hazard.

G Improve lighting where needed.

G Lock wheels and move footrests out of the way before helping residents into or out of wheelchairs.

G Lock bed wheels before helping a resident into and out of bed or when giving care.

G After completing care, return beds to their lowest position.

G Get help when moving residents. Do not assume you can do it alone. Keep residents' walking aids, such as canes or walkers, within their reach.

G Offer help with toileting often. Respond to requests for help immediately. Think about how you would feel if you had to wait for help to go to the bathroom.

G Leave furniture in the same place as you found it.

G Know which residents are at risk for falls. Pay attention so that you can give help often.

G If a resident starts to fall, be in a good position to help support her. Never try to catch a falling resident. Use your body to slide her to the floor. If you try to reverse a fall, you may hurt yourself and/or the resident.

G Whenever a resident falls, it must be reported to the nurse. Always complete an incident report, even if the resident says he or she feels fine.

Burns/Scalds

Burns can be caused by dry heat (e.g., a hot iron, stove, other electrical appliances), wet heat (e.g., hot water or other liquids, steam), or chemicals (e.g. lye, acids). Small children, older adults, or people with loss of sensation (such as from paralysis or diabetes) are at greatest risk of burns. **Scalds** are burns caused by hot liquids. It takes five seconds or less for a serious burn to occur when the temperature of liquid is 140°F. Coffee, tea, and other hot drinks are usually served at 160°F to 180°F. These temperatures can cause almost instant burns that require surgery. Preventing burns is very important.

Guidelines: Preventing Burns and Scalds

G Always check water temperature with a bath thermometer or on your wrist before using.

G Report frayed electrical cords or unsafe-looking appliances immediately. Do not use them. Remove them from the room.

G Let residents know you are about to pour or set down a hot liquid.

G Pour hot drinks away from residents.

G Keep hot drinks and liquids away from edges of tables. Put a lid on them.

G Make sure residents are sitting down before serving hot drinks.

G If plate warmers are used, monitor them carefully.

Resident Identification

Residents must always be identified before giving care or serving food. Failure to identify residents can cause serious problems, even death. Facilities have different methods of identification. Some have pictures to identify residents. Others have signs outside residents' doors (Fig. 2-13). NAs must identify each resident before beginning any procedure or giving any care. They should identify residents before placing meal trays or helping with feeding. The diet card should be checked against the resident's identification to make sure they match. The resident should be called by name.

Fig. 2-13. A resident's name may be displayed outside the room to identify who is living in that room. Before giving any care, nursing assistants must always identify residents.

Choking

Choking can occur when eating, drinking or taking medication. People who are weak, ill, or unconscious can choke on their own saliva. A person's tongue can also become swollen and obstruct the airway. To guard against choking, residents should eat sitting as upright as possible. Residents with swallowing problems may have a special diet with liquids thickened to the consistency of nectar, honey, or pudding. Thickened liquids are easier to swallow. More information about thickened liquids is in Chapter 8.

Poisoning

There are many harmful substances in facilities that should not be swallowed. These include cleaners, paints, medicines, toiletries, and glues.

These products should be stored or locked away from confused residents or those with limited vision. Cleaning products should not be left in residents' rooms. Residents with dementia may hide food and let it spoil in closets, drawers, or other places. NAs should investigate any odors they notice. The number for the Poison Control Center should be posted near all telephones.

Cuts/Abrasions

Cuts or abrasions typically occur in the bathroom at a facility. An **abrasion** is an injury that rubs off the surface of the skin. Sharp objects, including scissors, nail clippers, or razors, should be put away after use. NAs should take care when transferring residents into and out of beds, chairs, and wheelchairs. When moving residents in wheelchairs, NAs should push the wheelchair forward. Wheelchairs should not be pulled from behind. When using elevators, wheelchairs should be turned around before entering, so that residents are facing forward.

Safety Data Sheet (SDS)

The Occupational Safety and Health Administration (OSHA) (osha.gov) is a federal government agency that makes rules to protect workers from hazards on the job. OSHA requires that all dangerous chemicals have a Safety Data Sheet (SDS) (formerly called *Material Safety Data Sheet*, or *MSDS*). This sheet details the chemical ingredients, chemical dangers, and safe handling, storage, and disposal procedures for the product. Information about emergency response actions to be taken are also included. Some facilities use a toll-free number to access SDS information. SDSs must be accessible in work areas for all employees. Important information about the SDS includes the following:

- Employers must have an SDS for every chemical used.

- Employers must provide easy access to the SDS.

- NAs must know where the SDSs are kept and how to read them. They should ask for help if they do not know how to do this.

The list of hazardous chemicals that have to have an SDS will be updated as new chemicals are purchased.

Fire

All facilities have a fire safety plan, and all workers need to know this plan. Guidelines regarding fires and evacuations will be explained to all employees. Evacuation routes are posted in facilities. NAs should read and review them often. They should attend fire and disaster training when it is offered. A fast, calm, and confident response by the staff saves lives.

Guidelines: Reducing Fire Hazards and Responding to Fires

G Some facilities are non-smoking, while others allow residents to smoke. If residents smoke, make sure they are in the proper area for smoking. Be sure that cigarettes are extinguished. Empty ashtrays often. Before emptying ashtrays, make sure there are no hot ashes or hot matches in the ashtray. Burn-resistant aprons for smokers may be available. These aprons help protect a person from burns from hot ashes and lit cigarettes if they are dropped. If residents wear these aprons when smoking, make sure buckles and snaps are properly fastened and that the apron covers their torso and lap. Never leave any smoker unattended.

G Report frayed or damaged electrical cords immediately. Report electrical equipment in need of repair immediately.

G Fire alarms and exit doors should not be blocked. If they are, report this to the nurse.

G Every facility will have fire extinguishers (Fig. 2-14). The PASS acronym will help you understand how to use it:

Pull the pin.

Aim at the base of fire when spraying.

Squeeze the handle.

Sweep back and forth at the base of the fire.

Fig. 2-14. Nursing assistants should know where the extinguishers are stored and how to use them.

G In case of fire, the RACE acronym is a good rule to follow:

Remove residents from danger.

Activate alarm or call 911.

Contain fire if possible.

Extinguish, or fire department will extinguish.

Follow these guidelines for helping residents exit the building safely:

G Know the facility's fire evacuation plan.

G Stay calm.

G Follow the directions of the fire department.

G Know which residents need one-on-one help or assistive devices. Immobile residents can be moved in several ways. If they have a wheelchair, help them into it. You can also use other wheeled transporters, such as carts, bath chairs, stretchers, or beds. A blanket can be used as a stretcher or even pulled across the floor with someone on it.

G Residents who can walk will also need help getting out of the building. Those who are hearing impaired may not hear the warnings and instructions. Staff will need to tell them directly what to do while guiding them to a safe exit. People with vision problems should be moved out of the way of the wheelchairs, carts, etc., and helped to the exit. Confused and disoriented residents will also need guidance.

G Remove anything blocking a window or door that could be used as a fire exit.

G Do not use elevators.

G Stay low in a room to escape fire.

G If a door is closed, check for heat coming from it before opening it. If the door or doorknob feels hot, stay in the room if there is no safe exit. Plug the doorway (use wet towels or clothing) to prevent smoke from entering. Stay in the room until help arrives.

G Use the *stop, drop, and roll* fire safety technique to extinguish a fire on clothing or hair. Stop running or stay still. Drop to the ground, lying down if possible. Roll on the ground to try to extinguish the flames.

G Use a damp covering over the mouth and nose to reduce smoke inhalation.

G After leaving the building, move away from it.

Disaster Guidelines

Disasters can include fire, flood, earthquake, hurricane, tornado, or severe weather. Man-made dangers, such as acts of terrorism or bomb threats, are also considered disasters.

Nursing assistants need to be skilled and professional when a disaster occurs. Facilities have disaster plans, and NAs will be trained on these plans. Annual in-services and disaster drills are often held at facilities. NAs should take advantage of these sessions and pay close attention to instructions.

During disasters, a nurse or the administrator will give directions. NAs should listen carefully and follow instructions. Facilities may rely on local or state groups and the American Red Cross to assume responsibility for the ill and disabled. The following guidelines apply in any disaster situation:

• Remain calm.

• Know the locations of all exits and stairways.

• Know where the fire alarms and extinguishers are located.

• Know the appropriate action to take in any situation.

• Use the internet to stay informed, or keep the television or radio tuned to a local station to get the latest information.

In addition, NAs will be required to know specific guidelines for the area in which they work. The instructor's teaching material has more information on specific disasters and response guidelines.

5. Demonstrate how to recognize and respond to medical emergencies

Medical emergencies may be the result of accidents or sudden illnesses. This section discusses what to do in a medical emergency. Heart attacks, strokes, diabetic emergencies, choking, automobile accidents, and gunshot wounds are all medical emergencies. Falls, burns, and cuts can also be emergencies. In an emergency, responders should remain calm, act quickly, and communicate clearly. These steps show the correct response to emergencies:

Assess the situation. The responder should try to find out what has happened. She must make sure she is not in danger. She should notice the time.

Assess the victim. The responder should ask the injured or ill person what has happened. If the person is unable to respond, he may be unconscious. Being **conscious** means being mentally alert and having awareness of surroundings, sensations, and thoughts. Tapping the person and asking if he is all right helps to determine if a person is conscious. The responder should speak loudly and use the person's name if she knows it. If there is no response, she should assume the person is unconscious. This is an emergency situation. She should call for help right away or send someone else to call.

If a person is conscious and able to speak, then he is breathing and has a pulse. The responder should talk with him about what happened. She should get the person's permission to touch him. (Anyone who is unable to give consent for treatment, e.g., a child with no parent near or an unconscious or seriously injured person, may be treated with *implied consent*. This means that if the person were able or the parents were present, they would have given consent). The person should be checked for the following:

- Severe bleeding

- Changes in consciousness

- Irregular breathing

- Unusual color or feel to the skin

- Swollen places on the body

- Medical alert tags

- Anything the person says is painful

If any of these exists, professional medical help may be needed. A nursing assistant should always get help. She should call the nurse before doing anything else.

If the injured or ill person is conscious, he may be frightened. The responder should listen to the person and tell him what is being done to help him. A calm and confident response will help reassure him.

An NA will need to document the emergency and complete an incident report after it is over. It is important to include as many details as possible and report only facts.

First aid is emergency care given immediately to an injured person. **Cardiopulmonary resuscitation** (**CPR**) refers to medical procedures used when a person's heart or lungs have stopped working. CPR is used until medical help arrives.

Quick action is necessary. CPR must be started immediately to prevent or lessen brain damage. Brain damage can occur within four to six minutes after the heart stops beating and breathing stops. The person can die within 10 minutes.

Only properly trained people should perform CPR. Employers often arrange for NAs to be trained in CPR. If not, an NA can contact the American Heart Association (heart.org) or Red Cross (redcross.org) for more information. CPR is an important skill to learn. **If a person is not trained, he should not attempt to perform CPR.**

Nursing assistants need to know their facility's policies on initiating CPR if they have been trained to do so. Some employers do not allow NAs to begin CPR without direction of the nurse.

Choking

When something is blocking the tube through which air enters the lungs, the person has an **obstructed airway**. When people are choking, they usually put their hands to their throats (Fig. 2-15). As long as the resident can speak, breathe, or cough, the NA should only encourage her to cough as forcefully as possible to get the object out. The NA should stay with the resident until she stops choking or can no longer speak, breathe, or cough.

If a resident can no longer speak, breathe, or cough, the NA should get help immediately. She can use the call light or emergency cord. The choking victim should not be left alone.

Fig. 2-15. *People who are choking usually put their hands to their throats.*

Abdominal thrusts are a method of attempting to remove an object from the airway of someone who is choking. These thrusts work to remove the blockage upward, out of the throat. The NA should make sure the person needs help before starting to give abdominal thrusts. She must show signs of a severely obstructed airway. These signs include poor air exchange, an increase in trouble breathing, silent coughing, blue-tinged (**cyanotic**) skin, or inability to speak, breathe, or cough. The NA should ask, "Are you choking? I know what to do. Can I help you?" If the resident nods her head, "Yes," she has a severe airway obstruction and needs immediate help. The NA should begin giving abdominal thrusts. This procedure should never be performed on a person who is not choking. Abdominal thrusts risk injury to the ribs and internal organs.

Performing abdominal thrusts for the conscious person

1. Stand behind the person and bring your arms under her arms. Wrap your arms around the person's waist.

2. Make a fist with one hand. Place the flat, thumb side of the fist against the person's abdomen, above the navel but below the breastbone.

3. Grasp the fist with your other hand. Pull both hands toward you and up, quickly and forcefully (Fig. 2-16).

Fig. 2-16. *When giving abdominal thrusts, pull both hands toward you and up (inward and upward), quickly and forcefully.*

4. Repeat until the object is pushed out or the person loses consciousness.

5. Report and document the incident properly.

If the resident becomes unconscious while choking, she should be helped to the floor gently. She should be lying on her back with her face up. The NA should begin CPR for an unconscious person if trained and allowed to do so. The NA should make sure help is on the way. The resident may have a completely blocked airway and needs medical help immediately. The NA should stay with the victim until help arrives.

Shock

Shock occurs when organs and tissues in the body do not receive an adequate blood supply. Bleeding, heart attack, severe infection, and falling blood pressure can lead to shock. Shock can become worse when the person is frightened or in severe pain.

Shock is a dangerous, life-threatening situation. Signs of shock include pale or bluish (cyanotic) skin, staring, increased pulse and respiration rates, low blood pressure, and extreme thirst. An NA should always call for help if she suspects a resident is in shock.

Responding to shock

1. Notify the nurse immediately. Victims of shock should always receive medical care as soon as possible.

2. If you need to control bleeding, put on gloves first. This procedure is described later in the chapter.

3. Have the person lie down on her back. If the person is bleeding from the mouth or vomiting, place her on her side (unless you suspect that the neck, back, or spinal cord is injured).

4. Check pulse and respirations if possible (Chapter 7). Begin CPR if breathing and pulse are absent and if you are trained to do so.

5. Keep the person as calm and comfortable as possible.

6. Maintain normal body temperature. If the weather is cold, place a blanket around the person. If the weather is hot, provide shade.

7. Elevate the legs about eight to 12 inches unless the person has a head, neck, back, spinal, or abdominal injury, breathing difficulties, or fractures (Fig. 2-17). Elevating the legs allows blood to flow back to the brain (and other vital areas.) Elevate the head and shoulders if a head wound or breathing difficulties are present. Never elevate a body part if the person has a broken bone or if it causes pain.

Fig. 2-17. *If a person is in shock, elevate the legs eight to 12 inches unless she has a head, neck, back, spinal, or abdominal injury, breathing difficulties, or fractures.*

8. Do not give the person anything to eat or drink.

9. Report and document the incident properly.

Myocardial Infarction or Heart Attack

Myocardial infarction (MI), or heart attack, occurs when the heart muscle itself does not receive enough oxygen because blood vessels are blocked. A myocardial infarction is an emergency that can result in serious heart damage or death. The following are signs and symptoms of MI:

- Sudden, severe pain in the chest, usually on the left side or in the center, behind the breastbone

- Pain or discomfort in other areas of the body, such as one or both arms, the back, neck, jaw, or stomach

- Indigestion or heartburn

- Nausea and vomiting

- **Dyspnea**, or difficulty breathing

- Dizziness

- Bluish or gray (cyanotic) skin color, indicating lack of oxygen

- Perspiration

- Cold and clammy skin

- Weak and irregular pulse rate

- Low blood pressure

- Anxiety and a sense of doom

- Denial of a heart problem

The pain of a heart attack is commonly described as a crushing, pressing, squeezing, stabbing, piercing pain, or "like someone is sitting on my chest." The pain may go down the inside of the left arm. A person may also feel it in the neck and/or in the jaw. The pain usually does not go away.

As with men, women may experience chest pain or pressure. Women, though, can have heart attacks without chest pressure. Women are more likely to have shortness of breath, pressure or pain in the lower chest or upper abdomen, dizziness, lightheadedness, fainting, pressure in the upper back, or extreme fatigue. Some women's symptoms seem more flu-like, and women are more likely to deny that they are having a heart attack. NAs must take immediate action if a resident has any of these symptoms.

Responding to a heart attack

1. Notify the nurse immediately.

2. Place the person in a comfortable position. Encourage him to rest. Reassure him that you will not leave him alone.

3. Loosen the clothing around the person's neck (Fig. 2-18).

Fig. 2-18. Loosen clothing around the person's neck if you suspect he is having an MI.

4. Do not give the person liquids or food.

5. Monitor the person's breathing and pulse. If the person stops breathing or has no pulse, begin CPR if trained and allowed to do so.

6. Stay with the person until help arrives.

7. Report and document the incident properly.

Some states allow nursing assistants to offer heart medication, such as nitroglycerin, to a resident having a heart attack. If allowed to do this, NAs can only offer the medication. They cannot place it in the resident's mouth.

Bleeding

Severe bleeding can cause death quickly and must be controlled.

Controlling bleeding

1. Notify the nurse immediately.

2. Put on gloves. Take time to do this. If the resident is able, he can hold his bare hand over the wound until you can put on gloves.

3. Hold a thick sterile pad, clean cloth, handkerchief, or towel against the wound.

4. Press down hard directly on the bleeding wound until help arrives. Do not decrease pressure (Fig. 2-19). Put additional pads over the first pad if blood seeps through. Do not remove the first pad.

Fig. 2-19. Press down hard directly on the bleeding wound; do not decrease pressure.

5. If you can, raise the wound above the level of the heart to slow the bleeding. If the wound is on an arm, leg, hand, or foot, and there are no broken bones, prop up the limb. Use towels or other absorbent materials.

6. When bleeding is under control, secure the dressing to keep it in place. Check the person for symptoms of shock (pale skin, increased pulse and respiration rates, low blood pressure, and extreme thirst). Stay with the person until help arrives.

7. Remove and discard gloves. Wash hands thoroughly.

8. Report and document the incident properly.

Burns

Care of a burn depends on its depth, size, and location. Burns may require emergency help.

Treating burns

To treat a minor burn:

1. Notify the nurse immediately. Put on gloves.

2. Use cool, clean water to decrease the skin temperature and prevent further injury. Do not use ice or ice water, as ice may cause further skin damage. Dampen a clean cloth with cool water. Place it over the burn.

3. Once the pain has eased, you may cover the area with dry, sterile gauze or clean dressing.

4. Remove and discard gloves. Wash your hands.

5. Never use any kind of ointment, salve, or grease on a burn.

For more serious burns:

1. Remove the person from the source of the burn. If clothing has caught fire, have the person stop, drop, and roll, or smother the fire with a blanket or towel to put out flames. Protect yourself from the source of the burn.

2. Notify the nurse immediately. Put on gloves.

3. Check for breathing, pulse, and severe bleeding. If the person is not breathing and has no pulse, begin CPR if trained and allowed to do so.

4. Do not use any type of ointment, water, salve, or grease on the burn.

5. Do not try to pull away any clothing from burned areas. Cover the burn with thick, dry, sterile gauze, a clean cloth, or a clean white sheet. A dry, insulated cool pack may be used over the dressing. Take care not to rub the burned area.

6. Ask the person to lie down and elevate the affected part if this does not cause greater pain.

7. Wait for emergency medical help.

8. Remove and discard gloves. Wash your hands.

9. Report and document the incident properly.

Fainting

Fainting occurs as a result of decreased blood flow to the brain, causing a loss of consciousness. Fainting may be the result of hunger, fear, pain, fatigue, standing for a long time, poor ventilation, certain medications, pregnancy, or overheating. Signs and symptoms of fainting include dizziness, nausea, perspiration, pale skin, weak pulse, shallow respirations, and blackness in the visual field.

Responding to fainting

1. Notify the nurse immediately.

2. Have the person lie down or sit down before fainting occurs.

3. If the person is in a sitting position, have him bend forward (Fig. 2-20). He can place his head between his knees if he is able. If the person is lying flat on his back, elevate the legs.

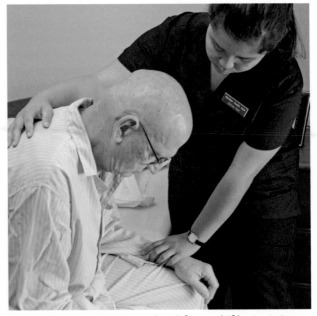

Fig. 2-20. Have the person bend forward if he is sitting.

4. Loosen any tight clothing.

5. Have the person stay in position for at least five minutes after symptoms disappear.

6. Help the person get up slowly. Continue to observe him for symptoms of fainting. Stay with him until he feels better. If you need help but cannot leave the person, use the call light.

7. If a person does faint, lower him to the floor or other flat surface. Position him on his back. Elevate his legs eight to 12 inches. Loosen any tight clothing. Check to make sure the person is breathing. He should recover quickly, but keep him lying down for several minutes. Report the incident to the nurse immediately.

8. Report and document the incident properly. Fainting may be a sign of a more serious medical condition.

Insulin Reaction and Diabetic Ketoacidosis

Insulin reaction and diabetic ketoacidosis are problems of diabetes that can be life-threatening. **Insulin reaction**, or hypoglycemia, can result from either too much insulin or too little food. It occurs when insulin is given and the person skips a meal or does not eat all the food required. Even when a regular amount of food is eaten, physical activity may rapidly absorb the food. This causes too much insulin to be in the body. Vomiting and diarrhea may also lead to insulin reaction in people who have diabetes.

The first signs of insulin reaction include feeling weak or different, nervousness, dizziness, and perspiration. These signal that the resident needs food in a form that can be rapidly absorbed. A lump of sugar, a hard candy, or a small glass of juice should be consumed right away. A diabetic should always have a quick source of sugar handy. The nurse should be notified if the resident has shown signs of insulin

reaction. Other signs and symptoms include the following:

*   Hunger
*   Weakness
*   Rapid pulse
*   Headache
*   Low blood pressure
*   Perspiration
*   Cold, clammy skin
*   Confusion
*   Trembling
*   Nervousness
*   Blurred vision
*   Numbness of the lips and tongue
*   Unconsciousness

Diabetic ketoacidosis (**DKA**), or hyperglycemia, is caused by having too little insulin. It can result from undiagnosed diabetes, going without insulin or not taking enough, eating too much, not getting enough exercise, infection, or physical or emotional stress. The signs of the onset of diabetic ketoacidosis include increased thirst and/or urination, abdominal pain, deep or labored breathing, and breath that smells sweet or fruity. The nurse should be notified immediately if the resident has shown signs of DKA. Other signs and symptoms include the following:

*   Hunger
*   Headache
*   Weakness
*   Rapid, weak pulse
*   Low blood pressure
*   Dry skin
*   Flushed cheeks
*   Drowsiness
*   Nausea and vomiting

- Air hunger, or resident gasping for air and being unable to catch his breath

- Unconsciousness

Chapter 4 has more information on diabetes.

Seizures

Seizures are involuntary, often violent, contractions of muscles. They can involve a small area or the entire body. Seizures are caused by an abnormality in the brain. They can occur in young children who have a high fever. Older children and adults who have a serious illness, fever, head injury, or a seizure disorder such as epilepsy may also have seizures.

The main goal during a seizure is to make sure the resident is safe. During a seizure, a person may shake severely and thrust arms and legs uncontrollably. He may clench his jaw, drool, and be unable to swallow. Most seizures only last a short time.

Responding to seizures

1. Note the time. Put on gloves.

2. Lower the person to the floor. Loosen clothing to help with breathing. Try to turn the person's head to one side to help lower the risk of choking. This may not be possible during a violent seizure.

3. Have someone call the nurse immediately or use the call light. Do not leave the person unless you must do so to get medical help.

4. Move furniture away to prevent injury. If a pillow is nearby, place it under his head.

5. Do not try to restrain the person or stop the seizure.

6. Do not force anything between the person's teeth. Do not place your hands in the person's mouth for any reason. You could be bitten.

7. Do not give the person liquids or food.

8. When the seizure is over, note the time. Gently turn the person to his left side if you do not suspect a head, neck, or spinal injury. This reduces the risk of choking on vomit or saliva. If the person begins to choke, get help immediately. Check for adequate breathing and pulse. Begin CPR if breathing and pulse are absent and if you are allowed and trained to do so. Do not begin CPR during a seizure.

9. Remove and discard gloves. Wash your hands.

10. Report and document the incident properly, including how long the seizure lasted.

CVA or Stroke

Cerebrovascular accident (CVA), or stroke, occurs when blood supply to a part of the brain is blocked or a blood vessel leaks or ruptures within the brain. A quick response to a suspected stroke is critical. Tests and treatment need to be given within a short time of the stroke's onset. Early treatment may be able to reduce the severity of the stroke.

A **transient ischemic attack (TIA)** is a warning sign of a CVA. It is the result of a temporary lack of oxygen in the brain. Symptoms may last up to 24 hours. They include difficulty speaking, weakness on one side of the body, temporary loss of vision, and numbness or tingling. These symptoms should not be ignored. They should be reported to the nurse immediately.

Signs that a CVA is occurring include

- Facial numbness, weakness, or drooping, especially on one side

- Arm or leg numbness or weakness, especially on one side

- Slurred speech or inability to speak

- Use of inappropriate words

- Inability to understand spoken or written words

- Redness in the face

- Noisy breathing

- Dizziness

- Blurred vision

- Trouble walking, loss of balance

- Ringing in the ears

- Severe headache

- Nausea/vomiting

- Seizures

- Loss of bowel and bladder control

- Paralysis on one side of the body

- Elevated blood pressure

- Slow pulse rate

- Loss of consciousness

In addition to the symptoms listed above, women may have these symptoms:

- Pain in the face, arms, and legs

- Hiccups

- Weakness

- Chest pain

- Shortness of breath

- Palpitations

Chapter 4 has more information on CVAs.

Vomiting

Vomiting, or **emesis**, is the act of ejecting stomach contents through the mouth and/or nose. It can be a sign of a serious illness or injury. Because an NA may not know when a resident is going to vomit, she may not have time to explain what she will do and assemble supplies ahead of time. The NA should talk to the resident soothingly as she helps him clean up. She should tell the resident what she is doing to help him.

1. Notify the nurse immediately.

2. Put on gloves.

3. Make sure the head is up or turned to one side. Place an emesis basin under the chin. Remove it when vomiting has stopped.

4. Remove soiled linens or clothes and set aside. Replace with fresh linens or clothes.

5. If resident's intake and output (I&O) is being monitored (Chapter 7), measure and note amount of vomitus.

6. Flush vomit down the toilet unless vomit is red, has blood in it, or looks like wet coffee grounds, or if medication/pills are in vomit. If these signs are observed, show this to the nurse before discarding the vomit. After disposing of vomit, wash, dry, and store basin.

7. Remove and discard gloves.

8. Wash your hands.

9. Put on fresh gloves.

10. Provide comfort to resident. Wipe face and mouth (Fig. 2-21). Position comfortably. Offer a drink of water. Provide oral care. It helps get rid of the taste of vomit in the mouth.

Fig. 2-21. Be calm and comforting when helping a resident who has vomited.

11. Put soiled linen in proper containers.

12. Remove and discard gloves.

13. Wash your hands again.

14. Report and document the incident properly. Document time, amount, color, odor, and consistency of vomitus.

---

6. Describe and demonstrate infection prevention practices

Infection prevention is the term for methods practiced in healthcare facilities to prevent and control the spread of disease. Preventing the spread of infection is the responsibility of all care team members. Nursing assistants must know and follow their facility's infection prevention policies. These policies help protect staff, residents, and others from disease.

A **microorganism** (**MO**) is a living thing or organism that is so small that it can be seen only under a microscope. A **microbe** is another name for a microorganism. Microorganisms are always present in the environment. **Infections** occur when harmful microorganisms, called **pathogens**, invade the body and multiply.

There are two main types of infections: localized and systemic. A **localized infection** is limited to a specific location in the body. It has local symptoms, which means the symptoms are near the site of infection. For example, if a wound becomes infected, the area around it may become red, hot, and painful. A **systemic infection** affects the entire body. This type of infection travels through the bloodstream and is spread throughout the body. It causes general symptoms, such as fever, chills, mental confusion, or lower than normal blood pressure.

A type of infection that can be localized or systemic is a healthcare-associated infection, formerly known as nosocomial infection. A **healthcare-associated infection** (**HAI**) is an infection acquired in a healthcare setting during the delivery of medical care. Healthcare settings include hospitals, long-term care facilities, and outpatient surgery centers, among others.

Preventing the spread of infection is important. To understand how to prevent disease, it is helpful to first understand how it is spread. The **chain of infection** is a way of describing how disease is transmitted from one being to another (Fig. 2-22). Definitions and examples of each of the six links in the chain of infection follow.

Fig. 2-22. The chain of infection.

Link 1: The **causative agent** is a pathogenic microorganism that causes disease. Causative agents include bacteria, viruses, fungi, and parasites. Normal flora are the microorganisms that live in and on the body. They normally do not cause harm as long as they remain in or at that particular area. When they enter a different part of the body, they may cause an infection.

Link 2: A **reservoir** is where the pathogen lives and grows. A reservoir can be a human, animal, plant, soil, or a substance. Microorganisms grow best in warm, dark, and moist places where food is present. Some microorganisms need oxygen to survive; others do not. Examples of reservoirs include the lungs, blood, and the large intestine.

Link 3: The **portal of exit** is any body opening on an infected person that allows pathogens to leave (Fig. 2-23). These include the nose, mouth, eyes, or a cut in the skin.

Link 4: The **mode of transmission** describes how the pathogen travels. Transmission can occur through the air or through direct or indirect contact. **Direct contact** happens by touching the infected person or his secretions. **Indirect contact** results from touching something contaminated by the infected person, such as a needle, dressing, or tissue. The primary route of disease transmission within the healthcare setting is on the hands of healthcare workers.

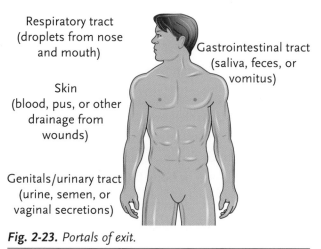

Respiratory tract (droplets from nose and mouth)

Gastrointestinal tract (saliva, feces, or vomitus)

Skin (blood, pus, or other drainage from wounds)

Genitals/urinary tract (urine, semen, or vaginal secretions)

Fig. 2-23. Portals of exit.

Link 5: The **portal of entry** is any body opening on an uninfected person that allows pathogens to enter (Fig. 2-24). These include the nose, mouth, eyes, and other mucous membranes, cuts in the skin, and cracked skin. **Mucous membranes** are the membranes that line body cavities that open to the outside of the body. These include the linings of the mouth, nose, eyes, rectum, and genitals.

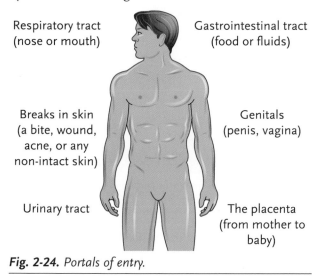

Respiratory tract (nose or mouth)

Gastrointestinal tract (food or fluids)

Breaks in skin (a bite, wound, acne, or any non-intact skin)

Genitals (penis, vagina)

Urinary tract

The placenta (from mother to baby)

Fig. 2-24. Portals of entry.

Link 6: A **susceptible host** is an uninfected person who could get sick. Examples include all healthcare workers and anyone in their care who is not already infected with that particular disease.

If one of the links in the chain of infection is broken, then the spread of infection is stopped. Infection prevention practices help stop pathogens from traveling (Link 4) and getting on a person's hands, nose, eyes, mouth, skin, etc. (Link 5). Immunizations (Link 6) reduce a person's chances of getting sick from diseases such as hepatitis B and influenza.

Transmission (passage or transfer) of most **infectious** diseases can be blocked by using proper infection prevention practices, such as handwashing. Handwashing is the most important way to stop the spread of infection. All caregivers should wash their hands often.

Handwashing is a part of medical asepsis. **Medical asepsis** refers to measures used to reduce and prevent the spread of pathogens. Medical asepsis is used in all healthcare settings. **Surgical asepsis**, or sterile technique, is the state of being free of all microorganisms, not just pathogens. Surgical asepsis is used for many types of procedures, such as changing catheters.

Standard Precautions and Transmission-Based Precautions

State and federal government agencies have guidelines and laws concerning infection prevention. The **Centers for Disease Control and Prevention (CDC)** (cdc.gov) is a government agency under the Department of Health and Human Services (HHS) (hhs.gov). It issues information to protect the health of individuals and communities. It promotes public health, as well as disease, injury, and disability prevention and control through education.

In 1996, the CDC recommended a new infection prevention system to reduce the risk of contracting infectious diseases in healthcare settings.

It has been updated since. There are two tiers of precautions within the infection prevention system: Standard Precautions and Transmission-Based Precautions.

Standard Precautions means treating blood, body fluids, non-intact skin (like abrasions, pimples, or open sores), and mucous membranes (linings of mouth, nose, eyes, rectum, and genitals) as if they were infected. Body fluids include saliva, **sputum** (mucus coughed up), urine, feces, semen, vaginal secretions, pus or other wound drainage, and vomit. They do not include sweat.

Standard Precautions must be used with every resident. This promotes safety. An NA cannot tell by looking at residents if they have a contagious disease such as tuberculosis, hepatitis, or influenza.

Standard Precautions and Transmission-Based Precautions are ways to stop the spread of infection. They interrupt the mode of transmission. In other words, these guidelines do not stop an infected person from giving off pathogens. However, by following these guidelines, NAs help prevent those pathogens from infecting them or those in their care:

- Standard Precautions must be practiced with every single person in an NA's care.

- Transmission-Based Precautions vary based on how an infection is transmitted. When indicated, they are used **in addition** to the Standard Precautions. More information about these precautions is located later in the chapter.

Guidelines: Standard Precautions

G   **Wash your hands** before putting on gloves. Wash your hands immediately after removing gloves. Be careful not to touch clean objects with your used gloves.

G   **Wear gloves** if you may come into contact with blood; body fluids or secretions; broken skin, such as abrasions, acne, cuts, stitches, or staples; or mucous membranes. Such contacts occur during mouth care; toilet assistance; perineal care; helping with a bedpan or urinal; ostomy care; cleaning up spills; cleaning basins, urinals, bedpans, and other containers that have held body fluids; and disposing of wastes.

G   **Remove gloves** immediately when finished with a procedure.

G   **Immediately wash all skin surfaces that have been contaminated** with blood and body fluids.

G   **Wear a disposable gown** that is resistant to body fluids if you may come into contact with blood or body fluids or when splashing or spraying blood or body fluids is likely.

G   **Wear a mask and protective goggles** if you may come into contact with blood or body fluids or when splashing or spraying blood or body fluids is likely.

G   **Wear gloves and use caution when handling razor blades, needles, and other sharps. Sharps** are needles or other sharp objects. Place sharps carefully in a biohazard container for sharps. Biohazard containers used for sharps are hard, leakproof containers. They are clearly labeled and warn of the danger of the contents inside (Fig. 2-25).

BIOHAZARD

Fig. 2-25. This label indicates that the material is potentially infectious.

G   **Never attempt to recap needles or sharps after use. You might stick yourself.** Dispose of them in a biohazard container for sharps.

G **Avoid nicks and cuts** when shaving residents.

G **Carefully bag all contaminated supplies.** Dispose of them according to your facility's policy.

G **Clearly label body fluids that are being saved for a specimen** with the resident's name, date of birth, room number, and date and a biohazard label. Keep them in a container with a lid. Put in a biohazardous specimen bag for transportation if required.

G **Dispose of contaminated wastes according to your facility's policy.** Waste containing blood or body fluids is considered biohazardous waste. Liquid waste can usually be disposed of through the regular sewer system as long as there is no splashing, spraying, or aerosolizing of the waste as it is being disposed. Appropriate PPE needs to be worn, followed by proper removal and handwashing. Follow instructions at your facility.

Nursing assistants must practice Standard Precautions on everyone for whom they care, regardless of their infection status. This greatly reduces the risk of transmitting infection.

Nursing assistants use their hands constantly while they work. Microorganisms are on everything they touch. The single most common way for healthcare-associated infections (HAIs) to be spread is via the hands of healthcare workers. Handwashing is the most important thing NAs can do to prevent the spread of disease.

The CDC has defined **hand hygiene** as washing hands with either plain or antiseptic soap and water or using alcohol-based hand rubs. Alcohol-based hand rubs (often called *hand sanitizers*) include gels, rinses, and foams that do not require the use of water.

Alcohol-based hand rubs have proven effective in reducing bacteria on the skin. However, they are not a substitute for proper handwashing. When hands are visibly soiled, they should be washed using antimicrobial soap and water. An **antimicrobial** agent destroys, resists, or prevents the development of pathogens. Once hands are clean, hand rubs can be used in addition to handwashing any time hands are not visibly soiled. When using a hand rub, the hands must be rubbed together until the product has completely dried. Hand lotion can help prevent dry, cracked skin.

NAs should avoid wearing rings while working. Rings may increase the risk of contamination. Fingernails should be short, smooth, and clean. Artificial nails or extenders should not be worn because they harbor bacteria and increase the risk of contamination. NAs should wash their hands at these times:

- When first arriving at work

- Whenever hands are visibly soiled

- Before, between, and after all contact with residents

- Before putting on gloves and after removing gloves

- After contact with any body fluids, mucous membranes, non-intact skin, or wound dressings

- After handling contaminated items

- After contact with objects in the resident's room (care environment)

- Before and after touching meal trays and/or handling food

- Before and after feeding residents

- Before getting clean linen

- After touching garbage or trash

- After picking up anything from the floor

- Before and after using the toilet

- After nose-blowing or coughing or sneezing into hands

- Before and after eating

- After smoking

- After touching areas on the body, such as the mouth, face, eyes, hair, ears, or nose

- Before and after applying makeup

- After any contact with pets and after contact with pet care items

- Before leaving the facility

Washing hands (hand hygiene)

Equipment: soap, paper towels

1. Turn on water at sink. Keep your clothes dry.

2. Wet hands and wrists thoroughly (Fig. 2-26).

Fig. 2-26. Keeping arms angled downward, wet hands and wrists thoroughly.

3. Apply soap to hands.

4. Keep your hands lower than your elbows and your fingertips down. Rub hands together and fingers between each other to create a lather. Lather all surfaces of wrists, hands, and fingers, using friction for at least 20 seconds (Fig. 2-27).
   Lather and friction loosen skin oils and allow pathogens to be rinsed away.

5. Clean your nails by rubbing them in palm of your other hand.
   Most pathogens on hands are under the nails.

6. Keep your hands lower than your elbows and your fingertips down. Being careful not to touch the sink, rinse thoroughly under running water. Rinse all surfaces of your wrists, hands, and fingers. Run water down from wrists to fingertips. Do not run water over unwashed arms down to clean hands.
   Water should run from cleanest to dirtiest. Wrists are cleanest, fingertips dirtiest.

Fig. 2-27. Using friction for at least 20 seconds, lather all surfaces of fingers and hands.

7. Use a clean, dry paper towel to dry all surfaces of your hands, wrists, and fingers. Do not wipe towel on unwashed forearms and then wipe clean hands. Dispose of towel into waste container without touching the container. If your hands touch the sink or wastebasket, start over.

8. Use a clean, dry paper towel to turn off the faucet (Fig. 2-28). Dispose of paper towel into waste container. Do not contaminate your hands by touching the surface of the sink or faucet.
   Hands will be recontaminated if you touch the dirty faucet or sink with clean hands.

Fig. 2-28. Use a clean, dry paper towel to turn off faucet so that you do not contaminate your hands.

Personal Protective Equipment

Personal protective equipment (**PPE**) is equipment that helps protect employees from serious injuries or illnesses resulting from contact with workplace hazards. In care facilities, PPE helps protect nursing assistants from contact with potentially infectious material. Employers are responsible for giving NAs the appropriate PPE to wear.

Personal protective equipment includes gowns, masks, goggles, face shields, and gloves. Gowns protect the skin and/or clothing. Masks protect the mouth and nose. Goggles protect the eyes. Face shields protect the entire face—the eyes, nose, and mouth. Gloves protect the hands. Gloves are used the most often by all caregivers.

Personal protective equipment must be worn if the NA could come into contact with body fluids, mucous membranes, or open wounds. Nursing assistants must wear, or **don**, gowns, masks, goggles, and face shields when splashing or spraying of body fluids or blood could occur.

Clean, non-sterile gowns protect exposed skin. They also prevent soiling of clothing. Gowns should fully cover the torso. They should fit comfortably over the body and have long sleeves that fit snugly at the wrist. When finished with a procedure, NAs should remove, or **doff**, the gown as soon as possible and wash their hands.

Putting on (donning) and removing (doffing) gown

1. Wash your hands.

2. Open gown. Hold out in front of you and allow gown to open/unfold. Do not shake it (Fig. 2-29). Facing the back opening of the gown, place your arms through each sleeve.

3. Fasten the neck opening.

4. Reach behind you. Pull the gown until it completely covers your clothing. Secure gown at waist (Fig. 2-30).

Fig. 2-29. Let the gown unfold without shaking it.

Fig. 2-30. Reaching behind you, secure the gown at the waist.

5. Use a gown only once and then remove and discard it. If gown becomes wet or soiled during care, remove it. Check clothing. Put on a new gown. OSHA requires non-permeable gowns—gowns that liquids cannot penetrate—when working in a bloody situation.

6. Put on your gloves after putting on gown. The cuffs of gloves should overlap the cuffs of the gown (Fig. 2-31).

Fig. 2-31. The cuff of the gloves should overlap the cuffs of the gown.

7. When removing a gown, remove and discard gloves properly (see procedure later in the chapter). Unfasten gown at neck and waist. Remove the gown without touching the outside of gown. Roll the dirty side in, while holding gown away from your body. Dispose of gown properly and wash your hands. *Rolling puts dirtiest surface inward, lessening the risk of contamination.*

Masks should be worn when caring for residents with respiratory illnesses. They should also be worn when it is likely that contact with blood or body fluids may occur. Sometimes special masks (respirators) are required for certain diseases, such as tuberculosis (TB). Masks should fully cover the nose and mouth and prevent fluid penetration. Masks should fit snugly over the nose and mouth. NAs must always change their masks when moving between residents. The same mask should not be worn from one resident to another. Goggles provide protection for the eyes. They are used when it is likely that blood or body fluids may be splashed or sprayed into the eye area or into the eyes. Eyeglasses alone do not provide proper eye protection. Goggles should fit snugly over and around the eyes or eyeglasses.

Putting on (donning) mask and goggles

1. Wash your hands.

2. Pick up mask by top strings or elastic strap. Do not touch mask where it touches your face.

3. Pull elastic strap over your head, or if mask has strings, tie top strings first, then bottom strings. Do not wear a mask hanging from only the bottom tie or strap. Masks must always be dry or they must be replaced.

4. Pinch the metal strip at the top of the mask (if part of mask) tightly around your nose so that it feels snug (Fig. 2-32).

Fig. 2-32. *Adjust the metal strip until the mask fits snugly around your nose.*

5. Put on the goggles over your eyes or eyeglasses. Use the headband to secure them to your head. Make sure they are on snugly.

6. Put on gloves after putting on mask and goggles.

When additional skin protection is needed (if part of facility policy), a face shield can be substituted for a mask or goggles. The face shield should cover the forehead, go below the chin, and wrap around the sides of the face. A headband secures it to the head.

Facilities have specific policies and procedures on when to wear gloves. NAs must learn and follow these rules. Gloves must always be worn for the following tasks:

- Anytime an NA might come into contact with blood or any body fluid, open wounds, or mucous membranes

- When performing or helping with mouth care or care of any mucous membrane

- When performing or helping with **perineal care** (care of the genitals and anal area)

- When performing personal care on **non-intact skin**—skin that is broken by abrasions, cuts, rashes, acne, pimples, lesions, surgical incisions, or boils

- When assisting with personal care when the NA has open sores or cuts on her hands

- When shaving a resident

- When disposing of soiled bed linens, gowns, dressings, and pads

- When touching surfaces or equipment that is either visibly contaminated or may be contaminated

Clean, non-sterile gloves are generally adequate. They may be latex, vinyl, or nitrile; however, some people are allergic to latex. An NA should let the nurse know if he is allergic to latex. Alternative gloves will be provided. An NA should also tell the nurse if he has dry, cracked, or broken skin. Non-intact areas should be covered with bandages or gauze before putting on gloves. Gloves should fit the hands comfortably and should not be too loose or too tight.

Disposable gloves can only be worn once. They cannot be washed or reused. Gloves should be changed immediately if they become soiled, torn, or damaged. Gloves should also be changed before contact with mucous membranes or broken skin. After removing gloves, the NA should wash his hands before donning new gloves.

Putting on (donning) gloves

1. Wash your hands.

2. If you are right-handed, slide one glove on your left hand (reverse if left-handed).

3. Using your gloved hand, slide the other hand into the second glove.

4. Interlace fingers. Smooth out folds and create a comfortable fit.

5. Carefully look for tears, holes, or spots. Replace the glove if needed.

6. If wearing a gown, pull the cuff of the gloves over the sleeves of the gown (Fig. 2-33).

Fig. 2-33. *Adjust gloves until they are pulled up over the sleeves of the gown.*

Gloves should be removed promptly after use and before caring for another resident. The NA should wash his hands. Gloves are worn to protect the skin from becoming contaminated. After giving care, gloves are contaminated. If the NA opens a door with a gloved hand, the doorknob becomes contaminated. Later, anyone who opens the door with an ungloved hand will be touching a contaminated surface. Before touching surfaces or leaving residents' rooms, the NA must remove gloves and wash his hands. Afterward, new gloves can be donned if needed.

Removing (doffing) gloves

1. Touch only the outside of one glove. With one gloved hand, grasp the other glove at the palm and pull the glove off (Fig. 2-34).

Fig. 2-34. *Grasp the glove at the palm and pull it off.*

2. With the fingertips of your gloved hand, hold the glove you just removed. With your ungloved hand, slip two fingers underneath cuff of the remaining glove at wrist. Do not touch any part of the outside of glove (Fig. 2-35). *The outside of the glove is contaminated.*

Fig. 2-35. *Reach inside glove at wrist, without touching any part of the outside of glove.*

3. Pull down, turning this glove inside out and over the first glove as you remove it.

4. You should now be holding one glove from its clean inner side. The other glove should be inside it.

5. Drop both gloves into the proper container without contaminating yourself.

6. Wash your hands.

This is the correct order that the NA should follow when donning (putting on) PPE:

1. Wash hands.

2. Put on gown.

3. Put on mask.

4. Put on goggles or face shield.

5. Put on gloves.

This is the correct order that the NA should follow when doffing (removing) PPE:

1. Remove and discard gloves.

2. Remove goggles or face shield.

3. Remove and discard gown.

4. Remove and discard mask.

5. Wash hands. Washing hands is always the final step after removing and discarding PPE.

Equipment and Linen Handling

In health care, an object is called **clean** if it has not been contaminated with pathogens. An object that is **dirty** has been contaminated with pathogens. Facilities have special rooms or areas for equipment, linen, and supplies. There are separate rooms for supplies that are considered clean and for supplies that are considered dirty or contaminated. NAs will be told where these rooms are located and what types of equipment and supplies are found in each room. NAs should perform hand hygiene before entering clean rooms and before leaving dirty rooms. This helps prevent the spread of pathogens.

Guidelines: Handling Equipment, Linen, and Clothing

G   Handle all equipment in a way that prevents

   • Skin/mucous membrane contact

   • Contamination of your clothing

   • Transfer of disease to other residents or areas

G   Do not use reusable equipment again until it has been properly cleaned and reprocessed. **Sterilization** is a cleaning measure that destroys all microorganisms, including pathogens. It uses steam under pressure, dry heat, or liquid or gas chemicals to sterilize. Items that need to be sterilized are ones that go directly into the bloodstream or into other normally sterile areas of the body (for example, surgical instruments). **Disinfection** is a process that kills pathogens but does not destroy all pathogens. It reduces the pathogen count to a level that is considered not infectious. Disinfection is carried out with pasteurization or chemical germicides. Examples of items that are usually disinfected are reusable oxygen tanks, wall mounted blood pressure cuffs, and any reusable resident care equipment.

G   Dispose of all single-use, or disposable, equipment properly. **Disposable** equipment is discarded after one use. Disposable razors and disposable thermometers are examples of disposable equipment.

G   Clean and disinfect

   • All environmental surfaces

   • Beds, bedrails, and all bedside equipment

   • All frequently touched surfaces (such as doorknobs and call lights)

G   Handle, transport, and process soiled linens and clothing in a way that prevents

   • Skin and mucous membrane exposure

- Contamination of clothing (hold linen and clothing away from your uniform) (Fig. 2-36)

- Transfer of disease to other residents and areas (do not shake linen or clothes; fold or roll linen so that dirtiest area is inside; do not put soiled linen on floor)

Fig. 2-36. Hold and carry dirty linen away from your uniform.

G Bag soiled linen at point of origin.

G Sort soiled linen away from resident care areas.

G Place wet linen in leakproof bags.

More information about cleaning equipment and supplies is in Chapter 7.

Spills

Spills can pose a serious risk of infection and can put residents and staff at risk for falls. Nursing assistants must clean spills using the proper solutions and equipment.

Guidelines: Cleaning Spills Involving Blood, Body Fluids, or Glass

G Apply gloves before starting. In some cases, industrial-strength gloves are best.

G First, absorb the spill with whatever product is used by the facility. It may be an absorbing powder.

G Scoop up the absorbed spill, and dispose of it in a designated container.

G Apply the proper disinfectant to the spill area and allow it to stand wet for a minimum of 10 minutes.

G Clean up spills immediately with the proper cleaning solution.

G Do not pick up any pieces of broken glass, no matter how large, with your hands. Use a dustpan and broom or other tools.

G Waste containing broken glass, blood, or body fluids should be properly bagged. Waste containing blood or body fluids may need to be placed in a special biohazard waste bag. Follow facility policy.

Transmission-Based Precautions

These precautions are used when caring for persons who are infected or suspected of being infected with a disease. These precautions are called **Transmission-Based Precautions**. When ordered, these precautions are used in addition to Standard Precautions. These precautions will always be listed in the care plan and on the assignment sheet. Following these precautions promotes the NA's safety, as well as the safety of others.

There are three categories of Transmission-Based Precautions:

- Airborne Precautions

- Droplet Precautions

- Contact Precautions

The category used depends on the disease and how it spreads to other people. They may also be used in combination for diseases that have multiple routes of transmission.

Airborne Precautions are used for diseases that are transmitted, or spread, through the air after being expelled (Fig. 2-37). The pathogens are so small that they can attach to moisture in the air. They can remain floating for some time. For certain care, NAs may be required to wear special masks, such as N95 or HEPA masks, to avoid being infected. Airborne diseases include tuberculosis, measles, and chickenpox.

Fig. 2-37. *Airborne Precautions are used for diseases that can be transmitted through the air.*

Droplet Precautions are used for diseases that are spread by droplets in the air. Droplets normally do not travel more than six feet. Coughing, sneezing, talking, laughing, or suctioning can spread droplets (Fig. 2-38). Droplet Precautions include wearing a face mask during care and restricting visits from uninfected people. Residents should wear masks, if possible, when being moved from room to room. NAs should cover their noses and mouths with a tissue when they sneeze or cough. They should ask others to do the same. Used tissues should be disposed of in the nearest waste container. Used tissues should not be placed in a pocket for later use. If a tissue is not available, NAs should cough or sneeze into their upper sleeve or elbow, not their hands. They should wash their hands immediately afterward. An example of a droplet disease is mumps.

Fig. 2-38. *Droplet Precautions are followed when the disease-causing microorganism does not remain in the air.*

Contact Precautions are used when there is a risk of spreading or contracting a microorganism by touching an infected object or person (Fig. 2-39). Conjunctivitis (pink eye) and

Clostridium difficile infection are examples of situations that require Contact Precautions. Transmission can occur with skin-to-skin contact during transfers or bathing. Contact Precautions include wearing PPE and resident isolation. Contact Precautions require washing hands with antimicrobial soap and not touching infected surfaces with ungloved hands or uninfected surfaces with contaminated gloves.

Fig. 2-39. *Contact Precautions are followed when the person is at risk of transmitting a microorganism by touching an infected object or person.*

Staff often refer to residents who need Transmission-Based Precautions as being in isolation. A sign should be on the door indicating *Isolation* or *Contact Precautions* and alerting people to see the nurse before entering the room.

Guidelines: Isolation

G When they are indicated, Transmission-Based Precautions are always used **in addition** to Standard Precautions.

G You will be told the proper PPE to wear for care of each resident in isolation. Make sure to put on the PPE properly and remove it safely. Remove PPE and place it in the appropriate container before exiting a resident's room. PPE cannot be worn outside the resident's room. Perform hand hygiene following removal of PPE and again after exiting the resident's room. In addition to handwashing areas within the resident's room, there may be an alcohol-based hand rub dispenser mounted on the wall inside the room as you exit.

G Do not share equipment between residents. Use disposable supplies that can be discarded after use whenever possible. Use dedicated (only for use by one resident) equipment when disposable is not an option. When using disposable supplies, discard them in the resident's room before leaving. Be careful not to contaminate reusable equipment by setting it on furniture or counters in the resident's room. When the resident no longer needs the additional precautions, properly dispose of dedicated equipment if required. If the dedicated equipment is to be used for other residents, it should be cleaned and disinfected after use.

G Wear the proper PPE, if indicated, when serving food and drink. Do not leave uneaten food uncovered in the resident's room. When the meal is completed, remove the meal tray. Take it to the proper area.

G Follow Standard Precautions when dealing with body waste removal. Wear gloves when touching or handling waste. Wear gowns and goggles when indicated. The waste must be disposed of in such a manner as to minimize splashing and spraying.

G If required to take a specimen from a resident in isolation, wear the proper PPE. Collect the specimen. Place it in the appropriate container without the outside of the container coming into contact with the specimen. Properly remove your PPE and dispose of it in the room. Perform hand hygiene before leaving the room. Take the specimen to the nurse.

G Residents need to feel that staff understand what they are going through. Listen to what residents are saying. Allow time to talk with residents about their concerns. Reassure them that it is the disease, not the person, that is being isolated. Explain why these steps are being taken. Relay any requests outside your scope of practice to the nurse.

Common Infectious Diseases

Bloodborne pathogens are microorganisms found in human blood. They can cause infection and disease in humans. They may also be in certain other body fluids, draining wounds, and mucous membranes. Bloodborne diseases can be transmitted by infected blood entering the bloodstream, or if infected semen or vaginal secretions contact mucous membranes. Having sexual contact with someone carrying the disease can also transmit a bloodborne disease. Sexual contact includes sexual intercourse (vaginal and anal), contact of the mouth with the genitals or anus, and contact of the hands with the genital area. Using a needle to inject drugs and sharing needles can also transmit bloodborne diseases. In addition, infected mothers may transmit bloodborne diseases to their babies in the womb or at birth.

In health care, contact with infected blood or body fluids is the most common way to be infected with a bloodborne disease. Infections can be spread through contact with contaminated blood or body fluids, needles or other sharp objects, or contaminated supplies or equipment. Standard Precautions, handwashing, isolation, and using PPE are all methods of preventing transmission of bloodborne diseases. Employers are required by law to help prevent exposure to bloodborne pathogens. Following Standard Precautions and other procedures helps protect caregivers from bloodborne diseases.

The major bloodborne diseases in the United States are acquired immune deficiency syndrome (AIDS) and the viral hepatitis family. Chapter 4 has more information about AIDS.

Hepatitis is inflammation of the liver caused by certain viruses and other factors, such as alcohol abuse, some medications, and trauma. Liver function can be permanently damaged by hepatitis. It can lead to other chronic, life-long illnesses. Several different viruses can cause hepatitis. The most common types of hepatitis are A, B, and C. Hepatitis B and C are blood-borne diseases that can cause death.

Hepatitis B (HBV) is spread through sexual contact, by sharing infected needles, and from a mother to her baby during delivery. It is also spread by exposure at work from accidental contact with infected needles or other sharps or from splashing blood. HBV is a threat to health-care workers. Employers must offer NAs a free vaccine to protect them from hepatitis B. The HBV vaccine can prevent hepatitis B. Prevention is the best option for dealing with this disease. NAs should take the vaccine when it is offered. Hepatitis C (HCV) is also transmitted through blood or body fluids and possibly by sexual intercourse. There is no vaccine for hepatitis C.

Other serious infections include the following:

Tuberculosis, or **TB**, is a highly contagious lung disease. It is caused by a bacterium that is carried on mucous droplets suspended in the air. When a person infected with TB talks, coughs, breathes, sings, laughs, or sneezes, he may release mucous droplets carrying the disease. TB usually infects the lungs, causing coughing, trouble breathing, fever, weight loss, and fatigue (Fig. 2-40). Usually TB can be cured by taking all of the prescribed medication. However, if left untreated, TB may cause death.

Fig. 2-40. A normal lung X-ray on the left, and an X-ray of a lung with TB on the right.

Symptoms of TB include prolonged coughing, pain in the chest, coughing up blood or sputum, fatigue, loss of appetite, weight loss, chills, fever, and night sweats.

When caring for residents who have TB, NAs should follow Standard Precautions and Airborne Precautions. They should use personal protective equipment as instructed. Special masks, such as N95, high efficiency particulate air (HEPA), or other masks must be used. NAs must take care when handling sputum. Residents will be placed in a special airborne infection isolation room (AIIR) (also called a *Negative Air Pressure Room* or *Acid-Fast Bacillus [AFB] isolation room*). The door to this type of room should not be opened or closed quickly. This pulls contaminated room air into the hallway. The door should remain closed as much as possible. NAs must follow isolation procedures if directed. They should help the resident remember to take all medication prescribed. Failure to do so is a major factor in the spread of TB.

Methicillin-resistant *Staphylococcus aureus* (**MRSA**) is an antibiotic-resistant infection often acquired in healthcare facilities. This type of MRSA is also known as *HA-MRSA*, which stands for hospital-associated MRSA. Community-associated methicillin-resistant *Staphylococcus aureus* (CA-MRSA) is a type of MRSA infection that occurs in people who have not recently been admitted to healthcare facilities and who have no past diagnosis of MRSA. Often CA-MRSA manifests as skin infections, such as boils or pimples. This type of infection is becoming more common.

MRSA is almost always spread by direct physical contact with infected people. This means if a person has MRSA on his skin, especially on the hands, and touches another person, he may spread MRSA. Spread also occurs through indirect contact by touching objects, such as sheets or wound dressings, contaminated by a person with MRSA.

NAs can help prevent MRSA by practicing proper hygiene. Handwashing, using soap and warm water, is the single most important measure to control the spread of MRSA. Cuts and abrasions should be kept clean and covered with a proper dressing (e.g., bandage) until healed. Contact with other people's wounds or material that is contaminated from wounds should be avoided.

VRE stands for vancomycin-resistant *enterococcus*. *Enterococci* are bacteria that live in the digestive and genital tracts. They normally do not cause problems in healthy people. Vancomycin is a powerful antibiotic used to treat bacterial infections. Vancomycin-resistant *enterococci* are bacteria that have developed resistance to antibiotics as a result of being exposed to vancomycin. VRE is spread through direct and indirect contact.

VRE infections are often difficult to treat and may require multiple medications. VRE infections can cause life-threatening infections in those with weak immune systems—the very young, the very old, and the very ill. Preventing VRE is much easier than trying to treat it. NAs should wash their hands often and wear PPE as directed. Items may need to be disinfected. That information should be listed in the care plan.

Clostridium difficile infection is commonly known as **C. diff or C. difficile**. It is a spore-forming bacterium which can be part of the normal intestinal flora. When the normal intestinal flora is altered, *C. difficile* can flourish in the intestinal tract. It produces a toxin that causes a watery diarrhea. Enemas, nasogastric tube insertion, and GI tract surgery increase a person's risk of developing the infection. The overuse of antibiotics may also alter the normal intestinal flora and increase the risk of developing *C. difficile*. It can also cause colitis, a more serious intestinal condition.

When released in the environment, *C. difficile* can form a spore that makes it difficult to kill. These spores can be carried on the hands of people who have direct contact with infected residents or with environmental surfaces (floors, bedpans, toilets, etc.) contaminated with *C. difficile*. Touching an object contaminated with *C. difficile* can transmit the infection. Alcohol-based hand sanitizers are not considered effective on *C. difficile*. Soap and water must be used each time hand hygiene is performed.

Proper handwashing with soap and water is vital in preventing the spread of the disease. Handling contaminated wastes properly can help prevent its spread. Cleaning surfaces with a proper disinfectant, such as bleach, can also help. Limiting the use of antibiotics helps lower the risk of developing *C. difficile*.

Employer-Employee Responsibilities

Employers' responsibilities for infection prevention include the following:

- Establish infection prevention procedures and an exposure control plan to protect workers
- Provide continuing in-service education on infection prevention, including bloodborne and airborne pathogens and updates on any new safety standards
- Have written procedures to follow should an exposure occur, including medical treatment and plans to prevent similar exposures
- Provide personal protective equipment (PPE) for employees to use and teach them when and how to properly use it
- Provide free hepatitis B vaccinations for all employees

Employees' responsibilities for infection prevention include the following:

- Follow Standard Precautions
- Follow all facility's policies and procedures
- Follow care plans and assignments
- Use provided PPE as indicated or as appropriate
- Take advantage of the free hepatitis B vaccination
- Immediately report any exposure to infection
- Participate in annual education programs covering the prevention of infection

3

Understanding Residents

1. Identify basic human needs

People have different genes, physical appearances, cultural backgrounds, ages, and social or financial positions. But all human beings have the same basic physical needs:

- Food and water

- Protection and shelter

- Activity

- Sleep and rest

- Comfort, especially freedom from pain

People also have **psychosocial needs**, which involve social interaction, emotions, intellect, and spirituality. Although they are not as easy to define as physical needs, psychosocial needs include the following:

- Love and affection

- Acceptance by others

- Safety and security

- Self-reliance and independence in daily living

- Contact with others (Fig. 3-1)

- Success and self-esteem

Health and well-being affect how well psychosocial needs are met. Stress and frustration occur when basic needs are not met. This can lead to fear, anxiety, anger, aggression, withdrawal, indifference, and depression. Stress can also cause physical problems that may eventually lead to illness.

Fig. 3-1. *Interaction with other people is a basic psychosocial need. Nursing assistants can encourage residents to be with friends or relatives. Social contact is important.*

Abraham Maslow was a researcher of human behavior. He wrote about human physical and psychosocial needs. He arranged these needs into an order of importance. He thought that physical needs must be met before psychosocial needs can be met. His theory is called *Maslow's Hierarchy of Needs* (Fig 3-2).

Humans are sexual beings. They continue to have sexual needs throughout their lives. Sexual urges do not end due to age or admission to a care facility. The ability to engage in sexual activity, such as intercourse and masturbation, continues unless a disease or injury occurs to prevent it. **Masturbation** means to touch or rub sexual organs in order to give oneself or another person sexual pleasure.

Fig. 3-2. Maslow's Hierarchy of Needs is a model developed by Abraham Maslow to show how physical and psychosocial needs are arranged in order of importance.

Residents have the right to choose how they express their sexuality. In all age groups, there is a variety of sexual behavior. This is also true of residents.

Guidelines: Respecting Sexual Needs

G   Always knock or announce yourself before entering residents' rooms. Listen and wait for a response before entering.

G   If you encounter a sexual situation between consenting adult residents, provide privacy and leave the room.

G   Be open and nonjudgmental about residents' sexual attitudes.

G   Respect residents' sexual orientation. No matter what your personal or religious feelings regarding sexuality may be, always treat residents with respect. Remember that every resident is a human being, first and foremost. Sexual identity is only one part of the resident's experience.

G   Honor *Do Not Disturb* signs. Be sensitive to privacy needs.

G   Do not view expression of sexuality by the elderly as disgusting or cute. That attitude is inappropriate. It deprives residents of their right to dignity and respect.

Residents' Rights

Sexual Abuse

Residents must be protected from unwanted sexual advances. If an NA sees sexual abuse happening, he should remove the resident from the situation and take the resident to a safe place. The NA should then report to the nurse immediately.

Helping residents meet their spiritual needs can help them cope with illness or disability. Spirituality is a sensitive area. NAs must not offend residents by making judgments or by pushing their beliefs on residents.

Guidelines: Respecting Spiritual Needs

G   Learn about residents' religions or beliefs. Listen carefully to what residents say.

G   Respect residents' decisions to participate in, or refrain from, food-related rituals.

G   If residents are religious, encourage participation in religious services.

G   Respect all religious items.

G   Report to the nurse (or social worker) if a resident expresses the desire to see clergy.

G   Allow privacy for clergy visits.

G   If asked, read religious materials aloud. If you are uncomfortable doing this, find another staff member who is not.

G   If a resident asks you, help find spiritual resources available in the area. Check the internet for churches, synagogues, and other houses of worship. You can also refer this request to the nurse or social worker.

G   You should never do any of the following:

   • Try to change someone's religion

   • Tell residents their belief or religion is wrong

   • Express judgments about a religious group

   • Insist residents join religious activities

   • Interfere with religious practices

2. Define *holistic care*

Holistic means considering a whole system, such as a whole person, rather than dividing the system up into parts. **Holistic care** means caring for the whole person—the mind as well as the body. This is the approach NAs should use when caring for residents. A simple example of holistic care is an NA talking with residents while helping them bathe. She is meeting the physical need with the bath and meeting the psychosocial need for interaction with others at the same time.

3. Explain why promoting independence and self-care is important

Any big change in lifestyle, such as moving into a long-term care facility, requires a huge emotional adjustment. Residents may be experiencing fear, loss, and uncertainty, along with their decline in health and independence. Other common reactions to illness are denial, withdrawal, anger, and depression. All of these feelings may cause residents to behave differently than they have before. Each person adjusts to illness and change in his or her own way and in his or her own time. It is important for NAs to be supportive and encouraging. NAs should be patient, understanding, and empathetic.

Moving to a care facility represents a tremendous loss of independence for a resident. Somebody else must now do what residents did for themselves all of their lives. It is also difficult for residents' friends and family members. For example, a resident may have been the main provider for his or her family. A resident may have been the person who did all of the cooking for the family. Other losses residents may be experiencing include the following:

- Loss of spouse, family members, or friends due to death

- Loss of workplace and its relationships due to retirement

- Loss of ability to go to favorite places

- Loss of ability to attend services and meetings at their faith communities

- Loss of home and personal possessions (Fig. 3-3)

- Loss of health and the ability to care for themselves

- Loss of ability to move freely

- Loss of pets

- Lesbian, gay, bisexual, or transgender (LGBT) residents may fear the loss of a comfortable and accepting environment.

Fig. 3-3. *Nursing assistants should understand and be sympathetic to the fact that many residents had to leave familiar places.*

Independence often means not having to rely on others for money, daily care, or participation in social activities. Activities of daily living (ADLs) are the personal care tasks a person does every day to care for himself. People may take these activities for granted until they can no longer do them for themselves. ADLs include bathing or showering, dressing, caring for teeth and hair, toileting, eating and drinking, and moving from place to place. When a person loses independence, these problems can result:

- Poor self-image

- Anger toward caregivers, others, and self

- Feelings of helplessness, sadness, and hopelessness

- Feelings of being useless

- Increased dependence
- Depression

To prevent these feelings, NAs should encourage residents to do as much as possible for themselves. Even if it seems easier for the NA to do a task for a resident, the resident should be allowed to do it independently. NAs must encourage self-care, regardless of how long it takes or how poorly residents are able to do it (Fig. 3-4). NAs should be patient.

Fig. 3-4. Even if tasks take a long time, residents should be encouraged to do what they can for themselves.

Allowing residents to make choices is another way to promote independence. For example, residents can choose where to sit while they eat. They can choose what they eat and in what order. NAs must respect a resident's right to make choices.

Residents' Rights

Dignity and Independence

Residents are adults; they should not be treated like children. NAs should encourage residents to do self-care without rushing them. Residents have the right to refuse care and to make their own choices. Promoting dignity and independence is part of protecting their legal rights. It is also the proper and ethical way for NAs to work.

4. Identify ways to accommodate cultural differences

The term **cultural diversity** refers to different groups of people with varied backgrounds and experiences living together in the world. Positive responses to cultural diversity include acceptance and knowledge, not prejudice. Each culture may have different knowledge, behaviors, beliefs, values, attitudes, religions, and customs. Nursing assistants will take care of residents with backgrounds and traditions different from their own. It is important that NAs respect and value each person as an individual. They should respond to differences and new experiences with acceptance.

There are so many different cultures that they cannot all be listed here. One might talk about American culture being different from Japanese culture. But within American culture there are thousands of different groups with their own cultures. Japanese Americans, African Americans, and Native Americans are just a few. Even people from a particular region, state, or city can be said to have a different culture (Fig. 3-5). The culture of the South is not the same as the culture of New York City.

Fig. 3-5. There are many different cultures in the United States.

Cultural background affects how friendly people are to strangers. It can affect how close they want others to stand to them when talking. It can affect how they feel about NAs performing care for them or discussing their health with them. NAs should be sensitive to residents' backgrounds. They may have to adjust their behavior around some residents. Regardless of background, all residents must be treated with respect and professionalism. NAs should expect to be treated respectfully as well.

A resident's primary language may not be English. If he or she speaks a different language, an interpreter may be necessary. It can be helpful if staff learn a few common phrases in a resident's language. Picture cards and flash cards can assist with communication.

Religious differences also influence the way people behave. Religion can be very important in people's lives, particularly when they are ill or dying. Nursing assistants must respect the religious beliefs and practices of residents, even if they are different from their own. They should not question residents' beliefs or discuss their beliefs with residents.

In addition to showing respect for different cultural and religious traditions, there may be specific practices that affect NAs' work. Many religious beliefs include dietary restrictions. These are rules about what and when followers can eat and drink. For example, many Jewish people do not eat pork. (Chapter 8 has more information about food preferences and special diets.)

Some people's backgrounds may make them less comfortable being touched. An NA should ask permission before touching residents. He should be sensitive to their feelings. NAs must touch residents in order to do their jobs. However, they should recognize that some residents feel more comfortable when there is little physical contact. The NA should learn about his residents and adjust care to their needs.

Residents' Rights

Culturally-Sensitive Care

Nursing assistants should focus on compassionate, respectful, and culturally-sensitive care. They should treat residents as they wish to be treated, not as NAs would want to be treated. This is part of person-directed care. Culture, age, family, and background shape each person's way of thinking. It is important for NAs to ask questions to find out what is appropriate and to always respect residents' choices, beliefs, and behaviors.

5. Describe the need for activity

Activity is an essential part of a person's life; it improves and maintains physical and mental health. Meaningful activities help promote independence, memory, self-esteem, and quality of life. In addition, physical activity can help manage illnesses, such as diabetes, high blood pressure, or high cholesterol. Regular physical activity can also help in these ways:

- Lessening the risk of heart disease, colon cancer, diabetes, and obesity
- Relieving symptoms of depression
- Improving mood and concentration
- Improving body function
- Lowering the risk of falls
- Improving sleep quality
- Improving the ability to cope with stress
- Increasing energy
- Increasing appetite and promoting better eating habits

Inactivity and immobility can result in physical and mental problems, such as the following:

- Loss of self-esteem
- Depression
- Boredom
- Pneumonia
- Urinary tract infection

63　　3

Understanding Residents

- Skin breakdown and pressure ulcers
- Constipation
- Blood clots
- Dulling of the senses

OBRA requires that facilities provide an activities program that is designed to meet the interests and the physical and psychosocial well-being of each resident. The activities are created to help residents socialize and keep them physically and mentally active. Daily schedules are normally posted with activities for that particular day. Activities include exercise, arts and crafts, board games, newspapers, magazines, books, TV and radio, pet therapy, gardening, and group religious events. When activities are scheduled, NAs should help residents with grooming beforehand, as needed and requested. They should assist with any personal care that residents require. NAs may need to help residents with walking and wheelchairs as well.

6. Discuss family roles and their significance in health care

Families play an important part in most people's lives. There are many different kinds of families (Fig. 3-6):

Fig. 3-6. Families come in all shapes and sizes.

- Nuclear families (two parents and one or more children)
- Single-parent families (one parent and one or more children)
- Married or committed couples of the same sex or opposite sex, with or without children
- Extended families (parents, children, grandparents, aunts, uncles, cousins, other relatives, and even friends)
- Blended families (divorced or widowed parents who have remarried and have children from previous relationships and/or the current marriage)

Often a family is defined more by supporting each other than by the particular people involved. Whatever kinds of families residents have, they have an important role to play. Family members help in many ways:

- Helping residents make care decisions
- Communicating with the care team
- Giving support and encouragement
- Connecting the resident to the outside world
- Offering assurance to dying residents that family memories and traditions will be valued and carried on

NAs should be respectful to friends and family members and allow privacy for visits. After any visitor leaves, the NA should observe the effect the visit had on the resident. Any noticeable effects should be reported to the nurse. Some residents have good relationships with their families. Others do not. NAs must immediately report any abusive behavior from a visitor toward a resident to the charge nurse.

Families are great sources of information about residents' personal preferences, history, diet, habits, and routines. The NA should ask them questions. Families often seek out nursing assistants because they are closest to the residents. This is an important responsibility. NAs should show families that they have time for them. They can communicate with family members, but cannot discuss a resident's care. Any questions about care should be reported to the nurse.

7. Describe the stages of human development

Throughout their lives, people change physically and psychologically. Everyone will go through the same stages of development. However, no two people will follow the exact pattern or rate of development. Each resident must be treated as an individual and a whole person who is growing and developing. He or she should not be treated as someone who is merely ill or disabled.

Infancy (Birth to 12 Months)

Infants grow and develop very quickly. In one year a baby moves from total dependence to the relative independence of moving around, communicating basic needs, and feeding himself. Physical development in infancy moves from the head down. For example, infants gain control over the muscles of the neck before the muscles in their shoulders. Control over muscles in the trunk area, such as the shoulders, develops before control of arms and legs (Fig. 3-7).

Fig. 3-7. *An infant's physical development moves from the head down.*

Toddler (Ages 1 to 3)

During the toddler years, children gain independence. One part of this independence is new control over their bodies. Toddlers learn to speak, gain coordination of their limbs, and learn to control their bladders and bowels (Fig. 3-8). Toddlers assert their new independence by exploring. Poisons and other hazards, such as sharp objects, must be locked away. Psychologically, toddlers learn that they are individuals, separate from their parents. Children of this age may try to control their parents. They may try to get what they want by throwing tantrums, whining, or refusing to cooperate. This is a key time for parents to set rules and standards.

Fig. 3-8. *Toddlers gain coordination of their limbs.*

Preschool (Ages 3 to 6)

Children in their preschool years develop new skills. These will help them become more independent and have social relationships (Fig. 3-9). They learn new words and language skills. They learn to play in groups. They become more physically coordinated and learn to care for themselves. Preschoolers also develop ways of relating to family members. They begin to learn right from wrong.

Fig. 3-9. *Children in preschool years develop social relationships.*

School-Age (Ages 6 to 10)

From ages 6 to about 10 years, children's development is centered on **cognitive** (related to thinking and learning) and social development. As children enter school, they also explore the world around them. They relate to other children through games, peer groups, and classroom activities. In these years, children learn to get along with each other. They also begin to behave in ways common to their gender. They begin to develop a conscience, morals, and self-esteem.

Preadolescence (Ages 10 to 13)

During the years between 10 and 13, children enjoy a growing sense of self-identity and a strong sense of identity with their peers. They tend to be very social. This is usually a relatively calm period, and preadolescents are often easy to get along with and able to handle more responsibility at home and school. Childhood fears of ghosts or monsters will give way to fears based in the real world. It is important that preadolescents feel able to trust in the attention and care of parents or other adults.

Adolescence (Ages 13 to 19)

Puberty is the stage of growth when secondary sex characteristics, such as body hair, appear. Reproductive organs begin to function. The body begins to secrete reproductive hormones. The start of puberty marks the beginning of adolescence. Although it varies, it generally occurs between the ages of 10 and 14 for girls and 12 and 16 for boys.

Many teenagers have a hard time adapting to the changes that occur in their bodies during puberty. Peer acceptance is important to them. Adolescents may be afraid that they are unattractive or abnormal. This concern for body image and acceptance, combined with changing hormones that influence moods, can cause rapid mood swings. Pressures develop as they remain dependent on their parents and yet need to express themselves socially and sexually (Fig. 3-10). This causes conflict and stress.

Fig. 3-10. *Adolescence is a time of adapting to change.*

Young Adulthood (Ages 19 to 40)

Physical growth has usually been completed by this time. Adopting a healthy lifestyle in these years can make life better now and prevent health problems in later adulthood. Psychological and social development continues, however. The tasks of these years include the following:

- Selecting an appropriate education
- Selecting an occupation or career
- Selecting a mate (Fig. 3-11)
- Learning to live with a mate or others
- Raising children
- Developing a satisfying sex life

Fig. 3-11. Young adulthood often involves finding mates.

Middle Adulthood (Ages 40 to 65)

In general, people in middle adulthood are more comfortable and stable than they were before. Many of their major life decisions have already been made. Physical changes related to aging also occur in middle adulthood. Adults in this age group may notice that they have difficulty maintaining their weight or notice a decrease in strength and energy. Metabolism and other body functions slow down. Wrinkles and gray hair appear. Many diseases and illnesses can develop in these years. These disorders can become chronic and life-threatening.

Late Adulthood (65 years and older)

Persons in late adulthood must adjust to the effects of aging. These changes can include the loss of strength and health, the death of loved ones, retirement, and preparation for their own death. The developmental tasks of this age may seem to deal entirely with loss. But solutions to these problems often involve new relationships, friendships, and interests.

Later adulthood covers an age range of as many as 25 to 35 years. People in this age category can have very different abilities, depending on their health. Some 70-year-old people enjoy active sports, while others are not active. Many 85-year-old people can still live alone. Others may live with family members or in long-term care facilities.

Ideas about older people are often false. They create prejudices against the elderly. These are as unfair as prejudices against racial, ethnic, or religious groups. On television or in the movies, older people are often shown as helpless, lonely, disabled, slow, forgetful, dependent, or inactive. However, research shows that most older people are active and engaged in work, volunteer activities, and learning and exercise programs. Aging is a normal process, not a disease. Most older people live independent lives and do not need assistance (Fig. 3-12). Prejudice toward, stereotyping of, and/or discrimination against older persons or the elderly is called **ageism**.

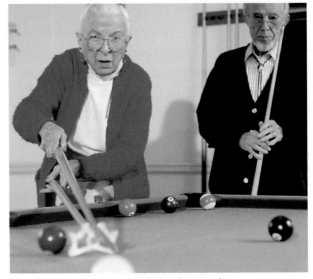
Fig. 3-12. Most older people lead active lives.

Nursing assistants are likely to spend much of their time working with elderly residents. They must be able to know what is true about aging and what is not true. Aging causes many changes. However, normal changes of aging do not mean an older person must become dependent, ill, or inactive. Knowing normal changes of aging from signs of illness or disability will allow NAs to better help residents. Normal changes of aging include the following:

- Skin is thinner, drier, more fragile, and less elastic.

- Muscles weaken and lose tone.

- Bones lose density and become more brittle.

- Sensitivity of nerve endings in the skin decreases.
- Responses and reflexes slow.
- Short-term memory loss occurs.
- Senses of vision, hearing, taste, touch, and smell weaken.
- Heart works less efficiently.
- Oxygen in the blood decreases.
- Appetite decreases.
- Urinary elimination is more frequent.
- Digestion takes longer and is less efficient.
- Levels of hormones decrease.
- Immunity weakens.
- Lifestyle changes occur.

There are also changes that are NOT considered normal changes of aging and should be reported to the nurse. These include the following:

- Signs of depression
- Loss of ability to think logically
- Poor nutrition
- Shortness of breath
- Incontinence

This is not a complete list. An NA's job includes reporting any change, normal or not.

8. Discuss developmental disabilities

Developmental disabilities are disabilities that are present at birth or emerge during childhood. A developmental disability is a chronic condition. It restricts physical and/or mental ability. These disabilities prevent a child from developing at a "normal" rate. Language, mobility, learning, and the ability to perform self-care may be affected. The care residents need will depend on the type and the extent of their disability.

An intellectual disability (formerly called *mental retardation*) is a type of developmental disability. It is neither a disease nor a mental illness.

People with an intellectual disability develop at a below-average rate. They have below-average mental functioning. They have difficulty learning, communicating, moving, and may have problems adjusting socially. Their ability to care for themselves may be affected.

Despite their special needs, people who have an intellectual disability have the same emotional and physical needs that others have. They experience the same emotions, such as anger, sadness, love, and joy, as others do, but their ability to express their emotions may be limited.

Guidelines: Intellectual Disability

G Treat adult residents as adults, regardless of their behavior.

G Praise and encourage often, especially positive behavior.

G Help teach ADLs by dividing a task into smaller units.

G Promote independence. Assist residents with activities and motor functions that are difficult.

G Encourage social interaction.

G Repeat words you use to make sure they understand.

G Be patient.

9. Describe some types of mental illness

Mental health and mental illness were first discussed in Chapter 2. There are many degrees of mental illness. It ranges from mild to severe.

Depression: Clinical depression is a serious mental illness. It may cause intense mental, emotional, and physical pain and disability. Depression also makes other illnesses worse. If left untreated, it may result in suicide. Clinical depression is not a normal reaction to stress. Sadness is only one symptom of this illness. Not all people who have depression complain of sadness or appear sad. These are other common symptoms of clinical depression:

- Pain, including headaches, stomach pain, and other body aches

- Low energy or fatigue

- **Apathy**, or lack of interest in activities

- Irritability

- Anxiety

- Loss of appetite or overeating

- Problems with sexual functioning and desire

- Sleeplessness, trouble sleeping, or excessive sleeping

- Lack of attention to basic personal care tasks (e.g., bathing, combing hair, changing clothes)

- Intense feelings of despair

- Guilt

- Trouble concentrating

- Withdrawal and isolation

- Repeated thoughts of suicide and death

There are different types and degrees of depression. **Major depressive disorder**, or major depression, may cause a person to lose interest in everything he once cared about. **Bipolar disorder**, also called manic-depressive illness, causes a person to swing from deep depression to extreme activity. These episodes can include high energy, little sleep, big speeches, rapidly changing thoughts and moods, high self-esteem, overspending, and poor judgment.

People cannot overcome depression through sheer will. It is an illness like any other illness. It can be treated successfully. People who suffer from depression need compassion and support. NAs should know the symptoms so they can recognize the beginning or worsening of depression. Any suicide threat should be taken seriously and reported immediately. It should not be regarded as an attempt to get attention.

Anxiety-related Disorders: Anxiety is uneasiness or fear, often about a situation or condition. When a person who is mentally healthy feels anxiety, he usually knows the cause. The anxiety fades once the cause is removed. A person who is mentally ill may feel anxiety all the time. He may not know the reason why. Physical signs and symptoms of anxiety-related disorders include shakiness, muscle aches, sweating, cold and clammy hands, dizziness, fatigue, racing heart, cold or hot flashes, a choking or smothering sensation, and a dry mouth.

A **phobia** is an intense form of anxiety or fear. Many people are very afraid of some things or situations. Examples are a fear of dogs or a fear of flying. For a person who has a mental illness, a phobia is a disabling terror. It keeps the person from doing normal things. For example, the fear of being in a confined space, **claustrophobia**, may make using an elevator terrifying. Other anxiety-related disorders include **panic disorder**, in which a person has repeated episodes of intense fear that something bad will occur. **Obsessive-compulsive disorder (OCD)** is an anxiety disorder characterized by obsessive behavior or thoughts. For example, a person may wash his hands over and over as a way of dealing with anxiety. Anxiety-related disorders may also be caused by a traumatic experience. This is known as **post-traumatic stress disorder**.

Schizophrenia: Schizophrenia is a brain disorder that affects a person's ability to think and communicate clearly. It also affects the ability to manage emotions, make decisions, and understand reality. It affects a person's ability to interact with other people. Treatment makes it possible for many people to lead relatively normal lives.

Some of the signs of schizophrenia are hallucinations and delusions. **Hallucinations** are false or distorted sensory perceptions. A person may see something that is not really there or hear a conversation that is not real. **Delusions** are persistent false beliefs. For example, a person may believe that other people are reading his thoughts. Paranoid schizophrenia is a form of the disease that centers mainly on hallucinations and delusions. Not all hallucinations or delusions are related to schizophrenia, though.

Guidelines: Mental Illness

G   Observe residents carefully for changes in condition or abilities. Document and report your observations.

G   Support the resident and his family and friends. Coping with mental illness can be very frustrating. Your positive, professional attitude can help the resident and his family.

G   Encourage residents to do as much as possible for themselves. Progress may be very slow. Be patient, supportive, and positive.

G   Mental illness can be treated. Medication and psychotherapy are common methods. Medication must be taken properly to promote benefits and reduce side effects. **Psychotherapy** is a method of treating mental illness that involves talking about one's problems with mental health professionals.

Observing and Reporting: Mental Illness

O/R   Changes in ability

O/R   Positive or negative mood changes, especially withdrawal (Fig. 3-13)

Fig. 3-13. Withdrawal is an important change to report.

O/R   Behavior changes, including changes in personality, extreme behavior, and behavior that does not seem to fit the situation

O/R   Comments, even jokes, about hurting oneself or others

O/R   Failure to take medicine or improper use of medicine

O/R   Real or imagined physical symptoms

O/R   Events, situations, or people that seem to upset or excite residents

Intellectual Disability and Mental Illness

Sometimes people confuse the terms *intellectual disability* and *mental illness*. They are not the same. An intellectual disability is a developmental disability that causes below-average mental functioning. It may affect a person's ability to care for himself, as well as to live independently. It is not a type of mental illness.

An intellectual disability affects mental ability. Mental illness may or may not affect mental ability. There is no cure for an intellectual disability, although persons who are intellectually disabled can be helped. Many mental illnesses can be cured with treatment, such as medications and therapy.

Although they are different conditions, persons who have either condition need emotional support, as well as care and treatment.

10. Explain how to care for dying residents

Death can occur suddenly without warning, or it can be expected. Older people or those with terminal illnesses may have time to prepare for death. A **terminal illness** is a disease or condition that will eventually cause death. Preparing for death is a process. It affects the dying person's emotions and behavior.

Dr. Elisabeth Kübler-Ross studied and wrote about the grief process. **Grief** is deep distress or sorrow over a loss. Her book, *On Death and Dying*, describes five stages that dying people and their loved ones may reach before death.

These five stages are listed below. Not all people go through all the stages. Some may stay in one stage until death occurs. Others may move back and forth between stages during the process.

Denial: People in the denial stage may refuse to believe they are dying. They often believe a mistake has been made. They may avoid discussion about their illnesses. They may simply act like it is not happening.

Anger: Once they start to face the possibility of their death, people may become angry that they are dying. They may be angry because they think they are too young or that they have always taken care of themselves.

Bargaining: Once people have begun to believe that they are dying, they may make promises to God, care providers, or others. They may somehow try to bargain for their recovery.

Depression: As dying people get weaker and symptoms get worse, they may become deeply sad or depressed. They may cry or withdraw or be unable to do even simple things.

Acceptance: Many people who are dying are eventually able to accept death and prepare for it. They may arrange with loved ones for the care of important people or things. They may make plans for their last days or for the ceremonies that may follow their death.

Advance directives are legal documents that allow people to choose what medical care they wish to have if they are unable to make those decisions themselves. Advance directives can also name someone to make decisions for a person if that person becomes ill or disabled. A living will and a durable power of attorney for health care are examples of advance directives.

A **living will** outlines the medical care a person wants, or does not want, in case he or she becomes unable to make those decisions. It is called a *living will* because it takes effect while the person is still living. It may also be called a *directive to physicians, health care declaration,* or *medical directive.* A living will is not the same

thing as a will. A will is a legal declaration of how a person wishes his or her possessions to be disposed of after death.

A **durable power of attorney for health care** (sometimes called a *health care proxy*) is a signed, dated, and witnessed legal document that appoints someone else to make medical decisions for a person in the event he or she becomes unable to do so. It can include instructions about medical treatment that the person wants to avoid.

A **do-not-resuscitate** (**DNR**) order is another tool that helps medical providers honor wishes about care. A DNR order tells medical professionals not to perform CPR. A DNR order means that medical personnel will not attempt emergency CPR if breathing or the heartbeat stops.

Residents' Rights

Advance Directives

By law, advance directives and DNR orders must be honored. Nursing assistants should respect each resident's decisions about advance directives. This is a very personal and private matter. NAs should not make comments about residents' choices to anyone, including family members, other residents, or staff.

Death is a very sensitive topic. Many people find it hard to discuss death. Feelings and attitudes about death can be formed by many factors:

- Experiences with death
- Personality type
- Religious beliefs
- Cultural background

Guidelines: Caring for the Dying Resident

G **Diminished senses**: Reduce glare and keep room lighting low (Fig. 3-14). Hearing is usually the last sense to leave the body. Speak in a normal tone. Tell the resident about any procedures that are being done or what is happening in the room. Do not expect an answer. Ask few questions. Observe body language to anticipate a resident's needs.

Fig. 3-14. Keep a dying resident's room softly lit without glare.

G **Care of the mouth and nose**: Give mouth care often. If the resident is unconscious, give mouth care every two hours. Apply lubricant, such as lip balm, to lips and nose.

G **Skin care**: Give bed baths and incontinence care as needed. Bathe perspiring residents often. Skin should be kept clean and dry. Change sheets and clothes for comfort. Keep sheets wrinkle-free. Skin care to prevent pressure ulcers is important. (Chapter 6 has more on pressure ulcers.)

G **Comfort**: Pain relief is critical. Residents may not be able to tell you that they are in pain. Observe for signs of pain. Report them. Frequent changes of position, back massage, skin care, mouth care, and proper body alignment may help.

G **Environment**: Put favorite objects and photographs where the resident can easily see them. Make sure the room is comfortable, appropriately lit, and well-ventilated. When leaving the room, place the call light within reach. Do this even if the resident is unaware of his surroundings.

G **Emotional and spiritual support**: Listening may be one of the most important things you can do for a dying resident. Pay attention to these conversations. Report any comments about fear to the nurse. Touch can also be important. Holding the resident's hand as you sit quietly can be very comforting. Do not avoid the dying person or his family or deny that death is approaching. Do not tell the resident that anyone knows how or when it will happen. Do give accurate information in a reassuring way. If other residents ask for information about the dying resident, refer their questions to the nurse.

Some residents may seek spiritual comfort from clergy. Give privacy for visits from clergy, family, and friends. Do not discuss your religious or spiritual beliefs with residents or their families or make recommendations.

NAs can treat residents with dignity when they are approaching death by respecting their rights and their preferences. There are some legal rights to remember when caring for people who are dying:

The right to refuse treatment. NAs must remember that whether they agree or disagree with a resident's decisions, the choice is not theirs. It belongs to the person involved and/or his family. NAs should be supportive of family members and not judge them. They are most likely following the resident's wishes.

The right to have visitors. When death is close, it is an emotional time for all those involved. Saying goodbye can be a very important part of dealing with a loved one's death. It may also be reassuring to the dying person to have someone in the room, even if the person does not seem to be aware of his surroundings.

The right to privacy. Privacy is a basic legal right, but privacy for visiting, or even when the person is alone, may be even more important now.

Other rights of a dying person are listed below in *The Dying Person's Bill of Rights*. This was created at a workshop, *The Terminally Ill Patient and the Helping Person*, sponsored by Southwestern Michigan In-Service Education Council, and appeared in the *American Journal of Nursing*, Vol. 75, January 1975, p. 99.

I have the right to:

• Be treated as a living human being until I die.

- Maintain a sense of hopefulness, however changing its focus may be.

- Be cared for by those who can maintain a sense of hopefulness, however changing this might be.

- Express my feelings and emotions about my approaching death in my own way.

- Participate in decisions concerning my care.

- Expect continuing medical and nursing attentions even though "cure" goals must be changed to "comfort" goals.

- Not die alone.

- Be free from pain.

- Have my questions answered honestly.

- Not be deceived.

- Have help from and for my family in accepting my death.

- Die in peace and dignity.

- Retain my individuality and not be judged for my decisions, which may be contrary to the beliefs of others.

- Discuss and enlarge my religious and/or spiritual experiences, whatever these may mean to others.

- Expect that the sanctity of the human body will be respected after death.

- Be cared for by caring, sensitive, knowledgeable people who will attempt to understand my needs and will be able to gain some satisfaction in helping me face my death.

Guidelines: Treating Dying Residents with Dignity

G Respect their wishes in all possible ways. Communication between staff is extremely important at this time so that everyone understands what the resident's wishes are. Listen carefully for ideas on how to provide simple gestures that may be special and appreciated.

G Do not isolate or avoid a resident who is dying. Enter his room regularly.

G Be careful not to make promises that cannot or should not be kept.

G Continue to involve the dying person in facility activities. Be person-centered. Do not talk with other staff members about your personal life when caring for a resident.

G Listen if a dying resident wants to talk but do not offer advice. Do not make judgmental comments.

G Do not babble or act especially cheerful or sad. Be professional.

G Keep the resident as comfortable as possible. The nurse needs to know immediately if pain medication is requested. Keep the resident clean and dry.

G Assure privacy when it is desired.

G Respect the privacy of the family and other visitors. They may be upset and not want to be social at this time. They may welcome a friendly smile, however, and should not be isolated, either.

G Help with the family's physical comfort. If requested, get them coffee, water, chairs, blankets, etc.

Common signs of approaching death include the following:

- Blurred and failing vision

- Unfocused eyes

- Impaired speech

- Diminished sense of touch

- Loss of movement, muscle tone, and feeling

- A rising or below-normal body temperature

- Decreasing blood pressure

- Weak pulse that is abnormally slow or rapid

- Alternating periods of slow, irregular respirations and rapid, shallow respirations, called **Cheyne-Stokes** respirations

- A rattling or gurgling sound as the person breathes

- Cold, pale skin

- Mottling (bruised appearance), spotting, or blotching of skin caused by poor circulation

- Perspiration

- Incontinence (both urine and stool)

- Disorientation or confusion

When death occurs, the body will not have heartbeat, pulse, respiration, or blood pressure. The muscles in the body become stiff and rigid. This is a temporary condition called *rigor mortis* which is Latin for *stiffness of death*. The eyelids may remain open or partially open with the eyes in a fixed stare. The mouth may remain open. The body may be incontinent of urine and stool. Though these things are a normal part of death, they can be frightening. NAs should inform the nurse immediately to help confirm the death.

Postmortem care is care of the body after death. It takes place after the resident has been declared dead by a nurse or doctor. NAs must be sensitive to the needs of the family and friends after death. Family members may wish to sit by the bed to say goodbye. They may wish to stay with the body for a while. They should be allowed to do these things. NAs should be aware of religious and cultural practices that the family wants to observe. NAs should follow their facility's policies and only perform assigned tasks.

Guidelines: Postmortem Care

G   Bathe the body. Be gentle to avoid bruising. Place drainage pads where needed. This is most often under the head and/or under the perineum. Follow Standard Precautions.

G   Do not remove any tubes or other equipment. A nurse or someone at the funeral home will do this.

G   If instructed, put dentures back in the mouth. Close the mouth. If not possible, place dentures in denture cup near the resident's head.

G   Close the eyes carefully.

G   Position the body on the back with legs straight. Fold arms across the abdomen. Put a small pillow under the head.

G   Follow facility policy on personal items. Check to see if you should remove jewelry. Always have a witness if personal items are removed or given to a family member. Document what was given to whom.

G   Strip the bed after the body has been removed. Open windows to air the room, as needed. Straighten up.

G   Document according to your facility's policy.

Dealing with grief after the death of a loved one is a process. Grieving is an individual process. No two people will grieve in exactly the same way. It is also a changing or adaptive process. Feelings may change from day to day, or even hour to hour. This is normal. Clergy, counselors, or social workers can help people who are grieving (Fig. 3-15). Family members or friends may have any of these reactions to the death of a loved one:

- Shock

- Denial

- Anger

- Guilt

- Regret

- Relief

- Sadness

- Loneliness

Fig. 3-15. Some people will speak with counselors to help them deal with their grief.

11. Define the goals of a hospice program

Hospice care is the term for the special care that a dying person needs. It is a compassionate way to care for dying people and their families. Hospice care uses a holistic approach. It treats the person's physical, emotional, spiritual, and social needs.

Hospice care can be given seven days a week, 24 hours a day. It is available with a doctor's order. Hospice care may be given in a hospital, at a care facility, or in the home. A hospice can be any location where a person who is dying is treated with dignity by caregivers. Any caregiver may give hospice care, but often specially-trained nurses and volunteers provide it.

Hospice care helps to meet all needs of the dying resident. The resident, as well as family and friends, are directly involved in care decisions. The resident is encouraged to participate in family life and decision-making as long as possible.

In long-term care, goals focus on recovery or on the resident's ability to care for herself as much as possible. In hospice care, however, the goals are the comfort and dignity of the resident. This type of care is called **palliative care**. This is an important difference. NAs will need to change their focus when caring for hospice residents. The focus should be on pain relief and comfort, rather than on teaching residents to care for themselves. Residents who are dying need to feel independent for as long as possible. Caregivers should allow residents to have as much control over their lives as possible. Eventually, caregivers may have to meet all of the person's basic needs.

Guidelines: Hospice Care

G Be a good listener. Some people, however, will not want to confide in their caregivers. Never push someone to talk.

G Respect privacy and independence.

G Be sensitive to individual needs. Ask family members or friends how you can help.

G Be aware of your own feelings. Know your limits and respect them.

G Recognize the stress. Talking with a counselor or support group may help. Remember, however, that specific information must be kept confidential.

G Take good care of yourself. Eating right, exercising, and getting enough rest are ways of taking care of yourself. Talk about and acknowledge your feelings. Take time to do things for yourself. Take a break when you need to.

G Allow yourself to grieve. You will develop close relationships with some residents. Know that it is normal to feel sad, angry, or lonely when residents die.

Community Resources

Here are a few of the many community resources available to help residents meet different needs:

- Eldercare Locator, a public service of the U.S. Administration on Aging (eldercare.gov or 800-677-1116)

- Ombudsman program (ltcombudsman.org or 202-332-2275)

- The National Resource Center on LGBT Aging (lgbtagingcenter.org or 212-741-2247)

- Alzheimer's Association (alz.org or 800-272-3900)

- American Cancer Society (cancer.org or 800-227-2345)

- AIDSinfo, a service of the U.S. Department of Health and Human Services (aidsinfo.nih.gov or 800-448-0440)

- Meals on Wheels Association of America (MOWAA) (mowaa.org or 888-998-6325)

- American Association on Intellectual and Developmental Disabilities (AAIDD) (aaidd.org or 202-387-1968)

- The National Institute of Mental Health (NIMH) (nimh.nih.gov or 866-615-6464)

- The National Hospice and Palliative Care Organization (NHPCO) (nhpco.org or 800-658-8898)

4

Body Systems and Related Conditions

Bodies are organized into body systems. Each system has a condition under which it works best. **Homeostasis** is the name for the condition in which all of the body's systems are working at their best. To be in homeostasis, the body's **metabolism**, or physical and chemical processes, must be working at a steady level. When disease or injury occurs, the body's metabolism is disturbed. Homeostasis is lost.

Each system in the body has its own unique structure and function. There are also normal, age-related changes for each body system. Knowing normal changes of aging will help nursing assistants better recognize any abnormal changes in residents. This chapter also includes tips on how NAs can help residents with their normal changes of aging.

The body's systems can be broken down in different ways. In this book the human body is divided into ten systems:

1. Integumentary (skin)
2. Musculoskeletal
3. Nervous
4. Circulatory or Cardiovascular
5. Respiratory
6. Urinary
7. Gastrointestinal
8. Endocrine
9. Reproductive
10. Immune and Lymphatic

Body systems are made up of organs. An organ has a specific function. Organs are made up of tissues. Tissues are made up of groups of cells that perform a similar task. For example, in the circulatory system, the heart is one of the organs. It is made up of tissues and cells. Cells are the building blocks of the body. Living cells divide, grow, and die, renewing the tissues and organs of the body.

Anatomical Terms of Location

Anatomical terms of location are terms to help identify positions or directions of the body. Here are some anatomical terms used to describe location in the human body:

- Anterior or ventral: the front of the body or body part
- Posterior or dorsal: the back of the body or body part
- Superior: toward the head
- Inferior: away from the head
- Medial: toward the midline of the body
- Lateral: to the side, away from the midline of the body
- Proximal: closer to the torso
- Distal: farther away from the torso

This chapter discusses the structure and function, age-related changes, and common diseases of each body system. Dementia and Alzheimer's disease, common diseases of the nervous system, will be discussed in Chapter 5.

1. Describe the integumentary system

The largest organ and system in the body is the skin. Skin is a natural protective covering, or integument. Skin prevents injury to internal organs. It protects the body against entry of bacteria. Skin also prevents the loss of too much water, which is essential to life. Skin is made up of layers of tissues. Within these layers are sweat glands, which secrete sweat to help cool the body when needed, and sebaceous glands, which secrete oil (sebum) to keep the skin lubricated. There are also hair follicles, many tiny blood vessels (capillaries), and tiny nerve endings (Fig. 4-1).

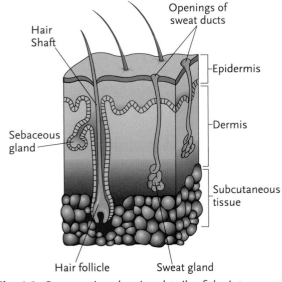

Fig. 4-1. Cross-section showing details of the integumentary system.

The skin is also a *sense organ*. It feels heat, cold, pain, touch, and pressure. It then tells the brain what it is feeling. Body temperature is regulated in the skin. Blood vessels **dilate**, or widen, when the outside temperature is too high. This brings more blood to the body surface to cool it off. The same blood vessels **constrict**, or narrow, when the outside temperature is too cold. By restricting the amount of blood reaching the skin, the blood vessels help the body retain heat.

Normal changes of aging include

- Skin is thinner, drier, and more fragile. It is more easily damaged.

- Skin is less elastic.

- Protective fatty tissue is lost, so person may feel colder.

- Hair thins and may turn gray.

- Wrinkles and brown spots, or "liver spots," appear.

- Nails are harder and more brittle.

- Dry, itchy skin may result from lack of oil from the sebaceous glands.

How the NA Can Help

Older adults perspire less and do not need to bathe as often. Most elderly people generally need a complete bath only twice a week, with sponge baths every day. Hair also becomes drier and needs to be shampooed less often. Using lotions as ordered helps to relieve dry skin. The NA should be gentle; elderly skin may be fragile and can tear easily. Gently brushing dry hair stimulates and distributes the natural oils. Clothing and bed covers can be layered for additional warmth. Bed linens should be kept wrinkle-free. The NA should not cut residents' toenails. Fluid intake should be encouraged.

Observing and Reporting: Integumentary System

During daily care, a resident's skin should be observed for changes that may indicate injury or disease. Observe and report these signs and symptoms:

O/R Pale, white, reddened, or purple areas

O/R Blisters or bruises

O/R Complaints of tingling, warmth, or burning

O/R Dry or flaking skin

O/R Rashes or any skin discoloration

O/R Swelling

O/R Cuts, boils, sores, wounds, abrasions

O/R Fluid or blood draining from the skin

O/R Broken skin

O/R Changes in moistness/dryness

O/R Changes in wound or ulcer (size, depth, drainage, color, odor)

O/R Redness or broken skin between toes or around toenails

O/R Scalp or hair changes

O/R Skin that appears different from normal or that has changed

O/R In darker complexions, any change in the feel of the tissue; any change in the appearance of the skin, such as an "orange-peel" look or a purplish hue; and extremely dry, crust-like areas that might be covering a tissue break

Pressure ulcers, a common disorder of the integumentary system, are covered in Chapter 6.

2. Describe the musculoskeletal system and related conditions

Muscles, bones, ligaments, tendons, and cartilage give the body shape and structure. They work together to move the body. The skeleton, or framework, of the human body has 206 bones (Fig. 4-2). Besides allowing the body to move, bones also protect organs. For example, the skull protects the brain. Two bones meet at a joint. Muscles are connected to bone by tendons. Muscles provide movement of body parts to maintain posture and to produce heat.

Fig. 4-2. The skeleton is composed of 206 bones that aid movement and protect organs.

Exercise is important for improving and maintaining physical and mental health. Inactivity and immobility can result in a loss of self-esteem, depression, pneumonia, and urinary tract infections. They can also lead to constipation, blood clots, dulling of the senses, and muscle atrophy or contractures. When **atrophy** occurs, the muscle wastes away, decreases in size, and becomes weak. When a **contracture** develops, the muscle or tendon shortens, becomes inflexible, and "freezes" in position. This causes permanent disability of the limb. Range of motion (ROM) exercises can help prevent these conditions. With ROM exercises, the joints are extended and flexed. Exercise increases circulation of blood, oxygen, and nutrients and improves muscle tone. Chapter 9 has information on ROM exercises.

Normal changes of aging include

- Muscles weaken and lose tone.

- Body movement slows.

- Bones lose density. They become more brittle, making them more susceptible to breaks.

- Joints may stiffen and become painful.

- Height is gradually lost.

How the NA Can Help

Falls can cause life-threatening complications, including fractures. The NA can help prevent falls by answering call lights immediately. She should keep pathways clear, clean up spills, and not move furniture. Walkers or canes need to be placed where residents can easily reach them. Residents should be wearing non-skid shoes with the laces tied. The NA should encourage regular movement and self-care. Residents should perform as many ADLs as possible. The NA can help with range of motion (ROM) exercises as needed.

Observing and Reporting: Musculoskeletal System

Observe and report these signs and symptoms:

O/R Changes in ability to perform routine movements and activities

O/R   Any changes in resident's ability to perform ROM exercises

O/R   Pain during movement

O/R   Any new or increased swelling of joints

O/R   White, shiny, red, or warm areas over a joint

O/R   Bruising

O/R   Aches and pains reported

Arthritis

Arthritis is a general term. It refers to **inflammation**, or swelling, of the joints. It causes stiffness, pain, and decreased mobility. Arthritis may be the result of aging, injury, or an **autoimmune illness**. An autoimmune illness causes the body's immune system to attack normal tissue in the body. Two common types of arthritis are rheumatoid arthritis and osteoarthritis.

Rheumatoid arthritis can affect people of all ages. Joints become red, swollen, and very painful. Deformities can result and may be severe and disabling (Fig. 4-3). Movement is eventually restricted. Fever, fatigue, and weight loss are also symptoms. Rheumatoid arthritis is considered an autoimmune disease.

Fig. 4-3. *Rheumatoid arthritis.* (PHOTO COURTESY OF DR. JAMES HEILMAN, WIKIPEDIA)

Osteoarthritis, also called degenerative joint disease (DJD) or degenerative arthritis, often affects older people. It may occur with aging or as the result of joint injury. Hips and knees, which are weight-bearing joints, are usually affected. Joints in the fingers, thumbs, and spine can also be affected. Pain and stiffness seem to increase in cold or damp weather.

Arthritis is often treated with the following:

- Anti-inflammatory medications such as aspirin or ibuprofen, or other medication

- Local applications of heat to reduce swelling and pain

- Range of motion exercises (Chapter 9)

- Regular exercise and/or activity routine

- Diet to reduce weight or maintain strength

Guidelines: Arthritis

G   Watch for stomach irritation or heartburn caused by aspirin or ibuprofen. Some residents cannot take these medications. Report signs of stomach irritation or heartburn immediately.

G   Encourage activity. Gentle activity can help reduce the effects of arthritis. Follow care plan instructions carefully. Use canes or other walking aids as needed.

G   Adapt activities of daily living (ADLs) to allow independence. Many devices are available to help residents bathe, dress, and feed themselves when they have arthritis (Chapter 9).

G   Choose clothing that is easy to put on and fasten. Encourage use of handrails and safety bars in the bathroom.

G   Treat each resident as an individual. Arthritis is very common among older residents. Do not assume that each resident has the same symptoms and needs the same care.

G   Help resident's self-esteem. Encourage self-care. Have a positive attitude. Listen to the resident's feelings. You can help him remain independent as long as possible.

Osteoporosis

Osteoporosis causes bones to become porous and brittle. Brittle bones can break easily. Weakness in the bones may be due to age, lack of hormones, lack of calcium in bones, excessive alcohol use, or lack of exercise. It occurs more commonly in women after **menopause** (the end of menstruation). Extra calcium and regular exercise can help prevent osteoporosis. Signs and symptoms of osteoporosis include low back pain, stooped posture, and becoming shorter over time.

To prevent or slow osteoporosis, nursing assistants should encourage residents to walk and do other light exercise as ordered. Exercise can strengthen bones as well as muscles. NAs must move residents with osteoporosis very carefully. Medication, calcium, and fluoride supplements are used to treat osteoporosis.

Hip Fracture and Knee Replacement

A fracture is a broken bone. It is caused by an accident or by osteoporosis. Preventing falls, which can lead to fractures, is very important. Fractures of arms, wrists, elbows, legs, and hips are the most common. Signs and symptoms of a fracture are pain, swelling, bruising, changes in skin color at the site, and limited movement.

Weakened bones make hip fractures more common. A sudden fall can result in a fractured hip that takes months to heal. Hip fractures can also occur when weakened bones fracture and then cause a fall. A hip fracture is a serious condition. The elderly heal slowly. They are also at risk for secondary illnesses and disabilities. Most fractured hips require surgery. Total hip replacement (THR) is the surgical replacement of the head of the long bone of the leg (femur) where it joins the hip. This surgery is often done for these reasons:

* Hip is fractured from an injury or fall that does not heal properly.

* Hip is weakened due to aging.

* Hip is painful and stiff because the joint is weak and the bones are no longer strong enough to bear the person's weight.

After the surgery, the person cannot stand on that leg while the hip heals. A physical therapist will assist after surgery. The goals of care include strengthening the hip muscles and getting the resident to bear weight on that leg.

The resident's care plan will state when the resident may begin putting weight on the hip. It will also give instructions on how much the resident is able to do. NAs should help with personal care and assistive devices, such as walkers or canes.

Guidelines: Hip Replacement

G   Keep often-used items, such as medications, telephone, tissues, call lights, and water, within easy reach. Avoid placing items in high places.

G   Dress the affected (weaker) side first.

G   Never rush the resident. Use praise and encouragement often. Do this even for small tasks.

G   Ask the nurse to give pain medication prior to moving if needed.

G   Have the resident sit to do tasks in order to save her energy.

G   Follow the care plan exactly, even if the resident wants to do more. Follow orders for weight-bearing. After surgery, the doctor's order will be written as *partial weight-bearing (PWB)* or *non-weight-bearing (NWB)*. **Partial weight-bearing** means the resident is able to support some body weight on one or both legs. **Non-weight-bearing** means the resident is unable to touch the floor or support any weight on one or both legs. Once the resident can bear full weight again, the doctor's order will be written for *full weight-bearing (FWB)*. **Full weight-bearing** means that both legs can bear 100 percent of the body weight on a step. Help as needed with cane, walker, or crutches.

G   Never perform ROM exercises on the operative leg unless directed by the nurse.

G Caution the resident not to sit with her legs crossed. The hip cannot be bent or flexed more than 90 degrees. It cannot be turned inward or outward.

G An abduction pillow will normally be used for six to 12 weeks after surgery while the resident is sleeping in bed. The abduction pillow immobilizes and positions the hips and lower extremities. The pillow is placed in between the legs. The legs are secured to the sides of pillow using straps (Fig. 4-4). Follow instructions for application and positioning.

Fig. 4-4. An abduction pillow is placed in between the legs to immobilize and position the hips and lower extremities. (PHOTO COURTESY OF NORTH COAST MEDICAL, INC., WWW.NCMEDICAL.COM, 800-821-9319)

G When transferring from a bed, use a pillow between the thighs to keep the legs separated. Raise the head of the bed. This allows the resident to move her legs over the side of the bed with the thighs still separated. Stand on the side of the unaffected hip. The strong side should lead in standing, pivoting, and sitting.

G With chair or toilet transfers, the operative leg should be straightened. The stronger leg should stand first (with a walker or crutches). Then the foot of the affected leg can be brought back to the walking position.

G Report any of these to the nurse:

- Redness, drainage, bleeding, or warmth in incision area

- An increase in pain

- Numbness or tingling

- Shortening and/or external rotation of affected leg

- Abnormal vital signs, especially a change in temperature

- Resident cannot use equipment properly and safely

- Resident is not following doctor's orders for activity and exercise

- Any problems with appetite

- Any improvements, such as increased strength and improved ability to walk

Total knee replacement (TKR) is the surgical replacement of the knee with a prosthetic knee. This surgery is performed to relieve pain. It also restores motion to a knee damaged by injury or arthritis. It can help stabilize a knee that buckles or gives out repeatedly. Care is similar to that for the hip replacement, but the recovery time is much shorter. These residents have more ability to care for themselves.

Guidelines: Knee Replacement

G To prevent blood clots, apply special stockings as ordered. One type is a compression stocking. It is a plastic, air-filled, sleeve-like device that is applied to the legs and hooked to a machine. This machine inflates and deflates on its own. It acts in the same way that the muscles usually do during normal activity. The sleeves are normally applied after surgery while the resident is in bed. Anti-embolic stockings are another type of special stocking. They aid circulation. Chapter 6 has more information on this type of stocking.

G Perform ankle pumps as ordered. These are simple exercises that promote circulation to the legs. Ankle pumps are done by raising the toes and feet toward the ceiling and lowering them again.

G Encourage fluids, especially cranberry and orange juices, which contain vitamin C, to prevent urinary tract infections (UTIs).

G Assist with deep breathing exercises as ordered.

G Ask the nurse to give pain medication prior to moving and positioning if needed.

G Report to the nurse if you notice redness, swelling, heat, or deep tenderness in one or both calves.

3. Describe the nervous system and related conditions

The nervous system is the control and message center of the body. It controls and coordinates all body functions. The nervous system also senses and interprets information from outside the human body. The nervous system has two main parts: the central nervous system (CNS) and the peripheral nervous system (PNS). The central nervous system is composed of the brain and spinal cord. The peripheral nervous system deals with the periphery, or outer part, of the body via the nerves that extend throughout the body (Fig. 4-5).

Fig. 4-5. The nervous system includes the brain, spinal cord, and nerves throughout the body.

Normal changes of aging include

• Responses and reflexes slow.

• Sensitivity of nerve endings in skin decreases.

• Person may show some memory loss, more often with short-term memory. Long-term memory, or memory for past events, usually remains sharp.

How the NA Can Help

Suggesting residents make lists or write notes about things they want to remember can help with memory loss. Placing a calendar nearby may also help. If residents enjoy reminiscing, the NA can take an interest in their past by asking to see photos or hear stories. The NA should allow time for decision-making and avoid sudden changes in schedule. The NA should allow plenty of time for movement; residents should not be rushed. Reading, thinking, and other mental activities should be encouraged.

Observing and Reporting: Central Nervous System

Observe and report these signs and symptoms:

O/R Fatigue or any pain with movement or exercise

O/R Shaking or trembling

O/R Inability to move one side of body

O/R Difficulty speaking or slurring of speech

O/R Numbness or tingling

O/R Disturbance or changes in vision or hearing

O/R Dizziness or loss of balance

O/R Changes in eating patterns and/or fluid intake

O/R Difficulty swallowing

O/R Bowel and bladder changes

O/R Depression or mood changes

O/R Memory loss or confusion

O/R Violent behavior

o/R Any unusual or unexplained change in behavior

o/R Decreased ability to perform ADLs

Dementia and Alzheimer's disease are common disorders of the nervous system. Chapter 5 has information on these diseases.

CVA or Stroke

The medical term for a stroke is a cerebrovascular accident (CVA). CVA, or stroke, occurs when blood supply to a part of the brain is blocked or a blood vessel leaks or ruptures within the brain. An ischemic stroke is the most common type of stroke (Fig. 4-6). With this type, the blood supply is blocked. Without blood, part of the brain does not receive oxygen. Brain cells begin to die. Additional damage can occur due to leaking blood, clots, and swelling of the tissues. Swelling can also cause pressure on other areas of the brain. Chapter 2 has information on the warning signs of a CVA.

Fig. 4-6. *An ischemic stroke is caused when the blood supply to the brain is blocked.*

Strokes can be mild or severe. After a stroke, a resident may experience any of the following:

• Paralysis on one side of the body, called **hemiplegia**

• Weakness on one side of the body, called **hemiparesis**

• Trouble communicating thoughts through speech or writing, called **expressive aphasia**

• Difficulty understanding spoken or written words, called **receptive aphasia**

• Loss of sensations such as temperature or touch

• Loss of bowel or bladder control

• Confusion

• Poor judgment

• Memory loss

• Loss of cognitive abilities

• Tendency to ignore one side of the body, called one-sided neglect

• Laughing or crying without any reason, or when it is inappropriate, called **emotional lability**

• Difficulty swallowing, called **dysphagia**

Each side of the brain controls different functions. Symptoms that a person has depend on which side of the brain is affected by the CVA. Weaknesses on the right side of the body show that the left side of the brain was affected. Weaknesses on the left side of the body show that the right side of the brain was affected.

If the stroke was mild, the resident may experience few, if any, complications. Physical therapy may help restore physical abilities. Speech and occupational therapy can also help with communication and performing ADLs.

Guidelines: CVA/Stroke

G Residents with paralysis, weakness, or loss of movement will usually have physical or occupational therapy. Range of motion exercises will help strengthen muscles and keep joints mobile. Residents may also need to perform leg exercises to aid circulation. Safety is always important when residents are exercising. Assist carefully with exercises as ordered.

G   Never refer to the weaker side as the "bad side." Do not talk about the "bad" leg or arm. The terms *weaker* or *involved* should be used to refer to the side with paralysis.

G   Residents with speech loss or communication problems may receive speech therapy. You may be asked to help. This includes helping residents recognize written or spoken words. Speech therapists will also evaluate a resident's swallowing ability. They will decide if swallowing therapy or thickened liquids are needed.

G   Being confused or having memory loss are upsetting. People often cry for no apparent reason after suffering a stroke. Be patient and understanding. Your positive attitude will be important. Keep a routine of care. This may help residents feel more secure.

G   Encourage independence and self-esteem. Let the resident do things for himself whenever possible, even if you could do a better or faster job. Make tasks less difficult for the resident to do. Notice and praise residents' efforts to do things for themselves even when they are unsuccessful. Praise even the smallest successes to build confidence.

G   Always check on the resident's body alignment. Sometimes an arm or leg can be caught and the resident is unaware.

G   Pay special attention to skin care and observe for changes in the skin if a resident is unable to move.

G   If residents have a loss of touch or sensation, check for potentially harmful situations (for example, heat and sharp objects). If residents are unable to sense or move part of the body, check and change positioning often to prevent pressure ulcers.

G   Adapt procedures when caring for residents with one-sided paralysis or weakness. Carefully assist with shaving, grooming, and bathing.

G   When helping with transfers or walking, always use a gait belt for safety. Stand on the weaker side. Support the weaker side. Lead with the stronger side (Fig. 4-7).

Fig. 4-7. *When helping a resident transfer, support the weaker side while leading with the stronger side.*

When assisting with dressing, remember to

G   Dress the weaker side first. Place the weaker arm or leg into the clothing first. This prevents unnecessary bending and stretching of the limb. Undress the stronger side first. Then remove the weaker arm or leg from clothing to prevent the limb from being stretched and twisted.

G   Use assistive equipment to help the resident dress himself. Encourage self-care.

When assisting with communication, remember to

G   Keep questions and directions simple.

G   Phrase questions so they can be answered with a "yes" or "no." For example, when helping a resident with eating, ask, "Would you like to start with a drink of milk?"

G   Agree on signals, such as shaking or nodding the head or raising a hand or finger for "yes" or "no."

G Give residents time to respond. Listen attentively.

G Use a pencil and paper if the resident can write. A thick handle or tape around the pencil may help the resident hold it more easily.

G Keep the call signal within reach of residents. They can let you know when you are needed.

G Use verbal and nonverbal communication to express your positive attitude. Let the resident know you have confidence in his or her abilities through smiles, touches, and gestures. Gestures and pointing can also help give information or allow the resident to speak to you.

G Use communication boards or special cards to aid communication (Fig. 4-8).

Guidelines for helping with eating for a person recovering from CVA are in Chapter 8.

Parkinson's Disease

Parkinson's disease is a progressive, incurable disease. Progressive means the disease gets worse with time. Parkinson's disease causes a section of the brain to degenerate. It affects the muscles, causing them to become stiff. It causes stooped posture and a shuffling **gait**, or walk. It can also cause pill-rolling. This is a circular movement of the tips of the thumb and the index finger when brought together, which looks like rolling a pill. Tremors or shaking make it hard for a person to perform ADLs such as eating and bathing. A person with Parkinson's may have a mask-like facial expression. Medications are commonly used to treat this disease. Surgery may be an option for some people.

Fig. 4-8. A sample communication board.

Guidelines: Parkinson's Disease

G   Residents are at a high risk for falls. Protect residents from any unsafe areas and conditions. Help with ambulation as needed.

G   Help with ADLs as needed.

G   Assist with range of motion exercises to prevent contractures and to strengthen muscles.

G   Encourage self-care. Be patient with self-care and communication.

Multiple Sclerosis (MS)

Multiple sclerosis (MS) is a progressive disease. It affects the central nervous system. When a person has MS, the protective covering for the nerves, spinal cord, and white matter of the brain breaks down over time. Without this covering, or sheath, nerves cannot send messages to and from the brain in a normal way. MS progresses slowly and unpredictably. Residents who have this disease will have widely varying abilities. Symptoms include blurred vision, fatigue, tremors, poor balance, and trouble walking. Weakness, numbness, tingling, incontinence, and behavior changes are also symptoms. MS can cause blindness, contractures, and loss of function in the arms and legs. MS is usually diagnosed when a person is in his or her early twenties to thirties. The exact cause is not known, but it may be an autoimmune disease. There is no cure for this disease; it is mostly treated with medication.

Guidelines: Multiple Sclerosis

G   Assist with ADLs as needed. Be patient with self-care and movement. Allow enough time for tasks. Offer rest periods as necessary.

G   Give the resident plenty of time to communicate. People with MS may have trouble forming their thoughts. Be patient. Do not rush them.

G   Prevent falls, which may be due to a lack of coordination, fatigue, or vision problems.

G   Stress can worsen the effects of MS. Be calm. Listen to residents when they want to talk.

G   Encourage a healthy diet with plenty of fluids.

G   Give regular skin care to prevent pressure ulcers.

G   Assist with range of motion exercises to prevent contractures and to strengthen muscles.

Head and Spinal Cord Injuries

Diving, sports injuries, falls, car and motorcycle accidents, industrial accidents, war, and criminal violence are common causes of head and spinal cord injuries. Head injuries can cause permanent brain damage. Residents who have had a head injury may have the following problems: intellectual disabilities; personality changes; breathing problems; seizures; coma; memory loss; loss of consciousness; paresis; and paralysis. Paresis is paralysis, or loss of muscle function, that affects only part of the body. Often, paresis describes a weakness or loss of ability on one side of the body.

The effects of spinal cord injuries depend on the force of impact and location of the injury. The higher the injury on the spinal cord, the greater the loss of function (Fig. 4-9). People with head and spinal cord injuries may have **paraplegia**. This is a loss of function of the lower body and legs. These injuries may also cause **quadriplegia**. This is loss of function in the legs, trunk, and arms.

Fig. 4-9. Loss of function depends on where the spine is injured.

Guidelines: Head or Spinal Cord Injury

G   Give emotional support, as well as physical help.

G   Safety is very important. Be very careful that residents do not fall or burn themselves. Because residents who are paralyzed have no sensation, they are unable to feel a burn.

G   Be patient with self-care. Allow as much independence as possible with ADLs.

G   Give careful skin care. It is important to prevent pressure ulcers.

G   Assist residents to change positions at least every two hours to prevent pressure ulcers. Be gentle when repositioning.

G   Perform range of motion exercises as ordered to prevent contractures and to strengthen muscles.

G   Immobility leads to constipation. Encourage fluids and a high-fiber diet if ordered.

G   Loss of ability to empty the bladder may lead to the need for a urinary catheter. Urinary tract infections are common. Encourage high intake of fluids. Give extra catheter care as needed.

G   Lack of activity leads to poor circulation and fatigue. Offer rest periods as necessary. Special stockings to help increase circulation may be ordered.

G   Difficulty coughing and shallow breathing can lead to pneumonia. Encourage deep breathing exercises as ordered.

G   Male residents may have involuntary erections. Provide for privacy and be sensitive to this. Be professional.

G   Assist with bowel and bladder training if needed.

The Nervous System: Sense Organs

The eyes, ears, nose, tongue, and skin are the body's major sense organs (Fig. 4-10 and Fig. 4-11). They are part of the central nervous system because they receive impulses from the environment. They relay these impulses to the nerves.

Fig. 4-10. *The parts of the eye.*

Fig. 4-11. *The outer ear, middle ear, and inner ear are the three main divisions of the ear.*

Normal changes of aging include

*   Vision and hearing decrease. Sense of balance may be affected.

*   Senses of taste, smell, and touch decrease.

*   Sensitivity to heat and cold decreases.

How the NA Can Help

Residents should use their eyeglasses. The NA can help by keeping them clean. Bright colors and proper lighting will also help. Hearing aids should be worn, and they should be kept clean. The NA should face the resident when speaking and speak slowly and clearly. Shouting should be avoided. The losses of senses of taste and smell may lead to decreased appetite. Providing oral care often and offering foods with a variety of tastes and textures may help. The loss of smell may make residents unaware of increased body odor. The NA should help as needed with regular bathing. Due to decreased sense of touch, residents may not be able to tell if something is too hot for them. The NA should be careful with hot drinks and hot bath water.

Observing and Reporting: Eyes and Ears

Observe and report these signs and symptoms:

o/R Changes in vision or hearing

o/R Signs of infection

o/R Dizziness

o/R Complaints of pain in eyes or ears

Vision Impairment

People over the age of 40 are at risk for developing certain serious vision problems. These include cataracts, glaucoma, and blindness. When a cataract develops, the lens of the eye, which is normally clear, becomes cloudy. This prevents light from entering the eye. Vision blurs and dims initially. Vision is eventually lost entirely. This disease can occur in one or both eyes. It is corrected with surgery, in which a permanent lens is usually implanted.

With glaucoma, the pressure in the eye increases. This eventually damages the retina and the optic nerve. It causes loss of vision and blindness. Glaucoma can occur suddenly, causing severe pain, nausea, and vomiting. It can also occur gradually, with symptoms that include blurred vision, tunnel vision, and blue-green halos around lights. Glaucoma is treated with eye drops and other medication and sometimes with surgery. More information about vision impairment is located in Chapter 2.

4. Describe the circulatory system and related conditions

The circulatory system is made up of the heart, blood vessels, and blood (Fig. 4-12). The heart

pumps blood through the blood vessels to the cells. The blood carries food, oxygen, and other substances cells need to function properly.

The circulatory system supplies food, oxygen, and hormones to cells. It supplies the body with infection-fighting blood cells. The circulatory system removes waste products from cells and also helps control body temperature.

Fig. 4-12. The heart, blood vessels, and blood are the main parts of the circulatory system.

Normal changes of aging include

- Heart pumps less efficiently.
- Blood flow decreases.
- Blood vessels narrow.

How the NA Can Help

Movement and exercise should be encouraged. Walking, stretching, and even lifting light weights can help maintain strength and promote circulation. ROM exercises are important for residents who cannot get out of bed. The NA should allow time to complete activities and try to prevent residents from tiring. Layering clothing helps keep residents warm. Socks, slippers, or shoes help keep the feet warm.

Observing and Reporting: Circulatory System

Observe and report these signs and symptoms:

%R Changes in pulse rate

%R Weakness, fatigue

%R Loss of ability to perform ADLs

%R Swelling of ankles, feet, fingers, or hands (edema)

%R Pale or bluish hands, feet, or lips

%R Chest pain

%R Weight gain

%R Shortness of breath, changes in breathing patterns, inability to catch breath

%R Severe headache

%R Inactivity (which can lead to circulatory problems)

Hypertension (HTN) or High Blood Pressure

When blood pressure is consistently 140/90 or higher, a person is diagnosed as having **hypertension** (**HTN**), or high blood pressure. People with HTN are often prescribed medications to lower blood pressure. Recent studies indicate, however, that blood pressure may measure as high as 150/90 in people over 60 without posing enough of a health risk to make it necessary to treat it with these medications. There is still some disagreement among doctors about this issue. A measurement of 140/90 or higher is still considered hypertension.

Hypertension may be caused by a hardening and narrowing of the blood vessels (Fig. 4-13). It can also result from kidney disease, tumors of the adrenal gland, pregnancy, and certain medications.

Hypertension can develop in people of any age. Signs and symptoms of hypertension are not always obvious, especially in the early stages. Often it is only discovered when a blood pressure measurement is taken. Persons may complain of headache, blurred vision, and dizziness.

Artery wall   Plaque

Fig. 4-13. *Arteries may become hardened or narrower because of a build-up of plaque. Hardened arteries are one cause of high blood pressure.*

Guidelines: Hypertension

G Hypertension can lead to serious problems such as CVA, heart attack, kidney disease, or blindness. Treatment to control it is vital. Residents may take medication that lowers blood pressure or cholesterol. They may take diuretics. **Diuretics** are a type of medication that reduces fluid in the body. Offer trips to the bathroom regularly. Answer call lights promptly.

G Residents may also have a prescribed exercise program or a special low-fat, low-sodium diet. Encourage residents to follow their diet and exercise programs.

Coronary Artery Disease (CAD)

Coronary artery disease occurs when the blood vessels in the coronary arteries narrow. This reduces the supply of blood to the heart muscle and deprives it of oxygen and nutrients. Over time, as fatty deposits block the artery, the muscle that was supplied by the blood vessel dies. CAD can lead to heart attack or stroke.

The heart muscle that is not getting enough oxygen causes chest pain, pressure, or discomfort, called **angina pectoris**. The heart needs more oxygen during exercise, stress, excitement, or to digest a heavy meal. In CAD, narrow blood vessels keep the extra blood with oxygen from getting to the heart (Fig. 4-14).

The pain of angina pectoris is usually described as pressure or tightness. It occurs in the left side or the center of the chest, behind the sternum or breastbone. Some people have pain moving down the inside of the left arm or to the neck and left side of the jaw. A person suffering from angina pectoris may sweat or look pale. The person may feel dizzy and have trouble breathing.

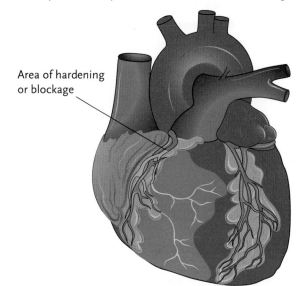

Fig. 4-14. *Angina pectoris results from the heart not getting enough oxygen.*

Guidelines: Angina Pectoris

G   Rest is extremely important. Rest reduces the heart's need for extra oxygen. It helps blood flow return to normal, often within three to 15 minutes. Encourage residents to rest.

G   Medication is also needed to relax the walls of the coronary arteries. This allows them to open and get more blood to the heart. This medication, nitroglycerin, is a small tablet that the resident places under the tongue. There it dissolves and is rapidly absorbed. Residents who have angina pectoris may keep nitroglycerin on hand to use as symptoms arise. Nursing assistants are not allowed to give medications. Tell the nurse if a resident needs help taking the medication. Nitroglycerin is also available as a patch. Do not remove the patch. Tell the nurse immediately if the patch comes off. Nitroglycerin may also come in the form of a spray that the resident sprays onto or under the tongue.

G   Residents may also need to avoid heavy meals, overeating, intense exercise, and cold or hot and humid weather.

Myocardial Infarction (MI) or Heart Attack

When blood flow to the heart muscle is blocked, oxygen and nutrients fail to reach the cells in that region (Fig. 4-15). Waste products are not removed. The muscle cells die. This is called a myocardial infarction (MI) or heart attack. A myocardial infarction is an emergency that can result in serious heart damage or death. Chapter 2 has a list of warning signs of an MI.

Area affected by complete lack of blood flow

Fig. 4-15. *A heart attack occurs when all or part of the blood flow to the heart is blocked.*

Guidelines: Myocardial Infarction

G   Most residents who have had an MI will be placed on a regular exercise program. Encourage residents to follow their exercise programs.

G   Residents may be on a diet that is low in fat and cholesterol and/or low in sodium. Encourage residents to follow their special diets.

G   Medications may be used to regulate heart rate and blood pressure.

G Quitting smoking will be encouraged. Be supportive.

G A stress management program may be started to help reduce stress levels. Help residents avoid stress and listen if they want to talk.

G Residents recovering from a heart attack may need to avoid cold temperatures.

Congestive Heart Failure (CHF)

Coronary artery disease, MI, hypertension, or other disorders may all damage the heart. When the heart muscle has been severely damaged, it fails to pump effectively. When the left side of the heart is affected, blood backs up into the lungs. When the right side of the heart is affected, blood backs up into the legs, feet, or abdomen. When one or both sides of the heart stop pumping blood properly, it is called congestive heart failure (CHF).

Guidelines: Congestive Heart Failure

G Although CHF is a serious illness, it can be treated and controlled. Medications can strengthen the heart muscle and improve its pumping.

G Medications help remove excess fluids. This means more trips to the bathroom. Answer call lights promptly.

G A low-sodium diet or fluid restrictions may be prescribed. Encourage residents to follow diet orders or restrictions.

G A weakened heart may make it hard for residents to walk, carry items, or climb stairs. Limited activity or bedrest may be prescribed. Allow for a period of rest after an activity.

G Measure intake and output of fluids as ordered.

G Resident may be weighed daily at the same time to watch for weight gain from fluid retention. Weigh residents as instructed.

G Apply elastic leg stockings as ordered to reduce swelling in feet and ankles.

G Range of motion (ROM) exercises improve muscle tone when activity and exercise are limited. Assist with ROM exercises.

G Extra pillows may help residents who have trouble breathing. Keeping the head of the bed elevated may also help with breathing.

G Help with personal care and ADLs as needed.

G A common side effect of medications for congestive heart failure is dizziness. This may result from a lack of potassium. High-potassium foods and drinks such as winter squash, baked sweet or regular potatoes, beans, raisins, apricots, prunes, bananas, prune juice, and orange juice can help this.

Peripheral Vascular Disease (PVD)

Peripheral vascular disease (PVD) is a disease in which the legs, feet, arms, or hands do not have enough blood circulation. This is due to fatty deposits in the blood vessels that harden over time. The legs, feet, arms, and hands feel cool or cold. Nail beds and/or feet become ashen or blue. Swelling occurs in the hands and feet. Ulcers of the legs and feet may develop and can become infected. Pain may be very severe when walking, but it is usually relieved with rest.

Risk factors for PVD include smoking, diabetes, high cholesterol, hypertension, inactivity, and obesity. Treatment includes quitting smoking, medications, exercise, and surgery.

5. Describe the respiratory system and related conditions

Respiration, the body taking in oxygen and removing carbon dioxide, involves breathing in, **inspiration**, and breathing out, **expiration**. The lungs accomplish this process (Fig. 4-16). The functions of the respiratory system are to bring oxygen into the body and to eliminate carbon dioxide produced as the body uses oxygen.

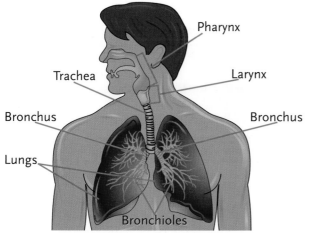

Fig. 4-16. *The respiratory process begins with inspiration through the nose or mouth. The air travels through the trachea and into the lungs via the bronchi, which then branch into bronchioles.*

Normal changes of aging include

• Lung strength decreases.

• Lung capacity decreases.

• Oxygen in the blood decreases.

• Voice weakens.

How the NA Can Help

Residents with acute or chronic upper respiratory conditions should not be exposed to cigarette smoke or polluted air. The NA should provide rest periods as needed and encourage exercise and regular movement. The NA should assist with deep breathing exercises as ordered. Residents who have difficulty breathing will usually be more comfortable sitting up, rather than lying down.

Observing and Reporting: Respiratory System

Observe and report these signs and symptoms:

O/R Change in respiratory rate

O/R Shallow breathing or breathing through pursed lips

O/R Coughing or wheezing

O/R Nasal congestion or discharge

O/R Sore throat, difficulty swallowing, or swollen tonsils

O/R The need to sit after mild exertion

O/R Pale, bluish, or gray color of the lips, arms, and/or legs

O/R Pain in the chest area

O/R Discolored sputum, mucus a person coughs up from the lungs (green, yellow, blood-tinged, or gray)

Chronic Obstructive Pulmonary Disease (COPD)

Chronic obstructive pulmonary disease (COPD) is a chronic disease. This means a person may live for years with it but never be cured. COPD causes trouble with breathing, especially in getting air out of the lungs. There are two chronic lung diseases that are grouped under COPD: chronic bronchitis and emphysema.

Bronchitis is an irritation and inflammation of the lining of the bronchi. Chronic bronchitis is a form of bronchitis that is usually caused by cigarette smoking. Symptoms include coughing that brings up sputum (phlegm) and mucus. Breathlessness and wheezing may be present. Treatment includes stopping smoking and possibly medications.

Emphysema is a chronic disease of the lungs that usually results from chronic bronchitis and cigarette smoking. People with emphysema have trouble breathing. Other symptoms are coughing, breathlessness, and a fast heartbeat. There is no cure for emphysema. Treatment includes managing symptoms and pain. Oxygen therapy, as well as medications, may be ordered. Quitting smoking is very important.

Over time, a person with either of these lung disorders becomes chronically ill and weakened. There is a high risk for acute lung infections, such as pneumonia. Pneumonia is an illness that can be caused by a bacterial, viral, or fungal infection. Acute inflammation occurs in lung tissue. The affected person develops a high fever, chills, cough, greenish or yellow sputum, chest pains, and rapid pulse. Treatment includes antibiotics, along with plenty of fluids. Recovery from pneumonia may take longer for older adults and persons with chronic illnesses.

When the lungs and brain do not get enough oxygen, all body systems are affected. Residents may have a constant fear of not being able to breathe. This can cause them to sit upright to try to improve their ability to expand the lungs. These residents can have poor appetites. They usually do not get enough sleep. All of this can add to feelings of weakness and poor health. They may feel they have lost control of their bodies, particularly their breathing. They may fear suffocation.

Residents with COPD may have these symptoms:

- Chronic cough or wheeze

- Trouble breathing, especially with inhaling and exhaling deeply

- Shortness of breath, especially during physical effort

- Pale, blue, reddish-purple skin

- Confusion

- General state of weakness

- Trouble completing meals due to shortness of breath

- Fear and anxiety

Guidelines: COPD

G Colds or viruses can make residents very ill quickly. Always observe and report signs of symptoms getting worse.

G Help residents sit upright or lean forward. Offer pillows for support (Fig. 4-17).

G Offer plenty of fluids and small, frequent meals.

G Encourage a well-balanced diet.

G Keep oxygen supply available as ordered.

Fig. 4-17. *It helps residents with COPD to sit upright and lean forward slightly.*

G Being unable to breathe or fearing suffocation can be very frightening. Be calm and supportive.

G Use infection prevention practices. Wash your hands often and encourage residents to do the same. Dispose of used tissues promptly.

G Encourage as much independence with ADLs as possible.

G Remind residents to avoid exposure to infections, especially colds and the flu.

G Encourage pursed-lip breathing. Pursed-lip breathing involves inhaling slowly through the nose and exhaling slowly through pursed lips (as if about to whistle). A nurse should teach residents how to do this.

G Encourage residents to save energy for important tasks. Encourage residents to rest.

G Report any of these to the nurse:

- Temperature over 101°F

- Changes in breathing patterns, including shortness of breath

- Changes in color or consistency of lung secretions

- Changes in mental state or personality

- Refusal to take medications as ordered

- Excessive weight loss

- Increasing dependence upon caregivers and family

6. Describe the urinary system and related conditions

The urinary system is composed of two kidneys, two ureters, one urinary bladder, a single ure-thra, and a meatus (Figs. 4-18 and 4-19). The urinary system has two important functions. Through urine, the urinary system eliminates waste products created by the cells. The urinary system also maintains the water balance in the body.

Fig. 4-18. *The male urinary system.*

Fig. 4-19. *The female urethra is shorter than the male urethra. This is one reason why the female bladder is more likely to become infected by bacteria traveling up the urethra. To help prevent infection, females should wipe from front to back after elimination.*

Normal changes of aging include

- The ability of kidneys to filter blood decreases.

- Bladder muscle tone weakens.

- Bladder holds less urine, which causes more frequent urination.

- Bladder may not empty completely, causing greater chance of infection.

How the NA Can Help

The NA should encourage fluids and offer frequent trips to the bathroom. If residents are incontinent, the NA should not show frustration or anger. **Urinary incontinence** is the inability to control the bladder, which leads to an involuntary loss of urine. Residents should be kept clean and dry.

Observing and Reporting: Urinary System

Observe and report these signs and symptoms:

O/R Weight loss or gain

O/R Swelling in upper or lower extremities

O/R Pain or burning during urination

O/R Changes in urine, such as cloudiness, odor, or color

O/R Changes in frequency and amount of urination

O/R Swelling in the abdominal/bladder area

O/R Complaints that bladder feels full or painful

O/R Urinary incontinence/dribbling

O/R Pain in the kidney or back/flank region

O/R Inadequate fluid intake

Urinary Incontinence

Urinary incontinence can occur in residents who are confined to bed, ill, elderly, paralyzed, or who have circulatory or nervous system diseases or injuries. Incontinence is not a normal part of aging. Nursing assistants should always report incontinence.

Guidelines: Urinary Incontinence

G Offer a bedpan, urinal, commode, or trip to the bathroom often. Follow toileting schedules in the care plan.

G Answer call lights and requests for help immediately.

G   Urinary incontinence is a major risk factor for pressure ulcers. Document all episodes of incontinence carefully and accurately.

G   Cleanliness and careful skin care are important. Urine is very irritating to the skin. It should be washed off immediately and completely. Keep residents clean, dry, and free from odor. Observe the skin carefully when bathing and giving perineal care.

G   Incontinent residents who are bedbound should have a waterproof bed protector placed under them to protect the bed. Place a draw sheet over it to absorb moisture and protect the skin.

G   Some residents will wear disposable incontinence pads or briefs for adults. They keep body wastes away from the skin. Change wet briefs immediately. Do not refer to an incontinence brief as a *diaper*. Residents are not children. Doing that is disrespectful.

G   Encourage residents to drink plenty of fluids.

G   Residents who are incontinent need reassurance and understanding. Be professional and kind when dealing with incontinence.

Urinary Tract Infection (UTI)

Urinary tract infection (UTI) causes inflammation of the bladder and the ureters. This results in painful burning during urination. It also causes a frequent feeling of needing to urinate. UTI, or cystitis, may be caused by a bacterial infection. Being bedbound can cause urine to stay in the bladder too long. This helps bacteria to grow. UTIs are more common in women. The urethra is much shorter in women (three to four inches) than in men (seven to eight inches). Bacteria can reach a woman's bladder more easily.

Guidelines: Preventing UTIs

G   Encourage residents to wipe from front to back after elimination (Fig. 4-20). When you give perineal care, make sure you do this too.

Fig. 4-20. *After elimination, wipe from front to back to prevent infection.*

G   Give careful perineal care when changing incontinence briefs.

G   Encourage plenty of fluids. Drinking plenty of fluids helps prevent UTIs. Drinking cranberry and blueberry juice acidifies urine. This helps to prevent infection. Vitamin C also has this effect.

G   Offer bedpan or a trip to the toilet at least every two hours. Answer call lights promptly.

G   Taking showers, rather than baths, helps prevent UTIs.

G   Report cloudy, dark, or foul-smelling urine, or if a resident urinates often and in small amounts.

7. Describe the gastrointestinal system and related conditions

The gastrointestinal (GI) system, also called the digestive system, is made up of the gastrointestinal tract and the accessory digestive organs (Fig. 4-21). The gastrointestinal system has two functions: digestion and elimination. **Digestion** is the process of preparing food physically and chemically so that it can be absorbed into the cells. **Elimination** is the process of expelling solid wastes (made up of the waste products of food) that are not absorbed into the cells.

Normal changes of aging include

•   Decreased saliva production affects the ability to chew and swallow.

•   Dulled sense of taste may result in poor appetite.

- Absorption of vitamins and minerals decreases.

- Process of digestion takes longer and is less efficient.

- Body waste moves more slowly through the intestines, causing more frequent constipation.

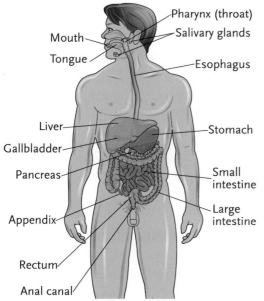

Fig. 4-21. The GI system consists of all the organs needed to digest food and process waste.

How the NA Can Help

Fluids and nutritious, appealing meals should be encouraged. The NA should allow time to eat and make mealtime enjoyable. Regular oral care should be provided. Dentures must fit properly and should be cleaned regularly. Residents who have trouble chewing and swallowing are at risk of choking. The NA should offer fluids during mealtime. Residents should eat a diet that contains fiber and drink plenty of fluids to help prevent constipation. Residents should be given the opportunity to have a bowel movement around the same time each day.

Observing and Reporting: Gastrointestinal System

Observe and report these signs and symptoms:

O/R Difficulty swallowing or chewing (including denture problems, tooth pain, or mouth sores)

O/R **Fecal incontinence** (inability to control the bowels, leading to involuntary passage of stool)

O/R Weight gain or weight loss

O/R Loss of appetite

O/R Abdominal pain and cramping

O/R Diarrhea

O/R Nausea and vomiting (especially vomitus that looks like coffee grounds)

O/R Constipation

O/R Flatulence

O/R Hiccups, belching

O/R Bloody, black, or hard stools

O/R Heartburn

O/R Poor nutritional intake

Constipation

Constipation is the inability to eliminate stool (have a bowel movement) or the infrequent, difficult, and often painful elimination of a hard, dry stool. Constipation occurs when the feces move too slowly through the intestine. This can result from decreased fluid intake, poor diet, inactivity, medications, aging, disease, or ignoring the urge to eliminate. Signs of constipation include abdominal swelling, gas, irritability, and a record of no recent bowel movement.

Treatment often includes increasing fiber and fluid intake, increasing activity level, and possibly medication. Accurate documentation of bowel movements is important. An enema or suppository may be ordered to help. An **enema** is a specific amount of water, with or without an additive, that is introduced into the colon to eliminate stool. A **suppository** is a medication given rectally to cause a bowel movement.

Fecal Impaction

A fecal impaction is a hard stool that is stuck in the rectum and cannot be expelled. It results from unrelieved constipation. Symptoms include no stool for several days, oozing of liquid stool, cramping, abdominal swelling, and rectal pain. When an impaction occurs, a nurse or doctor will insert one or two gloved fingers into the rectum and break the mass into fragments so that it can be passed. Prevention of fecal impactions includes a high-fiber diet, plenty of fluids, an increase in activity level, and possibly medication. Early assessments of constipation may also help prevent impactions.

Hemorrhoids

Hemorrhoids are enlarged veins in the rectum. They may also be visible outside the anus. Hemorrhoids can develop from an increase in pressure in the lower rectum due to straining during bowel movements. Chronic constipation, obesity, pregnancy, and sitting for long periods of time on the toilet are other causes. Signs and symptoms include rectal itching, burning, pain, and bleeding. Treatment may include medications, compresses, and sitz baths. Surgery may be necessary. When cleaning the anal area, NAs should be careful to avoid causing pain and bleeding from hemorrhoids.

Diarrhea

Diarrhea is the frequent elimination of liquid or semi-liquid feces. Abdominal cramps, urgency, nausea, and vomiting can accompany diarrhea, depending on the cause. Infections, microorganisms in food and water, irritating foods, and medications can cause diarrhea. Treatment usually involves medication, an increase in certain fluids, and a change of diet. A diet of bananas, rice, applesauce, and toast (BRAT diet) may be prescribed for short-term use.

Gastroesophageal Reflux Disease (GERD)

Gastroesophageal reflux disease, commonly referred to as *GERD*, is a chronic condition in which the liquid contents of the stomach back up into the esophagus. The liquid can inflame and damage the lining of the esophagus. It can

cause bleeding or ulcers. In addition, scars from tissue damage can narrow the esophagus and make swallowing difficult.

Heartburn is the most common symptom of GERD. Heartburn and GERD must be reported to the nurse. These conditions are usually treated with medications. Serving the evening meal three to four hours before bedtime may help. The resident should not lie down until at least two to three hours after eating. Extra pillows should be used to keep the body more upright during sleep. Serving the largest meal of the day at lunchtime, serving several small meals throughout the day, and reducing fast foods, fatty foods, and spicy foods may also help. Stopping smoking, not drinking alcohol, and wearing loose-fitting clothes are helpful as well.

Ostomies

An **ostomy** is the surgical creation of an opening from an area inside the body to the outside. The terms *colostomy* and *ileostomy* refer to the surgical removal of a portion of the intestines. In a resident with one of these ostomies, the end of the intestine is brought out of the body through an artificial opening in the abdomen. This opening is called a **stoma**. Stool, or feces, are eliminated through the ostomy rather than through the anus. An ostomy may be necessary due to bowel disease, cancer, or trauma.

The terms *colostomy* and *ileostomy* tell what part of the intestine was removed and the type of stool that will be eliminated. A colostomy is a surgically-created opening into the large intestine to allow stool to be expelled. With a colostomy, stool will generally be semi-solid. An ileostomy is a surgically-created opening into the end of the small intestine to allow stool to be expelled. Stool will be liquid and may be irritating to the resident's skin. Residents who have had an ostomy wear a disposable drainage bag that fits over the stoma to collect the feces (Fig. 4-22). The bag is attached to the skin by adhesive. A belt may also be used to secure it.

Fig. 4-22. *This photo shows the front and back of a two-piece system. The top is an ostomy drainage bag, and the bottom is a skin barrier.* (PHOTOS COURTESY OF HOLLISTER INCORPORATED, LIBERTYVILLE, ILLINOIS, HOLLISTER.COM)

Many people manage the ostomy appliance by themselves. Nursing assistants should receive training before providing ostomy care. NAs should give careful skin care. They should empty and clean or replace the ostomy bag whenever stool is eliminated. NAs should always wear gloves and wash hands carefully when providing ostomy care. They can help by teaching proper handwashing to residents with ostomies.

Residents' Rights

Ostomies

Many residents with ostomies feel they have lost control of a basic bodily function. They may be embarrassed or angry about the ostomy. NAs should be sensitive and supportive and should always provide privacy for ostomy care.

Caring for an ostomy

Equipment: protective pad, bath blanket, clean ostomy drainage bag and belt, disposable wipes, basin of warm water, soap, washcloth, skin cream as ordered, 2 towels, plastic disposable bag, gloves

1. Identify yourself by name. Identify the resident by name.
    Resident has right to know identity of his or her caregiver. Identifying resident by name shows respect and establishes correct identification.

2. Wash your hands.
    Provides for infection prevention.

3. Explain procedure to the resident. Speak clearly, slowly, and directly. Maintain face-to-face contact whenever possible.
    Promotes understanding and independence.

4. Provide for resident's privacy with curtain, screen, or door.
    Maintains resident's right to privacy and dignity.

5. Adjust bed to a safe level, usually waist high. Lock bed wheels.
    Prevents injury to you and to resident.

6. Put on gloves.
    Provides for infection prevention.

7. Place protective pad under resident. Cover resident with a bath blanket. Pull down the top sheet and blankets. Expose only the ostomy site. Offer resident a towel to keep clothing dry.
    Maintains resident's right to privacy and dignity.

8. Remove ostomy bag carefully. Place it in plastic bag. Note the color, odor, consistency, and amount of stool in the bag.
    Changes in stool can indicate a problem.

9. Wipe area around stoma with disposable wipes. Discard wipes in plastic bag.

10. Using a washcloth and warm, soapy water, wash the area in one direction, away from the stoma (Fig. 4-23). Rinse. Pat dry with another towel. Apply skin cream as ordered.
    Keeping skin clean and dry prevents skin breakdown.

Fig. 4-23. *Wash area gently, moving away from the stoma.*

11. Place the clean ostomy drainage bag on resident. Hold in place and seal securely. Make sure the bottom of the bag is clamped.

12. Remove protective pad and discard. Place soiled linens in proper container. Discard plastic bag properly.

13. Remove and discard gloves.

14. Wash your hands.
    Provides for infection prevention.

15. Return bed to lowest position. Remove privacy measures.
    Lowering the bed provides for safety.

16. Place call light within resident's reach.
    A call light allows resident to communicate with staff as necessary.

17. Report any changes in resident to the nurse. Note any changes in stoma and surrounding area. A normal stoma is red and moist and looks like the lining of the mouth. Call the nurse if the stoma is very red or blue or if swelling or bleeding is present.

18. Document procedure using facility guidelines.
    If you do not document the care you gave, legally it did not happen.

8. Describe the endocrine system and related conditions

The endocrine system is made up of glands in different areas of the body (Fig. 4-24). **Glands** are organs that produce and secrete chemicals called hormones. **Hormones** are chemical substances created by the body that control numerous body functions. The functions of the endocrine system are as follows:

- Maintains homeostasis

- Influences growth and development

- Regulates levels of sugar in the blood

- Regulates levels of calcium in the bones

- Regulates the body's ability to reproduce

- Determines how fast cells burn food for energy

Normal changes of aging include

- Levels of hormones, such as estrogen and progesterone, decrease.

- Insulin production lessens.

- Body is less able to handle stress.

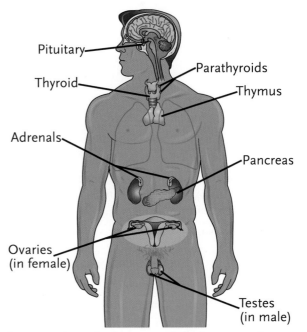

Fig. 4-24. *The endocrine system includes organs that produce hormones that regulate body processes.*

How the NA Can Help

The NA should encourage proper nutrition and try to eliminate or reduce stressors. Stressors are anything that causes stress. The NA can help by offering encouragement and listening to residents.

Observing and Reporting: Endocrine System

Observe and report these signs and symptoms:

O/R Headache

O/R Weakness

O/R Blurred vision

O/R Dizziness

O/R Irritability

O/R Sweating/excessive perspiration

O/R Change in "normal" behavior

O/R Confusion

O/R Change in mobility

O/R Change in sensation

○/ʀ Numbness or tingling in arms or legs

○/ʀ Weight gain or weight loss

○/ʀ Loss of appetite or increased appetite

○/ʀ Increased thirst

○/ʀ Frequent urination or any change in urine output

○/ʀ Hunger

○/ʀ Dry skin

○/ʀ Skin breakdown

○/ʀ Sweet or fruity breath

○/ʀ Sluggishness or fatigue

○/ʀ Hyperactivity

Diabetes

Diabetes mellitus, commonly called **diabetes**, occurs when the pancreas produces too little insulin or does not properly use insulin. **Insulin** is a hormone that converts **glucose**, or natural sugar, into energy for the body. Without insulin to process glucose, these sugars collect in the blood and cannot get to cells. This causes problems with circulation and can damage vital organs.

Diabetes is common in people with a family history of the illness, in the elderly, and in people who are obese. Diabetes is a chronic disease that has two major types: type 1 and type 2.

Type 1 diabetes is usually diagnosed in children and young adults. In type 1 diabetes, the pancreas does not produce any insulin. The condition will continue throughout a person's life. Type 1 diabetes is managed with daily injections of insulin or an insulin pump and a special diet. Regular blood glucose testing must be done.

Type 2 diabetes is the most common form of diabetes. In type 2 diabetes, either the body does not produce enough insulin or the body fails to properly use insulin. This is known as *insulin resistance*. Type 2 diabetes usually develops slowly. It is the milder form of diabetes.

It typically develops after age 35. The risk of getting it increases with age. However, the number of children with type 2 diabetes is growing rapidly. Type 2 diabetes often occurs in obese people or those with a family history of the disease. It can usually be controlled with diet and/or oral medications. Blood glucose levels should be tested regularly.

Pre-diabetes occurs when a person's blood glucose levels are above normal but not high enough for a diagnosis of type 2 diabetes. Research indicates that some damage to the body, especially the heart and circulatory system, may already be occurring during pre-diabetes.

Pregnant women who have never had diabetes before but who have high blood sugar (glucose) levels during pregnancy are said to have **gestational diabetes**.

People with diabetes may have these signs and symptoms:

- Excessive thirst
- Extreme hunger
- Frequent urination
- Weight loss
- High blood sugar levels
- Glucose (sugar) in the urine
- Sudden vision changes
- Tingling or numbness in hands or feet
- Feeling very tired much of the time
- Very dry skin
- Sores that are slow to heal
- More infections than usual

Diabetes can lead to further complications:

- Changes in the circulatory system can cause heart attack and stroke, reduced circulation, poor wound healing, and kidney and nerve damage.
- Damage to the eyes can cause vision loss and blindness.

- Poor circulation and impaired wound healing may cause leg and foot ulcers, infected wounds, and gangrene. Gangrene can lead to amputation.

- Insulin reaction and diabetic ketoacidosis can be serious complications of diabetes. Chapter 2 has more information.

Diabetes must be carefully controlled to prevent complications and severe illness. When working with people with diabetes, NAs must follow care plan instructions carefully.

Guidelines: Diabetes

G Follow diet instructions exactly. The intake of carbohydrates, including breads, potatoes, grains, pastas, and sugars, must be regulated. Meals must be eaten at the same time each day. The resident must eat all that is served. If a resident will not eat what is served, or if you suspect that he is not following the diet, tell the nurse.

G Encourage the resident to follow his exercise program. Regular exercise is important. Exercise affects how quickly bodies use food. Exercise also improves circulation. Exercise may include walking or other activities. It may also include passive range of motion exercises. Help with exercise as necessary. Be positive. Try to make it fun. A walk can be a chore or it can be the highlight of the day.

G Observe the resident's management of insulin. Doses are calculated exactly. They are given at the same time each day. Know when residents take insulin and when their meals should be served. There must be a balance between the insulin level and food intake.

G Perform urine and blood tests only as directed. A fingerstick blood glucose test is one type of blood test that may be used to check blood sugar. This is a simple test that is performed by quickly piercing the fingertip, then placing the blood on a chemically active disposable strip. The strip will indicate the result. Another type of test involves using strips, along with a blood glucose meter, a special glucose monitoring machine (Fig. 4-25). Sometimes the care plan will specify a daily blood or urine test for insulin levels. Not all states allow NAs to do this. Know your state's rules. Your facility will provide training if you are allowed to do these tests. Perform tests only as directed and allowed.

Fig. 4-25. *There are different types of equipment to measure glucose levels in the blood.*

G Proper foot care is vitally important for people with diabetes. Give foot care as directed. People with diabetes have poor circulation. Even a small sore on the leg or foot can grow into a large wound that may not heal. This can result in amputation. Careful foot care, including regular, daily inspection, is very important. The goals of diabetic foot care are to check for irritation or sores, to promote blood circulation, and to prevent infection.

G Encourage people with diabetes to wear comfortable, well-fitting leather shoes that do not hurt their feet. Leather shoes breathe and help prevent buildup of moisture. To avoid injuries to the feet, residents should never go barefoot. Cotton socks are best to absorb sweat. NAs should not trim or clip toenails. Only a nurse or doctor should do this.

9. Describe the reproductive system and related conditions

The reproductive system is made up of the reproductive organs. They are different in men and women (Figs. 4-26 and 4-27). The reproductive system allows human beings to **reproduce**, or create new human life. Reproduction begins when a male's and female's sex cells (sperm and ovum) join. These sex cells are formed in the male and female sex glands. These sex glands are called the **gonads**.

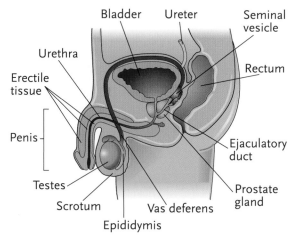

Fig. 4-26. The male reproductive system.

Fig. 4-27. The female reproductive system.

Normal changes of aging for males include

- Sperm production decreases.

- Prostate gland enlarges, which can interfere with urination.

Normal changes of aging for females include

- Menstruation ends. Menopause is when a female stops having menstrual periods.

- Decrease in estrogen may lead to a loss of calcium. This can cause brittle bones and, potentially, osteoporosis.

- Vaginal walls become drier and thinner.

How the NA Can Help

Sexual needs and desires continue as people age. The NA should provide privacy when necessary for sexual activity. The NA must respect residents' sexual needs and never judge any sexual behavior. However, any behavior that makes the NA uncomfortable or seems inappropriate should be reported. Inappropriate behavior is not a normal sign of aging and could be a sign of illness.

Observing and Reporting: Reproductive System

Observe and report these signs and symptoms:

- O/R Discomfort or difficulty with urination
- O/R Discharge from the penis or vagina
- O/R Swelling of the genitals
- O/R Blood in urine or stool
- O/R Breast changes, including size, shape, lumps, or discharge from the nipple
- O/R Sores on the genitals
- O/R Redness, rash on genitals
- O/R Genital itching
- O/R Resident reports of erectile dysfunction (ED) (trouble getting or keeping an erection)
- O/R Resident reports painful intercourse

Vaginitis

Vaginitis is an infection of the vagina. It may be caused by a bacteria, protozoa (one-celled animals), or fungus (yeast). It may also be caused by hormonal changes after menopause. Women who have vaginitis will notice a change in color, odor, and amount of vaginal discharge. This is accompanied by itching and burning. These symptoms should be reported to the nurse. Treatment of vaginitis includes oral medications, as well as vaginal creams or suppositories.

Benign Prostatic Hypertrophy (BPH)

Benign prostatic hypertrophy is a disorder that occurs in men as they age. The prostate becomes enlarged. This causes pressure on the urethra. The pressure leads to frequent urination, dribbling of urine, and difficulty in starting the flow of urine. Urinary retention (urine remaining in the bladder) may also occur, causing urinary tract infections. Urine can also back up into the ureters and kidneys, causing damage to these organs. Benign prostatic hypertrophy can be treated with medications or surgery. A test is also available to screen for cancer of the prostate. As men age, they are at increased risk for prostate cancer. Prostate cancer is usually slow-growing and responsive to treatment if detected early.

Residents' Rights

Sexual Expression and Privacy

Residents have the right to sexual freedom and expression. Residents have the right to privacy and the right to meet their sexual needs.

10. Describe the immune and lymphatic systems and related conditions

The immune system protects the body from disease-causing bacteria, viruses, and organisms in two ways. Nonspecific immunity protects the body from disease in general. Specific immunity protects against a particular disease that is invading the body at a given time.

The lymphatic system removes excess fluids and waste products from the body's tissues. It also helps the immune system fight infection. It is closely related to both the immune and the circulatory systems. The lymphatic system consists of lymph vessels and lymph capillaries in which a fluid called lymph circulates (Fig. 4-28). Lymph is a clear, yellowish fluid that carries disease-fighting cells called lymphocytes.

Normal changes of aging include

- Immune system weakens, increasing the risk of all types of infections.

- It may take longer for a person to recover from an illness.

- Number and size of lymph nodes decrease, which results in body being less able to produce a fever to fight infection.

- Response to vaccines decreases.

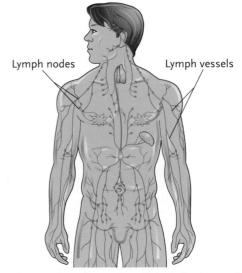

Fig. 4-28. *Lymph nodes work to fight infection and are located throughout the body.*

How the NA Can Help

Factors that weaken the immune system include not enough sleep, poor nutrition, chronic illness, and stress. Preventing infection is important. The NA should wash her hands often and keep the resident's environment clean. She can help with personal hygiene as needed. Proper nutrition and fluid intake should be encouraged. A slight temperature increase may indicate that a resident is fighting an infection. The NA should measure vital signs accurately.

Observing and Reporting: Immune and Lymphatic Systems

Observe and report these symptoms:

- °/R Recurring infections (such as fevers and diarrhea)

- °/R Swelling of the lymph nodes

- °/R Increased fatigue

HIV and AIDS

Acquired immune deficiency syndrome (AIDS) is a disease caused by the human immunodeficiency virus (HIV). HIV attacks the body's immune system. It gradually weakens and disables it. AIDS is the final stage of HIV infection in which infections, tumors, and symptoms appear due to a weakened immune system that is unable to fight infection. It can take years for HIV to develop into AIDS.

HIV is a sexually transmitted disease. It is also spread through the blood, from infected needles, or to a fetus from its mother.

In general, HIV affects the body in stages. The first stage shows symptoms like the flu, with fever, muscle aches, cough, and fatigue. These are signs of the immune system fighting the infection. As the infection worsens, the immune system overreacts. It attacks not only the virus, but also normal tissue.

When the virus weakens the immune system in later stages, a group of problems may appear. These include infections, tumors, and central nervous system symptoms. These would not occur if the immune system were healthy. This stage of the disease is known as AIDS. The diagnosis of AIDS is made when a person's CD4+ lymphocyte (a type of white blood cell) count falls to 200 or below. In the late stages of AIDS, damage to the central nervous system may cause memory loss, poor coordination, paralysis, and confusion. These symptoms together are known as AIDS dementia complex.

These are signs and symptoms of HIV infection and AIDS:

- Flu-like symptoms, including fever, cough, weakness, and severe or constant fatigue
- Appetite loss
- Weight loss
- Night sweats
- Swollen lymph nodes in the neck, underarms, or groin
- Severe diarrhea
- Dry cough
- Skin rashes

- Painful white spots in the mouth or on the tongue
- Cold sores or fever blisters on the lips and flat, white ulcers in the mouth
- Cauliflower-like warts on the skin and in the mouth
- Inflamed and bleeding gums
- Bruising that does not go away
- Low resistance to infection, particularly pneumonia, but also tuberculosis, herpes, bacterial infections, and hepatitis
- Kaposi's sarcoma, a form of skin cancer that appears as purple or red skin lesions
- Pneumocystis pneumonia, a lung infection
- AIDS dementia complex

Infections, such as pneumonia, tuberculosis, or hepatitis, invade the body when the immune system is weak and cannot defend itself. These illnesses worsen AIDS. They further weaken the immune system. It is hard to treat these infections. Over time, a person with AIDS may develop a resistance to some antibiotics. These infections can cause death in people with AIDS.

There is no cure for this disease, and there is no vaccine to prevent the disease. People who are infected with HIV are treated with drugs that slow the progress of the disease. Without medication, however, a weakened resistance to infections may lead to AIDS and eventually to death.

A combination of medications can help people with HIV live longer. The medicines must be taken at precise times. They have many unpleasant side effects. For some people, the medications work less well than for others. Other aspects of HIV treatment include relief of symptoms and prevention of infection.

Guidelines: HIV and AIDS

G   People with poor immune systems are more sensitive to infections. Wash your hands often. Keep everything clean. Follow Standard Precautions.

G Involuntary weight loss occurs in almost all people who develop AIDS. High-protein, high-calorie, and high-nutrient meals can help maintain a healthy weight.

G Some people with HIV/AIDS lose their appetites and have trouble eating. Encourage these residents to relax before meals and to eat in a pleasant setting. Familiar and favorite foods should be served. Report appetite loss or trouble eating to the nurse. If appetite loss continues, the doctor may prescribe an appetite stimulant.

G Residents with infections of the mouth may need food that is low in acid and neither cold nor hot. Spicy seasonings should be removed. Soft or pureed foods may be easier to swallow. Drinking liquid meals and fortified drinks may help ease the pain of chewing. Warm rinses may help painful mouth sores. Careful mouth care is vital.

G A person who has nausea or vomiting should eat small, frequent meals and should eat slowly. The person should avoid high-fat and spicy foods and eat a soft, bland diet. Residents should drink fluids in between meals. Proper intake of fluids to balance lost fluids is important.

G Residents with mild diarrhea may have small, frequent meals that are low in fat, fiber, and milk products. If diarrhea is severe, the doctor may order a BRAT diet (a diet of bananas, rice, applesauce, and toast). This diet is helpful for short-term use. Diarrhea rapidly depletes the body of fluids. Fluid replacement is necessary. Good rehydration fluids include water, juice, caffeine-free soda, and broth. Caffeinated drinks should be avoided.

G Numbness, tingling, and pain in the feet and legs is usually treated with medications. Wearing loose, soft slippers may be helpful. If blankets cause pain, a bed cradle can keep

sheets and blankets from resting on legs and feet (Fig. 4-29).

Fig. 4-29. *A bed cradle helps keep covers from resting on the feet.*

G Give emotional support, as well as physical care. Residents with HIV/AIDS may have anxiety and depression. In addition, they are often judged by family, friends, and society. Some people blame them for their illness. People with HIV/AIDS may feel tremendous stress. They may be uncertain about their illness, health care, and finances. They may also have lost friends who have died from AIDS. Treat residents with respect. Help give the emotional support they need. Residents with this disease need support from others. This may come from family, friends, religious and community groups, and support groups, as well as the care team.

G Withdrawal, avoidance of tasks, and mental slowness are early symptoms of HIV infection. Medications may also cause side effects of this type. AIDS dementia complex may cause further mental symptoms. There may also be muscle weakness and loss of muscle control, making falls a risk. Residents will need a safe environment and close supervision in their ADLs.

Residents' Rights

The Facts about HIV and AIDS

A handshake or a hug cannot spread HIV. The disease cannot be transmitted by telephones, doorknobs, tables, chairs, toilets, mosquitoes, or by breathing the same air as an infected person. NAs should spend time with residents who have HIV or AIDS. These residents need the same thoughtful, personal attention that NAs give to all residents.

Cancer

Cancer is a general term used to describe a disease in which abnormal cells grow in an uncontrolled way. Cancer usually occurs in the form of a tumor or tumors growing on or within the body. A **tumor** is a group of abnormally-growing cells. Benign tumors are considered non-cancerous. They usually grow slowly in local areas. Malignant tumors are cancerous. They can grow rapidly and invade surrounding tissues.

Cancer invades local tissue and can spread to other parts of the body. When it spreads from the site where it first appeared, it can affect other body systems. In general, treatment is more difficult and cancer is more deadly after this has occurred. Cancer often appears first in the breast, colon, rectum, uterus, prostate, lungs, or skin. There is no known cure for cancer, but some treatments are effective.

These risk factors may contribute to cancer:

- Age
- Race
- Gender
- Family history
- Tobacco use
- Alcohol use
- Poor diet/obesity
- Lack of physical activity
- Chemicals and food additives
- Radiation
- Exposure to sunlight

When diagnosed early, cancer can often be treated and controlled. The American Cancer Society has identified some warning signs of cancer:

- Unexplained weight loss
- Fever
- Fatigue
- Pain
- Skin changes
- Change in bowel or bladder function
- Sores that do not heal
- Unusual bleeding or discharge
- Thickening or lump in the breast, scrotum, or other parts of the body
- Indigestion or difficulty swallowing
- New mole or recent change in appearance of a mole or wart
- Nagging cough or hoarseness

People with cancer can live longer and sometimes recover if they are treated early. Often these treatments are combined:

- Surgery
- Chemotherapy
- Radiation

Guidelines: Cancer

G Each case is different. Cancer is a general term. It refers to many separate situations. Residents may live many years or only several months. Treatment affects each person differently. Do not make assumptions about a resident's condition.

G Residents may want to talk or may avoid talking. Respect their needs. Be honest. Never say, "Everything will be okay." Be sensitive. Remember that cancer is a disease. Its cause is unknown. Have a positive attitude (Fig. 4-30).

G Proper nutrition is important for residents with cancer. Follow the care plan carefully. Residents frequently have poor appetites. Encourage a variety of food and small portions. Liquid nutrition supplements may be used in addition to, not in place of, meals. If nausea or swallowing is a problem, foods such as soups, gelatin, or starches may appeal to the resident. Use plastic utensils for a resident receiving chemotherapy. It makes food taste better. Metal utensils cause a bitter taste.

Fig. 4-30. *Have a positive attitude and focus on concrete details. For example, comment if a resident seems stronger, or mention that the sun is shining outside.*

G   Cancer can cause great pain, especially in the late stages. Watch for signs of pain (Chapter 7). Report them to the nurse. Help with comfort measures, such as repositioning and providing conversation, music, or reading materials. Report if pain seems to be uncontrolled.

G   Give back rubs for comfort and to increase circulation. For residents who spend many hours in bed, moving to a chair for a period of time may improve comfort as well. Residents who are weak or immobile need to be repositioned at least every two hours.

G   Use lotion on dry or delicate skin. Do not apply lotion to areas receiving radiation therapy. Do not remove markings that are used in radiation therapy. Follow any skin care orders (for example: no hot or cold packs, no soap or cosmetics, no tight stockings).

G   Help residents brush and floss teeth regularly. Medications, nausea, vomiting, or mouth infections may cause pain and a bad taste in the mouth. You can help by using a soft-bristled toothbrush, rinsing with baking soda and water, or using a prescribed rinse. Do not use a commercial mouthwash. For residents with mouth sores, use oral swabs, rather than toothbrushes. Be gentle when giving care.

G   People with cancer may have a poor self-image because they are weak and their appearance has changed. For example, hair loss is a common side effect of chemotherapy. Help with grooming if desired.

G   If visitors help cheer your resident, encourage them. Do not intrude. If some times of day are better than others, suggest this. It may help a person with cancer to think of something else for a while. Pursue other topics. Get to know what interests your residents have.

G   Having a family member with cancer can be very difficult. Be alert to needs that are not being met or stresses created by the illness.

G   Report any of these to the nurse:

   •   Increased weakness or fatigue

   •   Weight loss

   •   Nausea, vomiting, or diarrhea

   •   Changes in appetite

   •   Fainting

   •   Signs of depression

   •   Confusion

   •   Blood in stool or urine

   •   Change in mental status

   •   Changes in skin

   •   New lumps, sores, or rashes

   •   Increase in pain, or unrelieved pain

   •   Blood in the mouth

Community resources for residents who are ill are located at the end of Chapter 3.

5
Confusion, Dementia, and Alzheimer's Disease

1. Discuss confusion and delirium

Confusion is the inability to think clearly. A confused person has trouble focusing his attention and may feel disoriented. Confusion interferes with the ability to make decisions. The person's personality may change. He may not know his name, the date, other people, or where he is. A confused person may be angry, depressed, or irritable.

Confusion may come on suddenly or gradually. It can be temporary or permanent. Confusion is more common in the elderly. It may occur when a person is in the hospital. Some causes of confusion include the following:

- Urinary tract infection (UTI)
- Low blood sugar
- Head trauma or head injury
- Dehydration
- Nutritional problems
- Fever
- Sudden drop in body temperature
- Lack of oxygen
- Medications
- Infections
- Brain tumor
- Diseases or illnesses
- Loss of sleep
- Seizures

Guidelines: Confusion

G Do not leave a confused resident alone.

G Stay calm. Provide a quiet environment.

G Speak in a lower tone of voice. Speak clearly and slowly.

G Introduce yourself each time you see the resident.

G Remind the resident of his or her location, name, and the date. A calendar can help.

G Explain what you are going to do, using simple instructions.

G Do not rush the resident.

G Talk to confused residents about plans for the day. Keeping a routine may help.

G Encourage the use of eyeglasses and hearing aids. Make sure they are clean and are not damaged.

G Promote self-care and independence.

G Report observations to the nurse.

Delirium is a state of severe confusion that occurs suddenly; it is usually temporary. Possible causes include infections, disease, fluid imbalances, and poor nutrition. Drugs and alcohol may also cause delirium. Signs and symptoms include the following:

- Agitation
- Anger
- Depression

- Irritability
- Disorientation
- Trouble focusing
- Problems with speech
- Changes in sensation and perception
- Changes in consciousness
- Decrease in short-term memory

NAs should report these signs and symptoms to the nurse. The goal of treatment is to control or reverse the cause. Emergency care may be needed, as well as a stay in a hospital.

Confusion and Delirium

When communicating with a person who is confused or disoriented, the NA should

- Keep her voice low
- Not raise her voice or shout
- Use the person's name, and speak clearly in simple sentences
- Use facial expressions and body language to aid in understanding
- Reduce distractions by taking action, such as turning down the TV
- Be gentle and try to decrease fears

2. Describe dementia and discuss Alzheimer's disease

As a person ages, some of the ability to think logically and clearly may be lost. This ability is called **cognition**. When some of this ability is lost, a person is said to have **cognitive impairment**. How much ability is lost depends on the individual. Cognitive impairment affects concentration and memory. Elderly residents may lose their memories of recent events. This can be frustrating for them. NAs can help by encouraging them to make lists of things to remember. Writing down names and phone numbers may also help. Other normal changes of aging in the brain are slower reaction time, trouble finding or using the right words, and sleeping less.

Dementia is a general term that refers to a serious loss of mental abilities such as thinking, remembering, reasoning, and communicating. As dementia advances, these losses make it hard to perform activities of daily living (ADLs) such as eating, bathing, dressing, and toileting. Dementia is not a normal part of aging (Fig. 5-1).

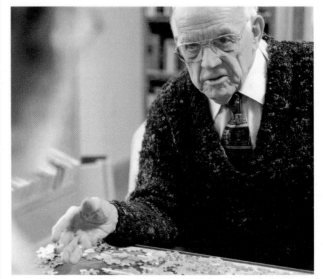

Fig. 5-1. *Some loss of cognitive ability is normal; however, dementia is not a normal part of aging.*

These are some common causes of dementia:

- Alzheimer's disease
- Multi-infarct or vascular dementia (a series of strokes causing damage to the brain)
- Lewy body dementia
- Parkinson's disease
- Huntington's disease

Alzheimer's disease (AD) is the most common cause of dementia in the elderly. The Alzheimer's Association (alz.org) estimates that as many as 5.2 million Americans are living with Alzheimer's disease. One in eight older Americans has Alzheimer's disease. Women are more likely than men to have Alzheimer's disease and dementia. The risk of getting AD increases with age, but it is not a normal part of aging.

Alzheimer's disease causes tangled nerve fibers and protein deposits to form in the brain. They eventually cause dementia. The disease gets worse, causing greater and greater loss of health and abilities. There is no known cause of AD, and there is no cure. Residents with AD will never recover. They will need more care as the disease progresses.

A diagnosis of dementia is difficult. It involves many physical and mental tests to rule out other causes. The only sure way to determine AD at this time is by autopsy (examination of the body after death). The length of time it takes AD to progress from onset to death varies greatly. It may take anywhere from three to 20 years.

Symptoms of AD appear gradually. It begins with memory loss. As AD progresses, the symptoms get worse. People with AD may get disoriented. They may be confused about time and place. Communication problems are common. They may lose their ability to read, write, speak, or understand. Mood and behavior changes. Aggressiveness, wandering, and withdrawal are all part of AD. The disease progresses to a complete loss of all ability to care for oneself. The person eventually requires constant care in most cases.

Each person with AD will show different symptoms at different times. For example, one resident with Alzheimer's may continue to read, but not be able to use the phone. Another may lose the ability to read, but can still do simple math. Skills a person has used over a lifetime are usually kept longer. Thus some people with Alzheimer's disease can play an instrument with some help long after they have lost much of their memory (Fig. 5-2).

Fig. 5-2. Even when a person loses much of her memory, she may still keep skills she has used her whole life.

It is important for NAs to encourage independence, regardless of what signs a person with AD shows. Residents with AD should be encouraged to do their ADLs. This helps keep their minds and bodies as active as possible. Working, socializing, reading, problem solving, and exercising should all be encouraged (Fig. 5-3). Having residents do as much as possible for themselves may even help slow the disease. Tasks should be challenging but not frustrating. NAs can help residents succeed in doing these tasks.

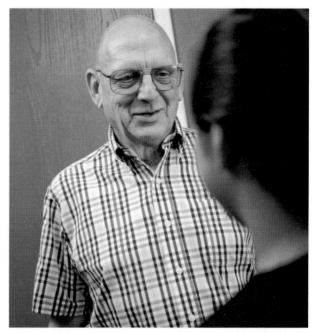

Fig. 5-3. Nursing assistants should encourage residents with AD to socialize, read, work, problem solve, and exercise to keep their minds and bodies active.

These attitudes help nursing assistants give the best possible care to residents with AD:

- Do not take things personally.

- Be empathetic.

- Work with the symptoms and behaviors noted.

- Work as a team.

- Be aware of difficulties associated with caregiving.

- Work with family members.

- Remember the goals of the care plan.

3. List strategies for better communication with residents with Alzheimer's disease

Communication with residents with AD may be helped if the NA does the following:

- Always approaches from the front and does not startle the resident.

- Determines how close the resident wants her to be.

- Communicates in a calm area with little background noise and distraction.

- Always identifies herself and uses the resident's name. She should continue to use the resident's name during the conversation.

- Speaks slowly, using a lower tone of voice. This is calming and easier to understand.

- Repeats herself. Uses the same words and phrases as often as needed.

- Uses signs, pictures, gestures, or written words to help communicate.

- Breaks complex tasks into smaller, simpler ones. Gives simple, step-by-step instructions as necessary.

In addition, residents with AD can be helped by using these techniques for specific situations:

If the resident is frightened or anxious, the NA should

- Try to keep the resident calm. Speak slowly in a low, calm voice. Get rid of noise and distractions, such as televisions.

- Try to see and hear herself as they might. She should always describe what she is going to do.

- Use simple words and short sentences. If helping with care, it is helpful to list steps one at a time.

- Check her body language. Make sure she is not tense or hurried.

If the resident forgets or shows memory loss, the NA should

- Repeat herself. Use the same words if she needs to repeat an instruction or question. However, she may be using a word the resident does not understand, such as *tired*. She can try other words like *nap*, *lie down*, or *rest*. Repetition can also be soothing. Many residents with AD will repeat words, phrases, questions, or actions. This is called **perseveration**. If a resident perseverates, the NA should not try to stop him. She should answer his questions, using the same words each time, until he stops.

- Keep messages simple. Break complex tasks into smaller, simpler ones.

If the resident has trouble finding words or names, the NA should

- Suggest a word that sounds correct. If this upsets the resident, the NA can learn from it. She should not try to correct a resident who uses an incorrect word. As words become more difficult, smiling, touching, and hugging can help show care and concern (Fig. 5-4). The NA should know, though, that some people find touch unwelcome.

Fig. 5-4. *Touch and smiles will be understood longer, even after a resident's speaking abilities decline.*

If the resident seems not to understand basic instructions or questions, the NA should

- Ask the resident to repeat her words. She should use short words and sentences and allow time to answer.

- Note the communication methods that are effective. Use them.

- Watch for nonverbal cues as the ability to talk declines. She can observe body language—eyes, hands, and face.

- Use signs, pictures, gestures, or written words. For example, a picture of a toilet on the bathroom door can remind a resident where the bathroom is. Combining verbal and nonverbal communication is helpful. For example, she can say, "Let's get dressed now," as she hold up clothes.

If the resident wants to say something but cannot, the NA should

- Ask the resident to point, gesture, or act it out.

- If the resident is upset but cannot explain why, she can offer comfort with a smile or try to distract him. Verbal communication may be frustrating.

If the resident does not remember how to perform basic tasks, the NA should

- Break each activity into simple steps. For example, she can say, "Let's go for a walk. Stand up. Put on your sweater. First the right arm..." She should always encourage the person to do what he can.

If the resident insists on doing something that is unsafe or not allowed, the NA should

- Try to limit the times she says "Don't." Instead, activities should be redirected.

If the resident hallucinates (sees or hears things that are not really happening) or is paranoid or accusing, the NA should

- Try not to take it personally.

- Try to redirect behavior or ignore it. Attention span is limited. This behavior often passes quickly.

If the resident is depressed or lonely, the NA should

- Take time, one-on-one, to ask how the resident is feeling. Really listen to the answer.

- Try to involve the resident in activities.

- Always report signs of depression to the nurse.

If the resident repeatedly asks to "go home," the NA should

- Ask the resident to tell her what his home was like and how he felt being there.

- Redirect or guide the conversation and/or the resident's activities to something he enjoys.

- Expect that the resident may continue to ask to go home and be patient and gentle in her responses.

If the resident is verbally abusive or uses bad language, the NA should

- Remember it is the dementia speaking, not the person. She should try to ignore the language and redirect his attention.

If the resident has lost most verbal skills, the NA should

- Use nonverbal skills. As speaking abilities decline, people with AD will still understand touch, smiles, and laughter for much longer. However, some people do not like to be touched. The NA should approach touching slowly and be gentle. Softly touching the hand or smiling can show affection and say that she wants to help.

- Remember that even after verbal skills are lost, signs, labels, and gestures can reach people with dementia.

- Assume people with AD can understand more than they can express. The NA should not talk about them as though they were not there.

4. List and describe interventions for problems with common activities of daily living (ADLs)

Nursing assistants should use the same procedures for personal care and ADLs for residents with Alzheimer's disease as they would with other residents. However, here are some general principles that will help them give the best care:

1. **Develop a routine and stick to it.** Being consistent is important for residents who are confused and easily upset.

2. **Promote self-care.** Helping residents care for themselves as much as possible will help them cope with this difficult disease.

3. **Take good care of themselves, both mentally and physically.** This will help NAs give the best care.

As Alzheimer's disease worsens, residents will have trouble doing their ADLs. Below are techniques that can help with these problems.

If a resident has problems with bathing, the NA should

- Schedule bathing when the resident is least agitated. She should be organized so the bath can be quick. Sponge baths can be given if the resident resists a shower or tub bath.

- Prepare the resident before bathing. Hand him the supplies (washcloth, soap, shampoo, towels). This serves as a visual aid.

- Take a walk down the hall with the resident. Stop at the tub or shower room, rather than asking directly about the bath.

- Make sure the bathroom is well-lit and is at a comfortable temperature.

- Provide privacy during the bath.

- Be calm and quiet when bathing a resident. Keep the process simple.

- Be sensitive when talking to the resident about bathing.

- Give the resident a washcloth to hold. This can distract him while the NA finishes the bath.

- Always follow safety precautions. Ensure safety by using non-slip mats, tub seats, and hand-holds.

- Be flexible about when to bathe the resident. A resident may not always be in the mood. Also, not everyone bathes with the same frequency. The NA should understand if a resident does not want to bathe.

- Be relaxed and allow the resident to enjoy the bath. The NA should offer praise.

- Let the resident do as much as possible during the bath.

- Check the skin regularly for signs of irritation during the bath.

If a resident has problems with grooming and dressing, the NA should

- Help with grooming to help residents feel attractive.

- Avoid delays or interruptions while dressing.

- Show the resident clothing to put on. This brings up the idea of dressing.

- Provide privacy and close doors and curtains. The resident should be dressed in his room.

- Encourage the resident to pick clothes to wear. Giving just a few choices is best. Clothing should be clean and appropriate. The NA should lay out clothes in the order in which they are put on (Fig. 5-5). Some people with AD layer clothing regardless of the weather.

- Break the task down into simple steps. The NA should introduce one step at a time. The resident should not be rushed.

- Use a friendly, calm voice when speaking. The NA should praise and encourage the resident at each step.

Fig. 5-5. Clothes should be laid out in the order in which they should be put on.

Underwear · T-shirt · Socks · Elastic-Waist Pants · Pullover Shirt

If a resident has problems with toileting, the NA should

- Encourage fluids. The NA should never withhold or discourage fluids because a resident is incontinent. She should tell the nurse if the resident is not drinking fluids.

- Mark the bathroom with a sign or a picture. This is a reminder of where it is and to use the toilet.

- Make sure there is enough light in the bathroom and on the way there.

- Note when the resident is incontinent over two to three days. He should be checked every 30 minutes. This can help determine "bathroom times." The NA should take the resident to the bathroom just before his bathroom time.

- Observe toilet patterns for two to three nights to try to determine nighttime bathroom times.

- Take the resident to the bathroom before and after meals and before bed. The NA should make sure the resident actually urinates before getting off the toilet.

- Put lids on trash cans, wastebaskets, or other containers if the resident urinates in them.

- Remember that family or friends may be upset by their loved one's incontinence. The NA should be professional when cleaning after episodes of incontinence. She should not show any disgust or irritation.

If a resident has problems with nutrition, the NA should

- Encourage nutritious foods. Food may not interest a resident with Alzheimer's disease at all. It may be of great interest, but he may only want to eat a few types of food. A resident with AD is at risk for malnutrition.

- Have meals at regular times each day. The NA may need to remind the resident that it is mealtime. Familiar, appetizing foods should be served.

- Make sure there is proper lighting.

- Keep noise and distractions low during meals.

- Keep the task of eating simple. If the resident is restless during meals, the NA can try smaller, more frequent meals. Finger foods (foods that are easy to pick up with the fingers) allow eating while moving around. They allow residents to choose the food they want to eat. Examples of finger foods that may be good to serve are sandwiches cut into fourths, chicken nuggets or small pieces of cooked boneless chicken, fish sticks, cheese cubes, halved hard-boiled eggs, and cut fresh fruit and soft vegetables.

- Avoid serving steaming or very hot foods or drinks.

- Use a simple place setting with a single eating utensil and remove other items from the table. Plain plates without patterns or colors work best (Fig. 5-6).

Fig. 5-6. *Plain white plates on a contrasting-colored surface may help avoid confusion and distraction.*

- Put only one item of food on the plate at a time. Multiple kinds of food on a plate or a tray may be overwhelming.

- Give simple, clear instructions. Residents with AD may not understand how to eat or use utensils. The NA should help the resident taste a sample first. She can place a spoon to the lips. This will encourage the resident to open his mouth. The NA can also ask him to open his mouth.

- Guide the resident through the meal. The NA should provide simple instructions. Offering regular drinks of water, juice, and other fluids helps prevent dehydration.

- Use adaptive equipment, such as special spoons and bowls, as needed.

- Feed the resident slowly, giving small pieces of food.

- Make mealtimes simple and relaxed. Allow time for eating. Give the resident time to swallow before each bite or drink.

- Seat residents who have AD with others at small tables. This encourages socializing.

- Observe and report eating or swallowing problems. The NA should also observe and report changes or problems in eating habits.

In addition, the NA should use the following tips when caring for residents with AD:

- Prevent infections and follow Standard Precautions.

- Observe the resident's physical health and report any potential problems. People with dementia may not notice their own health problems.

- Give careful skin care to prevent pressure ulcers.

- Watch for signs of pain. Nonverbal signs that a resident may be in pain include grimacing or clenching fists. Report possible signs of pain to the nurse.

- Maintain a daily exercise routine.

- Maintain self-esteem. Encourage independence in ADLs.

- Share in fun activities, looking at pictures, talking, and reminiscing.

- Reward positive and independent behavior with smiles and warm touches.

5. List and describe interventions for common difficult behaviors related to Alzheimer's disease

Below are some common difficult behaviors that NAs may face with residents with AD. Each resident is different, and NAs should work with each person as an individual.

Agitation: A resident who is excited, restless, or troubled is said to be agitated. Situations that lead to agitation are *triggers*. Triggers may include a change of routine or caregiver, new or frustrating experiences, or even television. If a resident is agitated, the NA should

- Try to remove triggers, keep a routine, and avoid frustration.

- Help the resident focus on a soothing, familiar activity. They can try sorting things or looking at pictures.

- Stay calm and use a low, soothing voice. This may reassure the resident.

- Place an arm around the shoulder or pat the resident. This may soothe some residents.

Sundowning: When a person gets restless and agitated in the late afternoon, evening, or night, it is called **sundowning**. Sundowning may be caused by hunger or fatigue, a change in routine or caregiver, or any new or frustrating situation. If a resident experiences this, the NA should

- Remove triggers, give snacks, and encourage rest.

- Avoid stressful situations during this time. Activities, appointments, and visits should be limited.

- Play soft music.

- Set a bedtime routine and keep it.

- Recognize when sundowning occurs. A calming activity can be done just before.

- Remove caffeine from the diet.

- Give a soothing back massage.

- Distract the resident with a simple, calm activity like looking at a magazine.

- Maintain a daily exercise routine.

Catastrophic Reactions: When a person with AD overreacts to something, it is called a **catastrophic reaction**. It may be triggered by any of the following:

- Fatigue

- Change of routine, environment, or caregiver

- Overstimulation (too much noise or activity)

- Difficult choices or tasks

- Physical pain

- Hunger

- Need for toileting

An NA can respond to catastrophic reactions as she would to agitation or sundowning. For example, she can remove triggers. She can help the resident focus on a soothing activity.

Violent Behavior: A resident who attacks, hits, or threatens someone is violent. Frustration or overstimulation may trigger violence. It can also be triggered by a change in routine, environment, or caregiver. If a resident is violent, the NA should

- Block blows but never hit back.

- Step out of reach.

- Call for help if needed.

- Avoid leaving the resident alone.

- Try to remove triggers.

- Use the same techniques to calm residents as for agitation or sundowning.

Pacing and Wandering: A resident who walks back and forth in the same area is **pacing**. A resident who walks aimlessly around the facility is **wandering** (Fig. 5-7). These are some causes of pacing and wandering:

- Restlessness

- Hunger

- Disorientation

- Need for toileting

- Constipation

- Pain

- Forgetting how or where to sit down

- Too much daytime napping

- Need for exercise

Fig. 5-7. A resident with AD who is walking aimlessly around the facility or facility grounds is wandering.

NAs should remove causes when they can. For example, give nutritious snacks, encourage an exercise routine, and maintain a toileting schedule. If residents pace and wander, they should do so in a safe and secure (locked) area. Staff should keep an eye on them. The NA can suggest another activity, such as going for a walk together. Marking rooms with signs or pictures may prevent residents from wandering into areas where they should not go.

Elopement

Residents with AD may try to **elope**, or leave a facility unsupervised and unnoticed. In order to guard against elopement, facilities often have secured areas so that residents with AD will not wander away. There may be a coded entry system. This system requires a code to be entered to open a door. The code is available to alert, oriented residents, visitors, and staff.

If a resident with AD elopes, the NA must notify the nurse immediately. Residents who elope are often found near where they were last seen. The earlier a search is begun, the more likely the resident is to be found nearby and safe.

Hallucinations or Delusions: A resident who sees, hears, smells, tastes, or feels things that are not there is having **hallucinations**. A resident who believes things that are not true is having **delusions**. If a resident is experiencing hallucinations and/or delusions, the NA should

- Ignore harmless hallucinations and delusions.

- Reassure a resident who seems agitated or worried.

- Not argue with a resident who is imagining things. The feelings are real to him. The NA should not tell the resident that she sees or hears his hallucinations. She should redirect the resident to other activities or thoughts.

- Be calm and reassure resident that she is there to help.

Depression: When residents become withdrawn, lack energy, or do not eat or do things they used to enjoy, they may be depressed. Depression may have many causes, including the following:

- Loss of independence

- Inability to cope

- Feelings of failure or fear

- Reality of facing a progressive, incurable illness

- Chemical imbalance

If a resident is depressed, the NA should

- Report signs of depression to the nurse immediately. It is an illness that can be treated with medication and/or therapy. Any threats of suicide should be reported immediately.

- Encourage independence, self-care, and activity.

- Talk about moods and feelings if the resident wants, and be a good listener.

- Encourage social interaction.

Perseveration or Repetitive Phrasing: A resident who repeats a word, phrase, question, or activity over and over is perseverating. Repeating a word or phrase is also called repetitive phrasing. This may be caused by disorientation or confusion. The NA should be patient and not try to silence or stop the resident. She should answer questions each time they are asked. She should use the same words each time.

Disruptiveness: Disruptive behavior is anything that disturbs others, such as yelling, banging on furniture, slamming doors, etc. Often this behavior is triggered by a wish for attention, by pain or constipation, or by frustration. When this behavior occurs, the NA should gain the resident's attention. She should be calm and friendly and try to find out what caused the behavior. There may be a physical reason, such as pain or discomfort. If a resident is being disruptive, the NA should

- Gently direct the resident to a private area.

- Notice and praise improvements in the resident's behavior. The NA should be sensitive while doing this to avoid treating the resident like a child.

- Tell the resident about any changes in schedules, routines, or the environment in advance. Involving the resident in developing routine activities and schedules may help.

- Encourage the resident to join in independent activities that are safe (for example, folding towels). This helps the resident feel in charge. It can prevent feelings of powerlessness. Independence is power.

- Help the resident find ways to cope. Focusing on activities the resident may still be able to do, such as knitting or crafts, can provide a diversion.

Inappropriate Social Behavior: Inappropriate social behavior may be cursing, name calling, or other behavior. As with violent or disruptive behavior, there may be many reasons why a resident is behaving this way. The NA should try not to take it personally. The resident may only be reacting to frustration or other stress, rather than to the NA. The NA should stay calm and be reassuring. She can try to find out what caused the behavior (such as too much noise, too many people, too much stress, pain, or discomfort). If the resident is disturbing others, the NA should gently direct him to a private area. The NA should respond positively to any appropriate behavior. Any physical abuse or serious verbal abuse should be reported to the nurse.

Inappropriate Sexual Behavior: Inappropriate sexual behavior, such as removing clothes, touching one's own genitals, or trying to touch others can embarrass those who see it. When dealing with such behavior, the NA should not overreact. This may reinforce the behavior. She should be sensitive to the nature of the problem. Is the behavior actually intentional? Is it consistent? If distracting the resident does not work, the NA can gently direct him to a private area. She should tell the nurse. A resident may be reacting to a need for physical stimulation or

affection. Ways to provide physical stimulation include backrubs, a soft doll or stuffed animal to cuddle, comforting blankets, or physical touch that is appropriate.

Pillaging and Hoarding: **Pillaging** is taking things that belong to someone else. A person with dementia may honestly think something belongs to him, even when it clearly does not. **Hoarding** is collecting and putting things away in a guarded way. Pillaging and hoarding should not be considered stealing. A person with Alzheimer's disease cannot and does not steal. Stealing is planned. It requires a conscious effort. In most cases, the person with AD is only collecting something that catches his attention. It is common for those with AD to wander in and out of rooms collecting things. They may carry these objects around for a while and then leave them in other places. This is not intentional. Residents with AD will often take their own things and leave them in another room, not knowing what they are doing. The NA can help lessen problems by

- Labeling all personal belongings with the resident's name and room number. This way there is no confusion about what belongs to whom.

- Placing a label, symbol, or object on the resident's door. This helps the resident find his own room.

- Not telling the family that their loved one is stealing from others.

- Preparing the family so they are not upset when they find items that do not belong to their family member.

- Asking the family to tell staff if they notice unfamiliar items in the room.

- Regularly checking areas where residents store items. They may store uneaten food in these places. Providing a rummage drawer—a drawer with items that are safe for the resident to take with him—can help.

Sleep Disturbances: Residents with AD may experience a number of sleep disturbances. If a resident experiences sleep problems, the NA should

- Make sure that the resident gets moderate exercise/activity throughout the day. The NA can encourage him to participate in activities he enjoys.

- Allow the resident to spend some time each day in natural sunlight if possible. Exposure to light and dark can help establish restful sleep patterns.

- Reduce light and noise as much as possible during nighttime hours.

- Discourage sleeping during the day.

Residents' Rights

Abuse and Alzheimer's Disease

People with Alzheimer's disease may be at a higher risk for abuse. One reason for this is that caring for someone with Alzheimer's disease is very difficult. There are many psychological and physical demands placed on caregivers.

To help manage the stress of caring for people with AD, NAs should take good care of themselves, both mentally and physically. This will help them give the best care. If needed, a supervisor can provide more resources to help an NA cope.

NAs must never abuse residents in any way. If an NA notices someone else abusing a resident, he is legally required to report it. All NAs are responsible for residents' safety and should take this responsibility seriously.

6. Describe creative therapies for residents with Alzheimer's disease

Although Alzheimer's disease cannot be cured, there are ways to improve life for residents with AD.

Reality orientation is using calendars, clocks, signs, and lists to help residents remember who and where they are. It is useful in early stages of AD when residents are confused but not totally disoriented. In later stages, reality orientation may frustrate residents.

Example: Each day when the NA goes into Mrs. Elkin's room, she shows her the calendar and points out what day of the week it is. On the calendar or another piece of paper, the NA lists all the things Mrs. Elkin will do that day. For example, she will take a shower, eat lunch, and go for a walk. When speaking to her, the NA calls her by her name: Mrs. Elkin. When helping with tasks, the NA explains why she does things as she does them. For example, "We use a shower chair in the shower so you don't have to stand up for so long, Mrs. Elkin."

Validation therapy is letting residents believe they live in the past or in imaginary circumstances. **Validating** means giving value to or approving. When using validation therapy, the NA should make no attempt to reorient the resident to actual circumstances (Fig. 5-8). She can explore the resident's beliefs. She should not argue with or correct him. Validating can give comfort and reduce agitation. It is useful in cases of moderate to severe disorientation.

Fig. 5-8. Validation therapy accepts a resident's fantasies without attempting to reorient him to reality.

Example: Mr. Baldwin tells the NA that he does not want to eat lunch today because he is going out to a restaurant with his wife. The NA knows his wife has been dead for many years and that Mr. Baldwin can no longer eat out. Instead of telling him that he is not going out to eat, the NA asks what restaurant he is going to and what he will have. She suggests that he eat a good lunch now because sometimes the service is slow in restaurants.

Reminiscence therapy is encouraging residents to remember and talk about the past. The NA can explore memories by asking about details (Fig. 5-9). He should focus on a time of life that was pleasant. It may help residents work through feelings about a hard time in the past. It is useful in many stages of AD, but especially with moderate to severe confusion.

Fig. 5-9. Reminiscence therapy encourages a resident to remember and talk about his past.

Example: Mr. Benton, an 83-year-old man with Alzheimer's disease, fought in the Korean War. In his room are many mementos of the war. He has pictures of his war buddies, a medal he was given, and more. The NA asks him to tell him where he was sent in the war. The NA asks him more detailed questions. Eventually the resident shares a lot: the friends he made in the service, why he was given the medal, times he was scared, and how much he missed his family.

Activity therapy uses activities that the resident enjoys to prevent boredom and frustration. These activities also promote self-esteem. The NA can help the resident take walks, do puzzles, listen to music, or do other things he or she enjoys (Fig. 5-10). Activities may be done in groups or one-on-one. Activity therapy is useful in most stages of AD.

Example: Mrs. Hoebel, a 70-year-old woman with AD, was a librarian for almost 45 years. She loves books and reading, but she cannot read much anymore. The NA obtains books from the facility that are filled with pictures. Mrs. Hoebel

sits with the books, sorting them, turning pages, and looking at pictures.

Fig. 5-10. Activities that are not frustrating can be helpful for residents with AD. They promote mental exercise.

Music Therapy

Music therapy involves using music to accomplish specific goals, such as managing stress and improving mood and cognition. This type of therapy has been used successfully with people who have Alzheimer's disease. Music is a form of sensory stimulation. Hearing familiar songs can cause a response in people with dementia who do not respond well or do not respond at all to other treatments. Music & Memory is a nonprofit organization that brings personalized music into the lives of the elderly. Their website, musicandmemory.org, provides more information.

6

Personal Care Skills

1. Explain personal care of residents

Personal care is different from other tasks that NAs may perform for residents, such as measuring vital signs or tidying a unit. The term *personal* refers to tasks that are concerned with the person's body, appearance, and hygiene. It suggests privacy may be important. **Hygiene** is the term used to describe ways to keep bodies clean and healthy. Bathing and brushing teeth are two examples. **Grooming** refers to practices like caring for fingernails and hair. Hygiene and grooming activities, as well as dressing, eating, transferring, and toileting are called *activities of daily living* (*ADLs*). NAs will help residents with these tasks every day. These activities are often called *a.m. care* or *p.m. care*. This refers to the time of day that they are done.

Assisting with a.m. care includes

- Offering a bedpan or urinal or helping the resident to the bathroom

- Helping the resident wash face and hands

- Assisting with hair care, dressing, and shaving

- Assisting with mouth care before or after breakfast

Assisting with p.m. care includes

- Offering a bedpan or urinal or helping the resident to the bathroom

- Helping the resident wash face and hands

- Giving a snack

- Assisting with mouth care

- Assisting with changing into nightclothes

- Giving a back rub

The way NAs help residents with personal care plays a large part in promoting their independence and dignity. The help NAs give will be different for each resident. It will depend on each resident's abilities. For example, a resident who has recently had a stroke will need more help than one who has a broken foot that is almost healed. Promoting independence is an important part of care.

Many people have been doing personal care tasks for themselves their entire lives. They may feel uncomfortable with having others do or help them do these tasks. Some residents may not like to be touched by someone else. NAs must be sensitive to these issues. They should be professional when helping with these tasks.

Before beginning a task, the NA should explain to the resident exactly what she will be doing. Having care explained is a resident's legal right. It may also help lessen anxiety. The NA should ask if he would like to use the bathroom or bedpan first. She should provide privacy by pulling the privacy curtain around the bed and closing the door. The resident should be allowed to make as many decisions as possible about when, where, and how a procedure is done (Fig. 6-1). This promotes dignity and independence. Other ways for NAs to promote respect, dignity, and privacy include the following:

- Encouraging residents to do as much as they are able to do and being patient

- Knocking and waiting for permission to enter the resident's room

- Not interrupting residents while they are in the bathroom

- Leaving the room when residents receive or make phone calls

- Respecting residents' private time and personal things

- Not interrupting residents while they are dressing

- Keeping residents covered whenever possible when helping with dressing

Fig 6-1. Nursing assistants should let the resident make as many decisions as possible about the personal care they will perform.

During personal care, the NA should look for any problems or changes that have occurred. Communication is very important during personal care. Some residents will share symptoms, feelings, and concerns with the NA. The NA should keep a small notepad in a pocket to note exactly how the resident describes these symptoms. These comments should be reported to the nurse and documented. NAs must also look for physical or mental changes. The resident's environment should be checked for anything unsafe. These issues should also be reported.

If the resident seems tired during a task, the NA should stop so the resident can take a short

rest. The resident should not be rushed. After care, the NA should always ask if the resident would like anything else. She should leave the resident's area clean and tidy. Before leaving, the NA must make sure the call light is left within the resident's reach. The room should be at a comfortable temperature. The walkways must be clear. The bed should be left in its lowest position unless the care plan instructs otherwise.

Observing and Reporting: Personal Care

O/R Skin color, temperature, redness

O/R Mobility

O/R Flexibility

O/R Comfort level or pain or discomfort

O/R Strength and the ability to perform ADLs

O/R Mental and emotional state

O/R Resident complaints

2. Identify guidelines for providing skin care and preventing pressure ulcers

Immobility reduces the amount of blood that circulates to the skin. Residents who are bedbound are at greater risk of skin deterioration at pressure points. **Pressure points** are areas of the body that bear much of its weight. Pressure points are mainly located at bony prominences. **Bony prominences** are areas of the body where the bone lies close to the skin. The skin here is at a much higher risk for skin breakdown. These areas include elbows, shoulder blades, tailbone, hips and knees (inner and outer parts), ankles, heels, toes, and the backs of the neck and head. Other areas at risk are the ears, the area under the breasts or scrotum, the area between the folds of the buttocks or abdomen, and skin between the legs (Fig. 6-2).

The pressure on these areas reduces circulation, decreasing the amount of oxygen the cells receive. Warmth and moisture also add to skin breakdown. Once the surface of the skin is weakened, pathogens can invade and cause infection. When infection occurs, the healing process slows.

Fig. 6-2. *Pressure ulcer danger zones.*

When skin begins to break down, it becomes pale, white, or a reddened color. Darker skin may look purple. The resident may also feel tingling or burning in the area. This discoloration does not go away, even when the resident's position is changed. If pressure is allowed to continue, the area will further break down. The resulting wound is called a **pressure ulcer**, pressure sore, bed sore, or decubitus ulcer. If caught early, a break in the skin can heal fairly quickly without other problems. Once a pressure ulcer forms, it can get bigger and deeper and become infected. Pressure ulcers are painful and difficult to heal. They can lead to life-threatening infections. Prevention is important. It is the key to skin health.

Four stages of pressure ulcers are (Fig. 6-3)

- **Stage I**: Skin is intact, but there is redness that is not relieved even after removing pressure. Darker skin may not look red, but

may appear to be a different color than the surrounding area. The area may be painful, firm, soft, and warmer or cooler when compared to the area around it.

- **Stage II**: There is partial skin loss involving the outer and/or inner layer of skin. The ulcer is superficial. It is usually tender or painful. It may appear red or pink. It looks like a scrape, blister, or shallow crater.

- **Stage III**: There is full skin loss involving damage or death of tissue that may extend down to, but not through the tissue that covers muscle. Fat may be visible, but not muscle, bone, or tendon. The ulcer can look like a shallow or deep crater.

- **Stage IV**: There is full skin loss with major destruction, tissue death, and damage to muscle, bone, or supporting structures.

Fig. 6-3. *The top photo is of a Stage I pressure ulcer on the buttocks. In the middle are two photos of Stage II pressure ulcers on the buttocks. On the bottom left is a photo of a Stage III pressure ulcer on the heel. On the bottom right is a Stage IV pressure ulcer on the foot.*
(PHOTOS COPYRIGHT © NATIONAL PRESSURE ULCER ADVISORY PANEL, NPUAP.ORG, USED WITH PERMISSION)

Observing and Reporting: Resident's Skin

Report any of these to the nurse:

O/R Pale, white, reddened, or purple areas

O/R Blisters or bruises

O/R Complaints of tingling, warmth, or burning of the skin

O/R Dry or flaking skin

O/R Itching or scratching

O/R Rash or any skin discoloration

O/R Swelling

O/R Fluid or blood draining from skin

O/R Broken skin

O/R Wounds or ulcers on the skin

O/R Changes in wound or ulcer (size, depth, drainage, color, odor)

O/R Redness or broken skin between toes or around toenails

In darker complexions, also look for

O/R Any change in the feel of the tissue; any change in the appearance of the skin, such as the "orange-peel" look; a purplish hue; or extremely dry, crust-like areas that might be covering a tissue break

Breaks in the skin can cause serious, even life-threatening, problems. It is better to prevent skin problems than it is to treat them.

Guidelines: Basic Skin Care

G Report any changes in a resident's skin.

G Provide regular, daily care for skin to keep it clean and dry. Check the skin daily, even when complete baths are not given or taken every day.

G Reposition immobile residents often (at least every two hours).

G Give frequent and thorough skin care as often as needed for incontinent residents.

Change clothing and linens often as well. Check on them every two hours or as needed.

G Do not scratch or irritate the skin in any way. Keep rough, scratchy fabrics away from the resident's skin. Report to the nurse if a resident wears shoes that cause blisters.

G Massage the skin often. Use light, circular strokes to increase circulation. Use little or no pressure on bony areas. Do not massage a white, red, or purple area or put any pressure on it. Massage the healthy skin and tissue around the area.

G Be gentle during transfers. Avoid pulling or tearing fragile skin.

G Residents who are overweight may have poor circulation and extra folds of skin. Pay careful attention to the skin under the folds. Keep it clean and dry. Report signs of skin irritation.

G Encourage well-balanced meals and plenty of fluids. Proper nutrition is important for keeping skin healthy.

G Keep plastic or rubber materials from coming into contact with the resident's skin. These materials prevent air from circulating, which causes the skin to sweat.

G Follow the care plan. It may include instructions about special skin care, such as washing the skin with a special soap.

For residents who are not mobile or cannot change positions easily:

G Keep the bottom sheet tight and free from wrinkles. Keep the bed free from crumbs. Keep clothing or gowns free of wrinkles, too.

G Do not pull the resident across sheets during transfers or repositioning. This causes shearing, which can lead to skin breakdown. **Shearing** is rubbing that results from the skin moving one way and the bone underneath it remaining fixed or moving in the opposite direction.

G Place a sheepskin or bed pad under the back and buttocks to absorb moisture that may build up. It can also protect the skin from irritating bed linens. Sheepskin covers are also available for wheelchairs.

G   Relieve pressure under bony prominences (Fig. 6-4). Use a pillow under the calves so that heels are elevated ("floating").

Fig. 6-4. *This foam boot suspends the heel to help reduce pressure.* (© MEDLINE INDUSTRIES, INC., 2014)

G   A bed or chair can be made softer with flotation pads.

G   Use a bed cradle to keep top sheets from rubbing the resident's skin.

G   Residents in chairs or wheelchairs need to be repositioned often, too. Reposition residents at least every hour if they are in a wheelchair or chair and cannot change positions easily.

Many positioning devices are available to help make residents safer and more comfortable.

Guidelines: Positioning Devices

G   Backrests provide support. They can be regular pillows or special wedge-shaped foam pillows.

G   Bed cradles or foot cradles are used to keep the bed covers from resting on a resident's legs and feet.

G   **Draw sheets**, or turning sheets, may be placed under residents who cannot help with turning, lifting, or moving up in bed. Draw sheets help prevent skin damage from shearing. A regular bed sheet folded in half can be used as a draw sheet.

G   Footboards are padded boards placed against the resident's feet to keep them properly aligned. They help prevent foot drop. **Foot drop** is a weakness of muscles in the feet and ankles that causes problems with the ability to flex the ankles and walk normally. Footboards are also used to keep bed covers off the feet. Rolled blankets or pillows can also be used as footboards.

G   Handrolls are cloth-covered or rubber items that keep the fingers from curling tightly (Fig. 6-5). A rolled washcloth, gauze bandage, or a rubber ball placed inside the palm may be used to keep the hand in a natural position. Handrolls can help prevent finger, hand, or wrist contractures.

Fig. 6-5. *Handrolls keep the fingers and hand in a natural position, helping to prevent contractures.* (REPRINTED WITH PERMISSION OF BRIGGS CORPORATION, 800-247-2343, WWW.BRIGGSCORP.COM)

G   An **orthotic device**, or **orthosis**, is a device that helps support and align a limb and improve its functioning. It may be prescribed to keep a resident's joints in the correct position. Orthoses also help prevent or correct deformities. Splints are a type of orthotic device (Fig. 6-6). Splints and the skin area around them should be cleaned at least once daily and as needed. Follow the care plan. Do not apply a splint unless you have been trained in its use.

G   Trochanter rolls are rolled towels or blankets used to keep a resident's hips from turning outward.

G   Pillows between the legs from knees to ankles, while in the lateral position, can help keep the spine, hips, and knees in the proper position. They ease pain in the back, leg, hip, and knee areas.

Fig. 6-6. *Different types of orthotic splints.* (PHOTOS COURTESY OF NORTH COAST MEDICAL, INC., WWW.NCMEDICAL.COM, 800-821-9319)

3. Describe guidelines for assisting with bathing

Bathing promotes health and well-being. It removes perspiration, dirt, oil, and dead skin cells from the skin. It helps to prevent skin irritation and body odor. Bathing can also be relaxing. The bed bath is an excellent time for moving arms and legs. It increases circulation. Bathing gives NAs an opportunity to observe residents' skin carefully.

Residents may have a bath in bed, or they may take a shower or have a tub bath. They may have a **partial bath**, which is a bath given on days when a complete bed bath, tub bath, or shower is not done. It includes washing the face, hands, axillae (underarms), and perineum. The **perineum** is the genital and anal area.

Guidelines: Bathing

G The face, hands, underarms, and perineum should be washed every day. A complete bath or shower can be taken every other day or less often.

G Older skin produces less perspiration and oil. Elderly people with dry, fragile skin should

bathe only once or twice a week. This prevents further dryness. Be gentle with the skin when bathing residents.

G Use only products approved by the facility or that the resident prefers.

G Before bathing a resident, make sure the room is warm enough.

G Be familiar with available safety and assistive devices.

G Gather supplies before giving a bath so the resident is not left alone.

G Before bathing, make sure the water temperature is safe and comfortable. Test the water temperature with a thermometer or against the inside of your wrist to make sure it is not too hot. Then have the resident test the water temperature. The resident is best able to choose a comfortable water temperature.

G Make sure all soap is removed from the skin before completing the bath.

G Keep a record of the bathing schedule for each resident. Follow the care plan.

Giving a complete bed bath

Equipment: bath blanket, bath basin, soap, bath thermometer, 2-4 washcloths, 2-4 bath towels, bed pads, clean clothes, 2 pairs of gloves, orangewood stick or nail brush, lotion, deodorant, brush or comb

When bathing, move resident's body gently and naturally. Avoid force and over-extension of limbs and joints.

1. Identify yourself by name. Identify the resident by name.
   Resident has right to know identity of his or her caregiver. Identifying resident by name shows respect and establishes correct identification.

2. Wash your hands.
   Provides for infection prevention.

3. Explain procedure to the resident. Speak clearly, slowly, and directly. Maintain face-to-face contact whenever possible.
   Promotes understanding and independence.

4. Provide for resident's privacy with curtain, screen, or door. Be sure the room is at a comfortable temperature and there are no drafts.
Maintains resident's right to privacy and dignity.

5. Adjust bed to a safe level, usually waist high. Lock bed wheels.
Prevents injury to you and to resident.

6. Place a bath blanket or towel over resident (Fig. 6-7). Ask him to hold onto it as you remove or fold back top bedding. Remove gown, while keeping resident covered with bath blanket (or top sheet). Place gown in proper container.

Fig. 6-7. Cover the resident with a bath blanket or towel before removing top bedding.

7. Fill the basin with warm water. Test water temperature with thermometer or against the inside of your wrist. Water temperature should not be over 105°F. Have resident check water temperature to see if it is comfortable. Adjust if necessary. The water will cool quickly. Change the water when it becomes too cool, soapy, or dirty.
Resident's sense of touch may be different than yours; therefore, resident is best able to identify a comfortable water temperature.

8. Put on gloves.
Protects you from contact with body fluids.

9. Ask the resident to participate in washing. Help him do this when needed.
Promotes independence.

10. Uncover only one part of the body at a time. Place a towel or bed pad under the part being washed.
Promotes resident's dignity and right to privacy. Also helps keep resident warm.

11. Wash, rinse, and dry one part of the body at a time. Start at the head. Work down, and complete the front first. When washing, use a clean area of the washcloth for each stroke.

Eyes, Face, Ears, and Neck: Wash face with wet washcloth (no soap). Begin with the eye farther away from you. Wash inner to outer area (Fig. 6-8). Use a different area of the washcloth for each stroke. Wash the face from the middle outward. Use firm but gentle strokes. Wash the ears and behind the ears. Wash the neck. Rinse and pat dry.

Fig. 6-8. Wash the eye from the inner to outer area, using a different area of the washcloth for each stroke.

Arms and Axillae: Remove one arm from under the towel. With a soapy washcloth, wash the upper arm and underarm. Use long strokes from the shoulder down to the wrist. Rinse and pat dry. Repeat for the other arm (Fig. 6-9).

Fig. 6-9. Support the wrist while washing the shoulder, arm, underarm, and elbow.

Hands: Wash one hand in a basin. Clean under the nails with an orangewood stick or nail brush (Fig. 6-10). Rinse and pat dry. Give nail care (see procedure later in this chapter). Repeat for the other hand. Put lotion on the resident's elbows and hands.

Fig. 6-10. Wash each hand in a basin. Thoroughly clean under the nails with a nail brush.

Fig. 6-12. Washing the feet includes cleaning between the toes.

Chest: Place the towel across the resident's chest. Pull the blanket down to the waist. Lift the towel only enough to wash the chest. Rinse it and pat dry. For a female resident, wash, rinse, and dry breasts and under breasts. Check the skin in this area for signs of irritation.

Abdomen: Keep towel across chest. Fold the blanket down so that it still covers the pubic area. Wash the abdomen, rinse, and pat dry. If the resident has an ostomy, give skin care around the opening (Chapter 4). Cover with the towel. Pull the cotton blanket up to the resident's chin. Remove the towel.

Legs and Feet: Expose one leg. Place a towel under it. Wash the thigh. Use long downward strokes. Rinse and pat dry. Do the same from the knee to the ankle (Fig. 6-11).

Fig. 6-11. Use long, downward strokes when washing the legs.

Place another towel under the foot. Move the basin to the towel. Place the foot into the basin. Wash the foot and between the toes (Fig. 6-12). Rinse foot and pat dry. Make sure areas between toes are dry. Apply lotion to the foot if ordered, especially at the heels. Do not apply lotion between the toes. Repeat steps for the other leg and foot.

Back: Help resident move to the center of the bed. Ask resident to turn onto his side so his back is facing you. If the bed has rails, raise the rail on the far side for safety. Fold the blanket away from the back. Place a towel lengthwise next to the back. Wash the back and neck with long, downward strokes (Fig. 6-13). Rinse and pat dry. Apply lotion if ordered.

Fig. 6-13. Wash the back with long downward strokes.

12. Place the towel under the buttocks and upper thighs. Help the resident turn onto his back. If the resident is able to wash his perineal area, place a basin of clean, warm water, a washcloth, and towel within reach. Hand items to the resident as needed. If the resident wants you to leave the room, remove and discard gloves. Wash your hands. Leave supplies and the call light within reach.

13. If the resident cannot provide perineal care, you will do it. Remove and discard your gloves. Wash your hands and put on clean gloves. Provide privacy at all times.

14. **Perineal area and buttocks**: Change the bath water. Place a towel or bed pad under the perineal area. Wash, rinse, and dry perineal area. Work from front to back (clean to dirty).

    For a female resident: Using water and a small amount of soap, wash the perineum from front to back. Use single strokes (Fig. 6-14). Do not wash from the back to the front. This may cause infection. Use a clean area of washcloth or a clean washcloth for each stroke.

Fig. 6-14. *Always work from front to back when performing perineal care. This helps prevent infection.*

First spread the labia majora, the outside folds of perineal skin that protect the urinary meatus and the vaginal opening. Wipe from front to back on one side with a clean washcloth. Then wipe the other side from front to back, using a clean part of the washcloth. Clean the perineum (area between vagina and anus) last with a front to back motion. Rinse the area thoroughly in the same way. Make sure all soap is removed.

Dry entire perineal area. Move from front to back, using a blotting motion with towel. Ask resident to turn on her side. Wash, rinse, and dry buttocks and anal area. Clean the anal area without contaminating the perineal area.

For a male resident: If the resident is uncircumcised, pull back the foreskin first. Gently push skin toward the base of penis. Hold the penis by the shaft. Wash in a circular motion from the tip down to the base (Fig. 6-15). Use a clean area of washcloth or clean washcloth for each stroke.

Fig. 6-15. *Wash the penis in a circular motion from the tip down to the base.*

Thoroughly rinse the penis and pat dry. If resident is uncircumcised, gently return foreskin to normal position. Then wash the scrotum and groin. The groin is the area from the pubis (area around the penis and scrotum) to the upper thighs. Rinse and pat dry. Ask the resident to turn on his side. Wash, rinse, and dry buttocks and anal area. Clean the anal area without contaminating the perineal area.

15. Cover the resident with the blanket.

16. Empty, rinse, and dry bath basin. Place basin in designated dirty supply area or return to storage, depending on facility policy.

17. Place soiled clothing and linens in proper containers.

18. Remove and discard gloves.

19. Wash your hands.

20. Provide deodorant. Brush or comb the resident's hair (see procedure later in this chapter). Help resident put on clean clothing. Help resident into comfortable position with proper body alignment.

21. Return bed to lowest position. Remove privacy measures.
    Lowering the bed provides for safety.

22. Place call light within resident's reach.
    Allows resident to communicate with staff as necessary.

23. Wash your hands.
    Provides for infection prevention.

24. Report any changes in resident to the nurse.
    Provides nurse with information to assess resident.

25. Document procedure using facility guidelines.
If you do not document the care, legally it did not happen.

A back rub can help residents relax. It can increase comfort and circulation. Back rubs are often given after baths. After giving a back rub, any changes in a resident's skin should be noted.

Giving a back rub

Equipment: cotton blanket or towel, lotion

1. Identify yourself by name. Identify the resident by name.
   Resident has right to know identity of his or her caregiver. Addressing resident by name shows respect and establishes correct identification.

2. Wash your hands.
   Provides for infection prevention.

3. Explain procedure to resident. Speak clearly, slowly, and directly. Maintain face-to-face contact whenever possible.
   Promotes understanding and independence.

4. Provide for resident's privacy with curtain, screen, or door.
   Maintains resident's right to privacy and dignity.

5. Adjust bed to a safe level, usually waist high. Lower the head of the bed. Lock bed wheels.
   Prevents injury to you and to resident.

6. Position resident lying on his side or stomach. Cover resident with a cotton blanket or towel. Fold back bed covers. Expose the back to the top of the buttocks. Back rubs can also be given with the resident sitting up.

7. Warm lotion by putting bottle in warm water for five minutes. Run your hands under warm water. Pour lotion on your hands. Rub them together. Always put lotion on your hands first, rather than on the resident's skin.
   Increases resident's comfort.

8. Place hands on each side of upper part of the buttocks. Use the full palm of each hand. Make long, smooth upward strokes with both hands. Move along each side of the spine, up to the shoulders (Figs. 6-16 and 6-17). Circle your hands outward. Move back along outer edges of the back. At buttocks, make another circle. Move your hands back up to the shoulders. Without taking your hands off resident's skin, repeat this motion for three to five minutes.
   Long upward strokes release muscle tension; circular strokes increase circulation in muscle areas.

Fig. 6-16. *Move along each side of the spine, up to the shoulders.*

Fig. 6-17. *Long, upward strokes help release muscle tension.*

9. Knead with the first two fingers and thumb of each hand. Place them at base of the spine. Move upward together along each side of the spine. Apply gentle downward pressure with fingers and thumbs. Follow the same direction as with the long smooth strokes, circling at shoulders and buttocks.

10. Gently massage bony areas (spine, shoulder blades, hip bones). Use circular motions of your fingertips. If any of these areas are pale, white, or red, massage around them rather than on them.
    Redness indicates that skin is already irritated and fragile. Include this information in your report to the nurse.

11. Let the resident know when you are almost through. Finish with some long, smooth strokes.

12. Dry the back if extra lotion remains on it.

13. Remove blanket or towel.

14. Help the resident get dressed. Help resident into comfortable position.

15. Store supplies. Place soiled clothing and linens in proper containers.

16. Return bed to lowest position. Remove privacy measures.
    Provides for resident's safety.

17. Place call light within resident's reach.
    Allows resident to communicate with staff as necessary.

18. Wash your hands.
    Provides for infection prevention.

19. Report any changes in resident to the nurse.
    Provides nurse with information to assess resident.

20. Document procedure using facility guidelines.
    If you do not document the care, legally it did not happen.

Hair care is an important part of cleanliness. Shampooing the hair removes dirt, bacteria, oils, and other materials from the hair. Residents who can get out of bed may have their hair shampooed in the sink, tub, or shower. For residents who cannot get out of bed, special troughs exist for shampooing hair in bed. There are also special types of shampoo that do not require the use of water (Fig. 6-18). Gloves should be worn if a resident has open sores on his scalp.

Shampooing hair in bed

Equipment: shampoo, hair conditioner (if requested), 2 bath towels, washcloth, bath thermometer, pitcher or handheld shower or sink attachment, waterproof pad, bath blanket, trough and catch basin, comb and brush, hair dryer

Fig. 6-18. *One type of shampoo that does not require water.* (REPRINTED WITH PERMISSION OF BRIGGS CORPORATION, 800-247-2343, WWW.BRIGGSCORP.COM)

1. Identify yourself by name. Identify the resident by name.
   Resident has right to know identity of his or her caregiver. Addressing resident by name shows respect and establishes correct identification.

2. Wash your hands.
   Provides for infection prevention.

3. Explain procedure to resident. Speak clearly, slowly, and directly. Maintain face-to-face contact whenever possible.
   Promotes understanding and independence.

4. Provide for resident's privacy with curtain, screen, or door. Be sure room is at a comfortable temperature and there are no drafts.
   Maintains resident's right to privacy and dignity.

5. Arrange the supplies within reach.

6. Test water temperature with thermometer or against the inside of your wrist. Water temperature should be no higher than 105°F. Have resident check water temperature. Adjust if necessary.
   Resident's sense of touch may be different than yours; therefore, resident is best able to identify a comfortable water temperature.

7. Remove all pillows and place the resident in a flat position. Adjust bed to a safe level, usually waist high. Lock bed wheels.
   Prevents injury to you and to resident.

8. Place the waterproof pad under the resident's head and shoulders. Cover the resident with

the bath blanket. Fold back the top sheet and regular blankets.
Protects bed linen.

9. Place the trough under resident's head. Connect trough to the catch basin. Place one towel across the resident's shoulders.

10. Protect resident's eyes with dry washcloth.

11. Use pitcher or attachment to wet hair thoroughly. Apply a small amount of shampoo to your hands and rub them together.

12. Lather and massage scalp with fingertips (not fingernails). Use a circular motion from front to back (Fig. 6-19). Do not scratch the scalp.

Fig. 6-19. *Use fingertips, not fingernails, to work shampoo into a lather. Be gentle so that you do not scratch the resident's scalp.*

13. Rinse hair until water runs clear. Use conditioner if resident wants it. Rinse as directed on container. Be sure to rinse the hair thoroughly to prevent the scalp from getting dry and itchy.

14. Wrap resident's hair in a clean towel. Dry his face and neck with the washcloth.

15. Remove trough and waterproof pad.

16. Raise the head of bed.

17. Gently rub the scalp and hair with the towel.

18. Comb or brush hair. Dry hair with a hair dryer on low setting if facility allows this. Style hair as resident prefers.

19. Return bed to lowest position. Remove privacy measures.
Lowering the bed provides for safety.

20. Place call light within resident's reach.
Allows resident to communicate with staff as necessary.

21. Empty, rinse, and wipe bath basin/pitcher. Take to proper area.

22. Clean comb or brush. Return hair dryer and comb or brush to proper storage.

23. Place soiled linen in proper container.

24. Wash your hands.
Provides for infection prevention.

25. Report any changes in resident to nurse.
Provides nurse with information to assess resident.

26. Document procedure using facility guidelines.
If you do not document the care, legally it did not happen.

Many people prefer showers or tub baths to bed baths (Fig. 6-20). NAs must check with the nurse first to make sure a shower or tub bath is allowed.

Fig. 6-20. *A common style of tub in long-term care facilities.*

Guidelines: Safety for Showers and Tub Baths

G Clean tub or shower before and after use.

G Make sure bathroom or shower room floor is dry.

G   Be familiar with available safety and assistive devices. Check that handrails, grab bars, and lifts are in working order.

G   Have resident use safety bars to get into or out of the tub or shower.

G   Place all needed items within reach.

G   Do not leave the resident alone.

G   Do not use bath oils, lotions, or powders in showers or tubs. They make surfaces slippery.

G   Test water temperature with thermometer or against the inside of your wrist before resident gets into tub or shower. Water temperature should be no higher than 105° F. Make sure temperature is comfortable for resident.

Residents' Rights

Privacy When Bathing

Privacy is very important when residents are taking showers or tub baths. Doors should be kept closed. Residents should be covered when possible. Their bodies should not be unnecessarily exposed. For facilities that have communal shower areas, make sure females only shower with other females, and males with other males.

Giving a shower or a tub bath

Equipment: bath blanket, soap, shampoo, bath thermometer, 2-4 washcloths, 2-4 bath towels, clean clothes, nonskid footwear, 2 pairs of gloves, lotion, deodorant, hair dryer

1. Wash your hands.
    Provides for infection prevention.

2. Place equipment in shower or tub room. Put on gloves. Clean shower or tub area and shower chair. Place bucket under shower chair (in case resident has a bowel movement). Turn on heat lamp to warm the room, if available.
    Cleaning reduces pathogens and prevents the spread of infection.

3. Remove and discard gloves. Wash your hands.
    Provides for infection prevention.

4. Go to resident's room. Identify yourself by name. Identify the resident by name.
    Resident has right to know identity of his or her caregiver. Addressing resident by name shows respect and establishes correct identification.

5. Wash your hands.
    Provides for infection prevention.

6. Explain procedure to resident. Speak clearly, slowly, and directly. Maintain face-to-face contact whenever possible.
    Promotes understanding and independence.

7. Provide for resident's privacy with curtain, screen, or door.
    Maintains resident's right to privacy and dignity.

8. Help resident to put on nonskid footwear. Transport resident to shower or tub room.
    Nonskid footwear helps lessen the risk of falls.

9. Put on clean gloves.

10. Help resident remove clothing and shoes.

For a shower:

11. If using a shower chair, place it close to resident. Lock wheels (Fig. 6-21). Safely transfer resident into shower chair.
    Chair may slide if resident attempts to get up.

Fig. 6-21. A shower chair is a sturdy chair designed to be placed in a bathtub or shower. It is water- and slip-resistant. A shower chair must be locked before transferring a resident into it. (PHOTO COURTESY OF NOVA MEDICAL PRODUCTS, WWW.NOVAMEDICALPRODUCTS.COM)

12. Turn on water. Test water temperature with thermometer or against the inside of your wrist. Water temperature should be no higher

than 105°F. Have resident check water temperature. Adjust if necessary. Check temperature throughout the shower.
Resident's sense of touch may be different than yours; therefore, resident is best able to identify a comfortable water temperature.

13. Unlock the shower chair and move it into the shower stall. Lock wheels.

14. Stay with resident during procedure.
Provides for resident's safety.

15. Let resident wash as much as possible. Help to wash his or her face.
Encourages resident to be independent.

16. Help resident shampoo and rinse hair.

17. Using soap, help to wash and rinse the entire body. Move from head to toe (clean to dirty).

18. Turn off water. Unlock shower chair wheels. Roll resident out of shower.

For a tub bath:

11. Residents may need help to get into the bath, depending on their level of mobility. Safely transfer resident onto chair or tub lift, or help resident into bath.

12. Fill the tub halfway with warm water. Test water temperature with thermometer or against the inside of your wrist. Water temperature should be no higher than 105°F. Have resident check water temperature. Adjust if necessary.

13. Stay with resident during procedure.
Provides for resident's safety.

14. Let resident wash as much as possible. Help to wash his or her face.
Encourages resident to be independent.

15. Help resident shampoo and rinse hair.

16. Using soap, help to wash and rinse the entire body. Move from head to toe (clean to dirty).

17. Drain the tub. Cover resident with bath blanket while the tub drains.
Maintains resident's dignity and right to privacy by not exposing body. Keeps resident warm.

18. Help resident out of tub and onto a chair.

Remaining steps for either procedure:

19. Give resident towel(s) and help to pat dry. Pat dry under the breasts, between skin folds, in the perineal area, and between toes.
Patting dry prevents skin tears and reduces chafing.

20. Apply lotion and deodorant as needed.

21. Place soiled clothing and linens in proper containers.

22. Remove and discard gloves.

23. Wash your hands.
Provides for infection prevention.

24. Help resident dress and comb hair before leaving shower or tub room. Offer a hair dryer if needed. Put on nonskid footwear. Return resident to room.
Combing hair in shower room allows resident to maintain dignity when returning to room.

25. Make sure resident is comfortable.

26. Place call light within resident's reach.
Allows resident to communicate with staff as necessary.

27. Report any changes in resident to nurse.
Provides nurse with information to assess resident.

28. Document procedure using facility guidelines.
If you do not document the care, legally it did not happen.

4. Describe guidelines for assisting with grooming

Grooming affects the way people feel about themselves and how they look to others (Fig. 6-22). When helping with grooming, NAs should always let residents do all they can for themselves. Residents should make as many choices as possible. Residents may have particular ways of grooming themselves. They may have routines. These routines remain important even when people are elderly, sick, or disabled. Some residents may be embarrassed, depressed, or anxious because they need help with grooming tasks. NAs should be sensitive to this.

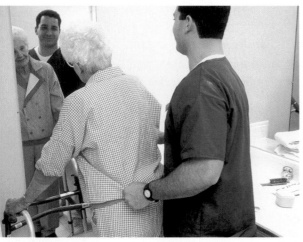

Fig. 6-22. *A well-groomed appearance helps a person feel good about herself.*

Fingernails can harbor bacteria. It is important to keep hands and nails clean to help prevent infection. Nail care should be given when nails are dirty or have jagged edges and whenever it has been assigned. Some facilities do not allow NAs to cut a resident's fingernails or toenails. Poor circulation can lead to infection if skin is accidentally cut while caring for nails. For a diabetic resident, such an infection can lead to a severe wound or even amputation. NAs should follow their facility's policies. The same nail equipment should not be used on more than one resident.

Providing fingernail care

Equipment: orangewood stick, emery board, lotion, basin, soap, washcloth, 2 towels, bath thermometer, gloves

1. Identify yourself by name. Identify the resident by name.
   Resident has right to know identity of his or her caregiver. Addressing resident by name shows respect and establishes correct identification.

2. Wash your hands.
   Provides for infection prevention.

3. Explain procedure to resident. Speak clearly, slowly, and directly. Maintain face-to-face contact whenever possible.
   Promotes understanding and independence.

4. Provide for resident's privacy with curtain, screen, or door.
   Maintains resident's right to privacy and dignity.

5. If resident is in bed, adjust bed to a safe level, usually waist high. Lock bed wheels.
   Prevents injury to you and to resident.

6. Fill the basin halfway with warm water. Test water temperature with thermometer or against the inside of your wrist. Ensure it is safe. Water temperature should be no higher than 105°F. Have resident check water temperature. Adjust if necessary. Place basin at a comfortable level for the resident.
   Resident's sense of touch may be different than yours; therefore, resident is best able to identify a comfortable water temperature.

7. Put on gloves.

8. Soak the resident's hands and nails in the basin of water. Soak all 10 fingertips for at least five minutes.
   Nail care is easier if nails are first softened.

9. Remove hands from water. Wash hands with soapy washcloth. Rinse. Pat hands dry with towel, including between fingers. Remove the hand basin.

10. Place resident's hands on the towel. Gently clean under each fingernail with orangewood stick (Fig. 6-23).
    Most pathogens on hands come from beneath the nails.

Fig. 6-23. *Be gentle when removing dirt from under the nails with an orangewood stick.*

11. Wipe orangewood stick on towel after each nail. Wash resident's hands again. Dry them thoroughly, especially between fingers.

12. Shape nails with an emery board or file. File in a curve. Finish with nails smooth and free of rough edges.
Filing in a curve smoothes nails and eliminates edges, which may catch on clothes or tear skin.

13. Apply lotion from fingertips to wrists. Remove excess, if any, with a towel.

14. Empty, rinse, and dry basin. Place basin in designated dirty supply area or return to storage, depending on facility policy.

15. Place soiled clothing and linens in proper containers.

16. Remove and discard gloves. Wash your hands.
Provides for infection prevention.

17. Return bed to lowest position. Remove privacy measures.
Lowering the bed provides for safety.

18. Place call light within resident's reach.
Allows resident to communicate with staff as necessary.

19. Report any changes in resident to the nurse.
Provides nurse with information to assess resident.

20. Document procedure using facility guidelines.
If you do not document the care, legally it did not happen.

Careful foot care is extremely important; it should be a part of daily care of residents.

Observing and Reporting: Foot Care

Report any of these to the nurse:

- O/R Dry, flaking skin
- O/R Non-intact or broken skin
- O/R Discoloration of the feet, such as reddened, gray, white, or black areas
- O/R Blisters
- O/R Bruises
- O/R Blood or drainage
- O/R Long, ragged toenails
- O/R Ingrown toenails
- O/R Swelling
- O/R Soft, fragile, or reddened heels
- O/R Differences in temperature of the feet

Providing foot care

Equipment: basin, bath mat, soap, lotion, washcloth, 2 bath towels, bath thermometer, clean socks, gloves

1. Identify yourself by name. Identify the resident by name.
Resident has right to know identity of his or her caregiver. Addressing resident by name shows respect and establishes correct identification.

2. Wash your hands.
Provides for infection prevention.

3. Explain procedure to resident. Speak clearly, slowly, and directly. Maintain face-to-face contact whenever possible.
Promotes understanding and independence.

4. Provide for resident's privacy with curtain, screen, or door.
Maintains resident's right to privacy and dignity.

5. If the resident is in bed, adjust bed to a safe level, usually waist high. Lock bed wheels.
Prevents injury to you and to resident.

6. Fill the basin halfway with warm water. Test water temperature with thermometer or against the inside of your wrist. Ensure it is safe. Water temperature should be no higher than 105° F. Have resident check water temperature. Adjust if necessary.
Resident's sense of touch may be different than yours; therefore, resident is best able to identify a comfortable water temperature.

7. Place basin on the bath mat or bath towel on the floor (if the resident is sitting in a chair) or on a towel at the foot of the bed (if the resident is in bed). Make sure basin is in a comfortable position for resident. Support the foot and ankle throughout the procedure.

8. Put on gloves.

9. Remove resident's socks. Completely submerge resident's feet in water. Soak the feet for 10 to 20 minutes. Add warm water to basin as necessary.

10. Put soap on wet washcloth. Remove one foot from water. Wash entire foot, including between the toes and around nail beds (Fig. 6-24).

Fig. 6-24. Soak the resident's feet before washing the entire foot, including the nail beds.

11. Rinse entire foot, including between the toes.

12. Dry entire foot, including between the toes.

13. Repeat steps 10 through 12 for the other foot.

14. Put lotion in hand. Warm lotion by rubbing hands together. Massage lotion into entire foot (top and bottom), except between the toes. Remove excess, if any, with a towel.

15. Help resident put on clean socks.

16. Empty, rinse, and dry basin. Place basin in designated dirty supply area or return to storage, depending on facility policy.

17. Place soiled clothing and linens in proper containers.

18. Remove and discard gloves. Wash your hands.
    Provides for infection prevention.

19. Return bed to lowest position. Remove privacy measures.
    Lowering the bed provides for safety.

20. Place call light within resident's reach.
    Allows resident to communicate with staff as necessary.

21. Report any changes in resident to the nurse.
    Provides nurse with information to assess resident.

22. Document procedure using facility guidelines.
    If you do not document the care, legally it did not happen.

Because hair thins as people age, pieces of hair can be pulled out of the head while combing or brushing it. NAs must handle residents' hair very gently.

Pediculosis is the medical term for an infestation of lice. Lice are tiny bugs that bite into the skin and suck blood to live and grow. Three types of lice are head lice, body lice, and crab or pubic lice. Head lice are usually found on the scalp. Lice are hard to see. Symptoms include itching, bite marks on the scalp, skin sores, and matted, bad-smelling hair and scalp. Lice eggs may be visible on the hair, behind the ears, and on the neck. They are small and round and may be brown or white. Lice droppings look like a fine black powder. They may be on sheets or pillows. If NAs notice any of these symptoms, they should tell the nurse immediately. Lice can spread very quickly. Special creams, shampoos, lotions, or sprays may be used to treat the lice. People who have lice spread it to others. To help prevent the spread of lice, residents' combs, brushes, clothes, wigs, or hats should not be shared with others.

Combing or brushing hair

Equipment: comb, brush, towel, mirror, hair care items requested by resident

Use hair care products that the resident prefers for his or her type of hair.

1. Identify yourself by name. Identify the resident by name.
   Resident has right to know identity of his or her caregiver. Addressing resident by name shows respect and establishes correct identification.

2. Wash your hands.
   Provides for infection prevention.

3. Explain procedure to resident. Speak clearly, slowly, and directly. Maintain face-to-face contact whenever possible.
Promotes understanding and independence.

4. Provide for resident's privacy with curtain, screen, or door.
Maintains resident's right to privacy and dignity.

5. If resident is in bed, adjust bed to a safe level, usually waist high. Raise head of bed so resident is sitting up. Lock bed wheels.
Prevents injury to you and to resident. Sitting upright puts resident in more natural position.

6. Place a towel under the head or around the shoulders.

7. Remove any hair pins, hair ties or clips.

8. Remove tangles first by dividing hair into small sections. Hold lock of hair just above the tangle so you do not pull at the scalp. Gently comb or brush through the tangle.
Reduces hair breakage, scalp pain, and irritation.

9. After tangles are removed, brush two-inch sections of hair at a time. Gently brush from roots to ends (Fig. 6-25).

Fig. 6-25. Gently brush hair after tangles are removed.

10. Neatly style hair as resident prefers. Avoid childish hairstyles. Each resident may prefer different styles. Offer mirror to the resident.
Each resident has the right to choose. Promotes resident's independence.

11. Return supplies to proper storage. Clean hair from comb or brush. Clean comb or brush.

12. Dispose of soiled linen in the proper container.

13. Return bed to lowest position. Remove privacy measures.
Lowering the bed provides for safety.

14. Place call light within resident's reach.
Allows resident to communicate with staff as necessary.

15. Wash your hands.
Provides for infection prevention.

16. Report any changes in resident to nurse.
Provides nurse with information to assess resident.

17. Document procedure using facility guidelines.
If you do not document the care, legally it did not happen.

The NA should make sure the resident wants her to shave him or help him shave. Personal preferences for shaving must be respected. NAs must wear gloves when shaving residents due to risk of exposure to blood. Razors should not be shared between residents. Different types of razors include the following:

- A **safety razor** has a sharp blade, which comes with a special safety casing to help prevent cuts. This type of razor requires shaving cream or soap.

- A **disposable razor** requires shaving cream or soap. It is discarded in a sharps container after use.

- An **electric razor** is the safest and easiest type of razor to use. It does not require soap or shaving cream.

Shaving a resident

Equipment: razor, basin filled halfway with warm water (if using a safety or disposable razor), 2 towels, washcloth, mirror, shaving cream or soap (if using a safety or disposable razor), after-shave lotion, gloves

1. Identify yourself by name. Identify the resident by name.
Resident has right to know identity of his or her caregiver. Addressing resident by name shows respect and establishes correct identification.

2. Wash your hands.
    Provides for infection prevention.

3. Explain procedure to resident. Speak clearly, slowly, and directly. Maintain face-to-face contact whenever possible.
    Promotes understanding and independence.

4. Provide for resident's privacy with curtain, screen, or door.
    Maintains resident's right to privacy and dignity.

5. If resident is in bed, adjust bed to a safe level, usually waist high. Lock bed wheels.
    Prevents injury to you and to resident.

6. Raise head of bed so resident is sitting up. Place towel across the resident's chest, under his chin.
    Sitting upright puts resident in a more natural position. Towel protects resident's clothing and bed linen.

7. Put on gloves.
    Shaving may cause bleeding. Wearing gloves promotes infection prevention and follows Standard Precautions.

Shaving using a safety or disposable razor:

8. Soften the beard with a warm, wet washcloth on the face for a few minutes before shaving. Lather the face with shaving cream or soap and warm water.
    Warm water and lather soften skin and hair and make shaving more comfortable.

9. Hold skin taut. Shave in the direction of hair growth. Shave beard in downward strokes on face and upward strokes on neck (Fig. 6-26). Rinse the blade often in the basin to keep it clean and wet.
    Maximizes hair removal by shaving in the direction of hair growth.

Fig. 6-26. *Holding the skin taut, shave in downward strokes on face and upward strokes on neck.*

10. When you have finished, wash and rinse the resident's face with a warm, wet washcloth. If he is able, let him use the washcloth himself. Use the towel to dry his face. Offer a mirror to resident.
    Removes soap, which may cause irritation. Promotes independence.

Shaving using an electric razor:

8. Use a small brush to clean the razor. Do not use an electric razor near any water source or when oxygen is in use.
    Electricity near water may cause electrocution. Electricity near oxygen may cause an explosion.

9. Turn on the razor and hold skin taut. Shave with smooth, even movements (Fig. 6-27). Shave beard with back and forth motion in direction of beard growth with foil shaver. Shave beard in circular motion with three-head shaver. Shave the chin and under the chin.

Fig. 6-27. *Shave, or have the resident shave, with smooth, even movements.*

10. Offer a mirror to resident.
    Promotes independence.

Final steps:

11. Apply after-shave lotion if resident wants it.
    Improves resident's self-esteem.

12. Remove the towel. Place the towel and washcloth in proper container.

13. Clean the equipment and store it. For safety razor, rinse the razor. For disposable razor, dispose of it in a sharps container. For electric razor, clean head of razor. Remove

whiskers from razor. Recap shaving head and return razor to case.

14. Remove and discard gloves. Wash your hands.
    Provides for infection prevention.

15. Make sure that resident and environment are free of loose hairs.

16. Return bed to lowest position. Remove privacy measures.
    Lowering the bed provides for safety.

17. Place call light within resident's reach.
    Allows resident to communicate with staff as necessary.

18. Report any changes in resident to the nurse.
    Provides nurse with information to assess resident.

19. Document procedure using facility guidelines.
    If you do not document the care, legally it did not happen.

5. List guidelines for assisting with dressing

Dressing and undressing residents is an important part of daily care. When helping with dressing, the NA should know what limitations the resident has. Residents may have a weaker side of the body due to stroke or injury. That side is called the **affected side**. It will be weaker. The NA should never refer to the weaker side as the "bad side," or talk about the "bad" leg or arm. The terms *weaker* or **involved** should be used to refer to the affected side. The weaker arm is placed through a sleeve first (Fig. 6-28). When a leg is weak, it is easier if the resident sits down to pull the pants over both legs.

Guidelines: Dressing and Undressing

G Ask and follow the resident's preferences. Let the resident choose clothing for the day. Check to see if it is clean, appropriate for the weather, and in good condition.

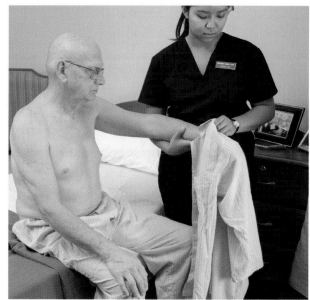

Fig. 6-28. When dressing, the NA should start with the affected (weaker) side first.

G Encourage the resident to dress in regular clothes rather than nightclothes. Clothing with elastic waistbands and clothing that is a size larger than normal are easier to put on.

G Let the resident do as much to dress or undress himself as possible. It may take longer, but it helps maintain independence. Assistive devices for dressing are available (Fig. 6-29). Use them as directed.

Fig. 6-29. Special dressing aids promote independence by helping residents dress themselves. (PHOTO COURTESY OF NORTH COAST MEDICAL, INC., WWW.NCMEDICAL.COM, 800-821-9319)

G Provide privacy and never expose more than what is needed.

G Roll or fold socks or stockings down when putting them on. Slip over the toes and foot, then unroll into place.

G For a female resident, make sure bra cups fit over the breasts. A front-fastening bra is easier for residents to work by themselves. A bra that fastens in back can be put around the waist and fastened first. After fastening, it should be rotated around and moved up. Arms can be put through the straps last. This can be done in reverse for undressing.

G Place the weaker arm or leg through the garment first. Then help with the stronger arm or leg. When undressing, do the opposite—start with the stronger, or unaffected, side.

Dressing a resident with an affected (weak) right arm

Equipment: clean clothes of resident's choice, nonskid footwear

When putting on items, move resident's body gently and naturally. Avoid force and over-extension of limbs and joints.

1. Identify yourself by name. Identify the resident by name.
   Resident has right to know identity of his or her caregiver. Addressing resident by name shows respect and establishes correct identification.

2. Wash your hands.
   Provides for infection prevention.

3. Explain procedure to resident. Speak clearly, slowly, and directly. Maintain face-to-face contact whenever possible.
   Promotes understanding and independence.

4. Provide for resident's privacy with curtain, screen, or door.
   Maintains resident's right to privacy and dignity.

5. Ask resident what she would like to wear. Dress her in outfit of choice.
   Promotes resident's right to choose.

6. Remove resident's gown or top. Do not completely expose resident. Take clothes off the stronger side first when undressing. Then remove from weaker side. Place gown in proper container.
   Maintains resident's dignity and right to privacy.

7. Help resident put the right (affected/weaker) arm through the right sleeve of the shirt, sweater, or slip before placing garment on left (unaffected/stronger) arm.

8. Help resident put on skirt, pants, or dress. Put the weaker leg through the skirt or pants first. Then place the stronger leg through the skirt or pants.

9. Place bed at the lowest position. Lock bed wheels.

10. Have resident sit down. Help to put on socks and nonskid footwear. Tie laces.
    Promotes resident's safety.

11. Finish with resident dressed appropriately. Make sure clothing is right-side-out and zippers and buttons are fastened.

12. Place gown in soiled linen container.

13. Keep bed in lowest position. Remove privacy measures.

14. Place call light within resident's reach.
    Allows resident to communicate with staff as necessary.

15. Wash your hands.
    Provides for infection prevention.

16. Report any changes in resident to the nurse.
    Provides nurse with information to assess resident.

17. Document procedure using facility guidelines.
    If you do not document the care, legally it did not happen.

IV is the abbreviation for **intravenous**, or into a vein. Medication, nutrition, or fluids drip from a bag suspended on a pole or are pumped by a portable pump through a tube and into the vein. Chapter 7 has more information on IV therapy.

Guidelines: Dressing a Resident with an IV

G Never disconnect IV lines or turn off the pump. The nurse will be responsible for unhooking IV tubing from the pump.

G Always keep the IV bag higher than the IV site on the body.

G First remove clothing from the side without the IV. Then gather the clothing on the side with the IV. Lift clothing over the IV site. Move it up the tubing toward the IV bag. Lift the IV bag off its pole. Carefully slide the clothing over the bag. Place the bag back on the pole.

G Apply clean clothing first to side with the IV. Slide the arm opening over the bag, then over the tubing, over the IV site, and onto the resident's arm. Place the IV bag back on the pole.

G Check that the IV is dripping properly. Make sure none of the tubing is dislodged. Check to see that the IV site dressing is in place. Make sure tubing is not kinked after you are finished.

For cases of poor circulation to the legs and feet, elastic stockings are ordered. These stockings help prevent swelling and blood clots and aid circulation. Elastic stockings are also known as *anti-embolic stockings* or *TED hose*. They are referred to as *anti-embolic* because they help prevent embolisms. An **embolism** is an obstruction of a blood vessel, usually by a blood clot. The embolism can travel from where it was formed to another part of the body, blocking blood flow. It can cause serious damage and even death.

Elastic stockings may either be knee-high or thigh-high. They need to be put on in the morning, before the resident gets out of bed. Legs are at their smallest size then. They are usually removed in the evening.

Applying knee-high elastic stockings

Equipment: elastic stockings

1. Identify yourself by name. Identify resident by name.
    Resident has right to know identity of his or her caregiver. Addressing resident by name shows respect and establishes correct identification.

2. Wash your hands.
    Provides for infection prevention.

3. Explain procedure to resident. Speak clearly, slowly, and directly. Maintain face-to-face contact whenever possible.
    Promotes understanding and independence.

4. Provide for resident's privacy with curtain, screen, or door.
    Maintains resident's right to privacy and dignity.

5. The resident should be in the supine position (on her back) in bed. With resident lying down, remove her socks, shoes, or slippers, and expose one leg. Expose no more than one leg at a time.

6. Turn stocking inside-out at least to heel area (Fig. 6-30).

Fig. 6-30. *Turning the stocking inside out allows the stocking to roll on gently.*

7. Gently place foot of stocking over toes, foot, and heel (Fig. 6-31). Make sure the heel is in the right place (heel of foot should be in heel of stocking).

Fig. 6-31. *Place the foot of the stocking over the toes, foot, and heel. Promote the resident's comfort and safety. Avoid force and over-extension of joints.*

8. Gently pull top of stocking over foot, heel, and leg.

9. Make sure there are no twists or wrinkles in stocking after it is on. It must fit smoothly and be comfortable (Fig. 6-32). Make sure the heel of stocking is over the heel of foot. If the stocking has an opening in the toe area, make sure the opening is either over or under the toe area. This depends on the manufacturer's instructions. Adjust if needed.

Fig. 6-32. *Make stocking smooth. Twists or wrinkles cause the stocking to be too tight, which reduces circulation.*

10. Repeat for other leg.

11. Place call light within resident's reach.
    Allows resident to communicate with staff as necessary.

12. Wash your hands.
    Provides for infection prevention.

13. Report any changes in resident to nurse.
    Provides nurse with information to assess resident.

14. Document procedure using facility guidelines.
    If you do not document the care, legally it did not happen.

6. Identify guidelines for proper oral hygiene

Oral care, or care of the mouth, teeth, and gums, is done at least twice each day. Oral care should be done after breakfast and after the last meal or snack of the day. It may also be done before a resident eats. Oral care includes brushing teeth, tongue, and gums; flossing teeth; caring for lips; and caring for dentures (Fig. 6-33).

When giving oral care, NAs must wear gloves. They should follow Standard Precautions.

Fig. 6-33. *Some supplies needed for oral care.*

When an NA performs oral care, he should observe the resident's mouth carefully.

Observing and Reporting: Oral Care

Report any of these to the nurse:

O/R Irritation

O/R Raised areas

O/R Coated or swollen tongue

O/R Ulcers, such as canker sores or small, painful, white sores

O/R Flaky, white spots

O/R Dry, cracked, bleeding, or chapped lips

O/R Loose, chipped, broken or decayed teeth

O/R Swollen, irritated, bleeding, or whitish gums

O/R Breath that smells bad or fruity

O/R Resident reports of mouth pain

Providing oral care

Equipment: toothbrush, toothpaste, emesis basin, gloves, clothing protector or towel, glass of water, lip moisturizer

1. Identify yourself by name. Identify the resident by name.
    Resident has right to know identity of his or her caregiver. Addressing resident by name shows respect and establishes correct identification.

2. Wash your hands.
    Provides for infection prevention.

3. Explain procedure to resident. Speak clearly, slowly, and directly. Maintain face-to-face contact whenever possible.
Promotes understanding and independence.

4. Provide for resident's privacy with curtain, screen, or door.
Maintains resident's right to privacy and dignity.

5. If resident is in bed, adjust bed to a safe level, usually waist high. Raise the head of the bed to have resident in an upright sitting position. Lock bed wheels.
Prevents injury to you and to resident. Prevents fluids from running down resident's throat, causing choking.

6. Put on gloves.
Brushing may cause gums to bleed.

7. Place a clothing protector or towel across resident's chest.
Protects resident's clothing and bed linen.

8. Wet toothbrush. Put on small amount of toothpaste.
Water helps distribute toothpaste.

9. Clean entire mouth, including tongue and all surfaces of teeth and the gumline. Use gentle strokes. First brush inner, outer, and chewing surfaces of the upper teeth. Then do the same with the lower teeth. Use short strokes. Brush back and forth. Brush tongue.
Brushing upper teeth first lessens production of saliva in lower part of mouth.

10. Give the resident water to rinse the mouth. Place emesis basin under the resident's chin, with the inward curve under the chin. Have resident spit water into emesis basin (Fig. 6-34). Wipe resident's mouth and remove towel. Apply lip moisturizer.

11. Rinse toothbrush and place in proper container. Empty, rinse, and dry basin. Place basin and toothbrush in designated dirty supply area or return to storage, depending on facility policy.

12. Place soiled clothing and linens in proper containers.

Fig. 6-34. Rinsing and spitting removes food particles and toothpaste.

13. Remove and discard gloves. Wash your hands.
Provides for infection prevention.

14. Return bed to lowest position. Remove privacy measures.
Lowering the bed provides for safety.

15. Place call light within resident's reach.
Allows resident to communicate with staff as necessary.

16. Report any problems with teeth, mouth, tongue, and lips to nurse. This includes odor, cracking, sores, bleeding, and any discoloration.
Provides nurse with information to assess resident.

17. Document procedure using facility guidelines.
If you do not document the care, legally it did not happen.

Even though residents who are unconscious cannot eat, breathing through the mouth causes saliva to dry in the mouth. Oral care needs to be performed more frequently to keep the mouth clean and moist.

With unconscious residents, NAs must use as little liquid as possible when giving mouth care. Because the person's swallowing reflex is weak, he or she is at risk for aspiration. **Aspiration** is the inhalation of food, fluid, or foreign material into the lungs. Aspiration can cause pneumonia or death. Turning unconscious residents on their sides before giving oral care can also help prevent aspiration. For these residents, only swabs soaked in tiny amounts of fluid should be used to clean the mouth.

Providing oral care for the unconscious resident

Equipment: sponge swabs, tongue depressor, towel, emesis basin, gloves, glass of water, lip moisturizer, cleaning solution (check the care plan)

1. Identify yourself by name. Identify the resident by name. Even residents who are unconscious may be able to hear you. Always speak to them as you would to any resident.
   Resident has right to know identity of his or her caregiver. Addressing resident by name shows respect and establishes correct identification.

2. Wash your hands.
   Provides for infection prevention.

3. Explain procedure to resident. Speak clearly, slowly, and directly. Maintain face-to-face contact whenever possible.
   Promotes understanding. The resident may be able to hear and understand even though he is unconscious.

4. Provide for resident's privacy with curtain, screen, or door.
   Maintains resident's right to privacy and dignity.

5. Adjust bed to a safe level, usually waist high. Lock bed wheels.
   Prevents injury to you and to resident.

6. Put on gloves.
   Protects you from coming into contact with body fluids.

7. Turn resident on his side or turn his head to the side. Place a towel under his cheek and chin. Place an emesis basin next to the cheek and chin for excess fluid.
   Protects resident's clothing and bed linen.

8. Hold mouth open with tongue depressor.
   Enables you to safely clean mouth.

9. Dip sponge swab in cleaning solution. Squeeze excess solution to prevent aspiration. Wipe teeth, gums, tongue, and inside surfaces of mouth. Remove debris with the

swab. Change swab often. Repeat this until the mouth is clean (Fig. 6-35).
Stimulates gums and removes mucus.

Fig. 6-35. *Wipe all inside surfaces of the mouth to clean the mouth, stimulate the gums, and remove mucus.*

10. Rinse with clean swab dipped in water. Squeeze swab first to remove excess water.
    Removes solution from mouth.

11. Remove the towel and basin. Pat lips or face dry if needed. Apply lip moisturizer.
    Prevents lips from drying and cracking. Improves resident's comfort.

12. Empty, rinse, and dry basin. Place basin in designated dirty supply area or return to storage, depending on facility policy.

13. Place soiled linens in the proper container.

14. Remove and discard gloves. Wash your hands.
    Provides for infection prevention.

15. Return bed to lowest position. Remove privacy measures.
    Lowering the bed provides for safety.

16. Place call light within resident's reach.
    Allows resident to communicate with staff as necessary.

17. Report any problems with teeth, mouth, tongue, and lips to nurse. This includes odor, cracking, sores, bleeding, and any discoloration.
    Provides nurse with information to assess resident.

18. Document procedure using facility guidelines.
    If you do not document the care, legally it did not happen.

Flossing the teeth removes plaque and tartar buildup around the gum line and between the teeth. Teeth may be flossed immediately after or before they are brushed, as the resident prefers. NAs should follow the care plan's instructions for flossing.

Flossing teeth

Equipment: dental floss, glass of water, emesis basin, gloves, towel

1. Identify yourself by name. Identify the resident by name.
   Resident has right to know identity of his or her caregiver. Addressing resident by name shows respect and establishes correct identification.

2. Wash your hands.
   Provides for infection prevention.

3. Explain procedure to resident. Speak clearly, slowly, and directly. Maintain face-to-face contact whenever possible.
   Promotes understanding and independence.

4. Provide for resident's privacy with curtain, screen, or door.
   Maintains resident's right to privacy and dignity.

5. If resident is in bed, adjust bed to a safe level, usually waist high. Raise the head of the bed to have resident in an upright sitting position. Lock bed wheels.
   Prevents fluids from running down resident's throat, causing choking.

6. Put on gloves.
   Flossing may cause gums to bleed.

7. Wrap the ends of floss securely around each index finger (Fig. 6-36).

Fig. 6-36. *Before beginning, wrap floss securely around each index finger.*

8. Start with the back teeth. Place floss between teeth. Move it down the surface of the tooth. Use a gentle sawing motion (Fig. 6-37).

Fig. 6-37. *Being gentle protects the gums.*

Continue to the gum line. At the gum line, curve the floss. Slip it gently into the space between the gum and tooth. Then go back up, scraping that side of the tooth (Fig. 6-38). Repeat this on the side of the other tooth.
Removes food and prevents tooth decay.

Fig. 6-38. *Floss gently in the space between the gum and tooth.*

9. After every two teeth, unwind floss from your fingers. Move it so you are using a clean area. Floss all teeth.

10. Offer water to rinse the mouth. Ask the resident to spit it into the basin.
    Flossing loosens food. Rinsing removes it.

11. Offer resident a face towel when done flossing all teeth.
    Promotes dignity.

12. Discard floss. Discard water and rinse and dry the basin. Place basin in designated dirty supply area or return to storage, depending on facility policy.

13. Place soiled linen in the proper container.

14. Remove and discard gloves. Wash your hands.
    Provides for infection prevention.

15. Return bed to lowest position. Remove privacy measures.
    Lowering the bed provides for safety.

16. Place call light within resident's reach.
    Allows resident to communicate with staff as necessary.

17. Report any problems with teeth, mouth, tongue, and lips to nurse. This includes odor, cracking, sores, bleeding, and any discoloration.
    Provides nurse with information to assess resident.

18. Document procedure using facility guidelines.
    If you do not document the care, legally it did not happen.

Dentures are artificial teeth. They are expensive. It is important to take good care of them. Dentures must be handled carefully to avoid breaking or chipping them. If a resident's dentures break, he or she cannot eat. NAs must wear gloves when handling and cleaning dentures. Dentures and denture brushes should not be placed on contaminated surfaces. The NA should notify the nurse if a resident's dentures do not fit properly, are chipped, or are missing.

Dentures should be stored in a denture cup labeled with the resident's name and room number. They should not be removed from the resident's room. Care must be taken to prevent them from being lost. Dentures should be stored in solution or in clean moderate/tepid water when not in the resident's mouth.

Residents' Rights

Denture Care

Denture care is very personal. The NA should pull the privacy curtain and close the door before beginning. Many people who have dentures do not want to be seen without their teeth in place. When the NA removes the teeth, he should clean and return them immediately.

Cleaning and storing dentures

Equipment: denture brush or toothbrush, denture cleanser or toothpaste, labeled denture cup, 2 towels, gloves

1. Wash your hands.
   Provides for infection prevention.

2. Put on gloves.
   Prevents you from coming into contact with body fluids.

3. Line the sink or basin with a towel(s) and partially fill sink with water.
   Prevents dentures from breaking if dropped.

4. Handle dentures carefully. Hold them over the sink. Rinse dentures in moderate temperature running water before brushing them. Do not use hot water.
   Hot water may warp dentures.

5. Apply toothpaste or denture cleanser to brush.

6. Brush dentures on all surfaces (Fig. 6-39). This includes the inner, outer, and chewing surfaces of dentures, as well as the groove that will touch gum surfaces.

Fig. 6-39. *Brush dentures on all surfaces to properly clean them.*

7. Rinse all surfaces of dentures under moderate temperature running water. Do not use hot water.
   Hot water may warp dentures.

8. Rinse denture cup before placing clean dentures in the cup.
   Removes pathogens.

9. Place dentures in clean, labeled denture cup with solution or moderate temperature water.

Place lid on cup. Return denture cup to storage. Some residents will want to wear dentures all of the time. They will only remove them for cleaning. If the resident wants to continue wearing dentures, return them to him or her. Do not place them in the denture cup.

10. Rinse brush. Dry and return equipment to storage. Drain sink. Place soiled linens in the proper container.

11. Remove and discard gloves. Wash your hands.
    Provides for infection prevention.

12. Document procedure using facility guidelines. Report any change in appearance of dentures to the nurse.
    If you do not document the care, legally it did not happen.

7. Explain guidelines for assisting with toileting

Residents who are unable to get out of bed to use the toilet may be given a bedpan, a fracture pan, or a urinal. A **fracture pan** is a bedpan that is flatter than the regular bedpan. It is used for residents who cannot assist with raising their hips onto a regular bedpan (Fig. 6-40). Women will generally use a bedpan for urination and bowel movements. Men will generally use a urinal for urination and a bedpan for bowel movements (Fig. 6-41).

Elimination equipment is usually kept in the bathroom between uses. Residents who share bathrooms may need to have urinals and bedpans labeled. This equipment must never be placed on overbed tables or on top of side tables.

Urine and feces are considered infectious wastes. NAs must always wear gloves when handling bedpans, urinals, or basins that contain wastes, including dirty bath water. NAs should be careful not to spill or splash wastes, and wastes should be discarded in the toilet.

Immediately after use, containers used for elimination should be placed in the proper area for cleaning, or they should be cleaned and stored according to facility policy.

Fig. 6-40. *On the left is a standard pan and on the right is a fracture pan.*

Fig. 6-41. *A urinal.* (PHOTO COURTESY OF NOVA MEDICAL PRODUCTS, WWW.NOVAMEDICALPRODUCTS.COM)

Assisting resident with use of bedpan

Equipment: bedpan, bedpan cover, protective pad, bath blanket, toilet paper, disposable wipes, towel, 2 pairs of gloves

1. Identify yourself by name. Identify the resident by name.
   Resident has right to know identity of his or her caregiver. Addressing resident by name shows respect and establishes correct identification.

2. Wash your hands.
   Provides for infection prevention.

3. Explain procedure to resident. Speak clearly, slowly, and directly. Maintain face-to-face contact whenever possible.
   Promotes understanding and independence.

4. Provide for resident's privacy with curtain, screen, or door.
   Maintains resident's right to privacy and dignity.

5. Adjust bed to a safe level, usually waist high. Before placing bedpan, lower the head of the bed. Lock bed wheels.
   When bed is flat, resident can be moved without working against gravity.

6. Put on gloves.
Prevents contact with body fluids.

7. Cover the resident with the bath blanket. Ask him to hold it while you pull down the top covers underneath. Do not expose more of the resident than you need to.
Maintains resident's right to privacy and dignity.

8. Place a protective pad under the resident's buttocks and hips. To do this, have the resident roll toward you. If the resident cannot do this, you must turn him toward you (see later in this chapter). Be sure resident cannot roll off the bed. Move to empty side of bed. Place protective pad on the area where the resident will lie on his back. The side of protective pad nearest the resident should be fanfolded (folded several times into pleats) and tucked under the resident.

   Ask resident to roll onto his back, or roll him as you did before. Unfold rest of protective pad so it completely covers area under and around the resident's hips (Fig. 6-42).
   Prevents linen from being soiled.

Fig. 6-42. *Unfold the rest of the protective pad so it completely covers area under and around the resident's hips.*

9. Ask resident to remove undergarments or help him do so.
Promotes independence.

10. Place bedpan near his hips in the correct position. A **standard bedpan** should be positioned with the wider end aligned with the resident's buttocks. A **fracture pan** should be positioned with handle toward foot of bed.

11. If resident is able, ask him to raise hips by pushing with feet and hands at the count of three (Fig. 6-43). Slide the bedpan under his hips.

Fig. 6-43. *On the count of three, slide the bedpan under the resident's hips. The wider end of bedpan should be aligned with the resident's buttocks.*

If a resident cannot help you in any way, keep the bed flat and roll the resident away from you. Slip the bedpan under his hips and gently roll the resident back onto the bedpan. Keep the bedpan centered underneath.

12. Remove and discard gloves. Wash your hands.
Provides for infection prevention.

13. Raise the head of the bed. Prop the resident into a semi-sitting position using pillows.
Puts resident in comfortable position for voiding.

14. Make sure the bath blanket is still covering the resident. Place toilet paper and disposable wipes within resident's reach. Ask resident to clean his hands with a wipe when finished if he is able.

15. Place the call light within resident's reach. Ask resident to signal when done. Leave the room and close the door.
Ensures ability to communicate need for help.

16. When called by the resident, return and put on clean gloves.

17. Lower the head of the bed. Make sure resident is still covered.
Places resident in proper position to remove pan. Promotes dignity.

18. Remove bedpan carefully and cover bedpan.
Promotes infection prevention and odor control.
Provides dignity for resident.

19. Give perineal care if help is needed. Wipe female residents from front to back. Dry the perineal area with a towel. Help the resident put on undergarment. Cover the resident and remove the bath blanket.
Wiping from front to back prevents spread of pathogens that may cause urinary tract infection.

20. Place the towel and bath blanket in a hamper or bag. Remove and discard protective pad and disposable supplies.

21. Take bedpan to the bathroom. Empty bedpan carefully into the toilet unless a specimen is needed or urine is being measured for intake/output monitoring. Note color, odor, and consistency of contents before flushing. If you notice anything unusual about the stool or urine (for example, the presence of blood), do not discard it. Inform the nurse.
Changes may be the first sign of a medical problem.

22. Turn the faucet on with a paper towel. Rinse the bedpan with cold water and empty it into the toilet. Flush the toilet. Place bedpan in proper area for cleaning or clean it according to policy.

23. Remove and discard gloves. Wash your hands.
Provides for infection prevention.

24. Return bed to lowest position. Remove privacy measures.
Lowering the bed provides for resident's safety.

25. Place call light within resident's reach.
Allows resident to communicate with staff as necessary.

26. Report any changes in resident to the nurse.
Provides nurse with information to assess resident.

27. Document procedure using facility guidelines.
If you do not document the care, legally it did not happen.

Assisting a male resident with a urinal

Equipment: urinal, protective pad, disposable wipes, 2 pairs of gloves

1. Identify yourself by name. Identify the resident by name.
Resident has right to know identity of his or her caregiver. Addressing resident by name shows respect and establishes correct identification.

2. Wash your hands.
Provides for infection prevention.

3. Explain procedure to resident. Speak clearly, slowly, and directly. Maintain face-to-face contact whenever possible.
Promotes understanding and independence.

4. Provide for resident's privacy with curtain, screen, or door.
Maintains resident's right to privacy and dignity.

5. Adjust bed to a safe level, usually waist high. Lock bed wheels.
Prevents injury to you and to resident.

6. Put on gloves.
Prevents you from coming into contact with body fluids.

7. Place a protective pad under the resident's buttocks and hips, as in earlier procedure.
Prevents linen from being soiled.

8. Hand the urinal to the resident. If the resident is not able to help himself, place urinal between his legs and position the penis inside the urinal (Fig. 6-44). Replace covers.
Promotes independence, dignity and privacy.

Fig. 6-44. *Position the penis inside the urinal if the resident cannot do it himself.*

9. Remove and discard gloves. Wash your hands.

10. Place disposable wipes within resident's reach. Ask the resident to clean his hands with a hand wipe when finished if he is able. Place the call light within resident's reach. Ask resident to signal when done. Leave the room and close the door.
Ensures ability to communicate need for help.

11. When called by the resident, return and put on clean gloves.

12. Discard disposable wipes.

13. Remove urinal or have resident hand it to you. Empty contents into toilet unless specimen is needed or urine is being measured for intake/output monitoring. Note color, odor, and qualities (for example, cloudiness) of contents.
Changes may be the first sign of medical problem.

14. Turn the faucet on with a paper towel. Rinse the urinal with cold water. Empty rinse water into the toilet. Flush the toilet. Place urinal in proper area for cleaning or clean it according to facility policy.

15. Remove and discard protective pad. Remove and discard gloves. Wash your hands.

16. Return bed to lowest position. Remove privacy measures.
Lowering the bed provides for resident's safety.

17. Place call light within resident's reach.
Allows resident to communicate with staff as necessary.

18. Report any changes in resident to the nurse.
Provides nurse with information to assess resident.

19. Document procedure using facility guidelines.
If you do not document the care, legally it did not happen.

Some residents are able to get out of bed, but may still need help walking to the bathroom and using the toilet. Others who are able to get out of bed but cannot walk to the bathroom may use a portable commode, or bedside commode (BSC). A **portable commode** is a chair with a toilet seat and a removable container underneath (Fig. 6-45).

Fig. 6-45. *The top photo shows a regular portable commode, and the bottom photo shows a bariatric portable commode, which can be used for people who are overweight or obese.* (PHOTO COURTESY OF NOVA MEDICAL PRODUCTS, WWW.NOVAMEDICALPRODUCTS.COM)

Assisting a resident to use a portable commode or toilet

Equipment: portable commode with basin, toilet paper, disposable wipes, towel, 3 pairs of gloves

1. Identify yourself by name. Identify the resident by name.
Resident has right to know identity of his or her caregiver. Addressing resident by name shows respect and establishes correct identification.

2. Wash your hands.
Provides for infection prevention.

3. Explain procedure to resident. Speak clearly, slowly, and directly. Maintain face-to-face contact whenever possible.
Promotes understanding and independence.

4. Provide for resident's privacy with curtain, screen, or door.
Maintains resident's right to privacy and dignity.

5. Lock bed wheels. Make sure resident is wearing nonskid shoes and that the laces are tied. Help resident out of bed and to the portable commode or bathroom.

6. Put on gloves.
Prevents contact with body fluids.

7. If needed, help resident remove clothing and sit comfortably on toilet seat. Put toilet paper and disposable wipes within reach. Ask resident to clean his hands with a wipe when finished if he is able.

8. Remove and discard gloves. Wash your hands.

9. Provide privacy. Place the call light within resident's reach. Ask resident to signal when done. Leave the room and close the door.
Ensures ability to communicate need for help.

10. When called by the resident, return and put on clean gloves. Give perineal care if help is needed. Wipe female residents from front to back. Dry the perineal area with a towel. Help the resident put on clothing.
Wiping from front to back prevents spread of pathogens that may cause urinary tract infection.

11. Place the towel in a hamper or bag. Discard disposable supplies.

12. Remove and discard gloves. Wash your hands.

13. Help resident back to bed.

14. Put on clean gloves.

15. Remove waste container. Empty into toilet unless a specimen is needed or the urine is being measured for intake/output monitoring. Note color, odor, and consistency of contents.
Changes may be first sign of medical problem.

16. Turn the faucet on with a paper towel. Rinse the container with cold water. Empty rinse water into the toilet. Flush the toilet. Place container in proper area for cleaning or clean it according to facility policy.

17. Remove and discard gloves. Wash your hands.
Provides for infection prevention.

18. Make sure bed is in lowest position. Remove privacy measures.

19. Place call light within resident's reach.
Allows resident to communicate with staff as necessary.

20. Report any changes in resident to the nurse.
Provides nurse with information to assess resident.

21. Document procedure using facility guidelines.
If you do not document the care, legally it did not happen.

---

8. Explain the guidelines for safely positioning and moving residents

Residents who spend a lot of time in bed often need help getting into comfortable positions. They also need to change positions periodically to avoid muscle stiffness and skin breakdown or pressure ulcers. Too much pressure on one area for too long can cause a decrease in circulation. This can lead to pressure ulcers. **Positioning** means helping residents into positions that promote comfort and health. Bedbound residents should be repositioned at least every two hours. Residents in wheelchairs or chairs should be repositioned at least every hour. Each time there is a change, NAs should document the position and the time. NAs should also check the skin for signs of irritation each time they reposition residents. These are the five basic body positions:

1. **Supine** or lying flat on the back (Fig. 6-46)

Fig. 6-46. *A person in the supine position is lying flat on his or her back.*

2. **Lateral** or lying on either side (Fig. 6-47)

Fig. 6-47. A person in the lateral position is lying on his or her side.

3. **Prone** or lying on the stomach (Fig. 6-48)

Fig. 6-48. A person in the prone position is lying on his or her stomach.

4. **Fowler's** or semi-sitting position (45 to 60 degrees) (Fig. 6-49)

Fig. 6-49. A person lying in the Fowler's position is partially reclined.

5. **Sims'** or lying on the left side with one leg drawn up (Fig. 6-50)

Fig. 6-50. A person lying in the Sims' position is lying on his or her left side with one leg drawn up.

Helping a resident move up in bed helps prevent skin irritation that can lead to pressure ulcers. An NA should get help if she thinks it is not safe to move the resident by herself.

Moving a resident up in bed

1. Identify yourself by name. Identify the resident by name.
   Resident has right to know identity of his or her caregiver. Addressing resident by name shows respect and establishes correct identification.

2. Wash your hands.
   Provides for infection prevention.

3. Explain procedure to resident. Speak clearly, slowly, and directly. Maintain face-to-face contact whenever possible.
   Promotes understanding and independence.

4. Provide for resident's privacy with curtain, screen, or door.
   Maintains resident's right to privacy and dignity.

5. Adjust bed to a safe level, usually waist high. Lock bed wheels.
   Prevents injury to you and to resident.

6. Lower the head of bed to make it flat. Move pillow to the head of the bed.
   When bed is flat, resident can be moved without working against gravity. Pillow prevents injury should resident hit the head of bed.

7. If the bed has side rails, raise the rail on the far side of the bed.

8. Stand by bed with feet apart. Face the resident.

9. Place one arm under resident's shoulder blades. Place other arm under resident's thighs. Use good body mechanics.
   Putting your arm under resident's neck could cause injury.

10. Ask resident to bend her knees, place her feet on the mattress, and push her feet and hands on the count of three (Fig. 6-51).
    Enables resident to help as much as possible and reduces strain on you.

11. On three, shift your body weight. Help move resident while she pushes with her feet.
    Communicating helps resident help you.

Fig. 6-51. *Keep your back straight and your knees bent.*

12. Place pillow under resident's head.
    Provides for resident's comfort.

13. Return bed to lowest position. Remove privacy measures.
    Lowering the bed provides for resident's safety.

14. Place call light within resident's reach.
    Allows resident to communicate with staff as necessary.

15. Wash your hands.
    Provides for infection prevention.

16. Report any changes in resident to the nurse.
    Provides nurse with information to assess resident.

17. Document procedure using facility guidelines.
    If you do not document the care, legally it did not happen.

Moving a resident to the side of the bed

Equipment: draw sheet

1. Identify yourself by name. Identify the resident by name.
   Resident has right to know identity of his or her caregiver. Addressing resident by name shows respect and establishes correct identification.

2. Wash your hands.
   Provides for infection prevention.

3. Explain procedure to resident. Speak clearly, slowly, and directly. Maintain face-to-face contact whenever possible.
   Promotes understanding and independence.

4. Provide for resident's privacy with curtain, screen, or door.
   Maintains resident's right to privacy and dignity.

5. Adjust the bed to a safe level, usually waist high. Lock bed wheels.
   Prevents injury to you and to resident.

6. Lower the head of bed.
   When bed is flat, resident can be moved without working against gravity.

7. Stand on the same side of the bed to where you are moving the resident. Stand with feet apart and knees bent.

8. **With a draw sheet**: Roll the draw sheet up to the resident's side and grasp the sheet with your palms up. One hand should be at the resident's shoulders, the other about level with the resident's hips. Apply one knee against the side of the bed, and lean back with your body. On the count of three, slowly pull the draw sheet and resident toward you.

   Without a draw sheet: Gently slide your hands under the resident's head and shoulders and move them toward you (Fig. 6-52). Gently slide your hands under her midsection and move it toward you. Gently slide your hands under the hips and legs and move them toward you (Fig. 6-53).
   Being gentle while sliding helps protect resident's skin.

9. Return bed to lowest position. Remove privacy measures.
   Lowering the bed provides for resident's safety.

10. Place call light within resident's reach.
    Allows resident to communicate with staff as necessary.

11. Wash your hands.
    Provides for infection prevention.

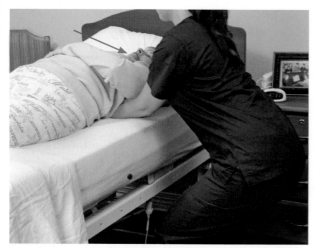

Fig. 6-52. *Gently move the resident's head and shoulders toward you.*

Fig. 6-53. *Gently move the hips and legs toward you.*

12. Report any changes in resident to the nurse.
    Provides nurse with information to assess resident.

13. Document procedure using facility guidelines.
    If you do not document the care, legally it did not happen.

Turning a resident

1. Identify yourself by name. Identify the resident by name.
   Resident has right to know identity of his or her caregiver. Addressing resident by name shows respect and establishes correct identification.

2. Wash your hands.
   Provides for infection prevention.

3. Explain procedure to resident. Speak clearly, slowly, and directly. Maintain face-to-face contact whenever possible.
   Promotes understanding and independence.

4. Provide for resident's privacy with curtain, screen, or door.
   Maintains resident's right to privacy and dignity.

5. Adjust bed to a safe level, usually waist high. Lock bed wheels.
   Prevents injury to you and to resident.

6. Lower the head of bed.
   When bed is flat, resident can be moved without working against gravity.

7. Stand on side of bed opposite where resident will be turned. If the bed has side rails, raise the far side rail. Lower side rail nearest you if it is up.

8. Move resident to side of bed nearest you using previous procedure.
   Positions resident for turn.

9. **Turning resident away from you:**

In some cases, if there is another person present or the bed has side rails, you can turn the resident away from you. Follow facility policy.

a. Cross resident's arm over her chest. Move arm on side resident is being turned to out of the way. Cross leg nearest you over the far leg (Fig. 6-54).

Fig. 6-54. *Cross leg nearest you over far leg.*

b. Stand with feet shoulder-width apart, with one foot slightly in front of the other. Bend your knees.
   Reduces your risk of injury. Promotes proper body mechanics.

c. Place one hand on the resident's shoulder. Place the other hand on the resident's nearest hip.

d. Gently roll resident onto side as one unit, toward the other side of bed (toward raised side rail if present). Shift your weight from your back leg to your front leg (Fig. 6-55).

Fig. 6-55. Gently push resident as you shift your weight from your back leg to your front leg.

Turning resident toward you:

a. Cross resident's arm over his chest. Move arm on side resident is being turned to out of the way. Cross leg furthest from you over the near leg.

b. Stand with feet shoulder-width apart. Bend your knees.
Reduces your risk of injury. Promotes proper body mechanics.

c. Place one hand on the resident's far shoulder. Place the other hand on the far hip.

d. Gently roll the resident onto side as one unit, toward you (Fig. 6-56). Your body will block resident and help prevent him from rolling out of bed.

Fig. 6-56. Gently roll resident toward you.

10. Position the resident properly:

- Head supported by pillow (resident's face should not be obstructed by pillow)

- Shoulder adjusted so resident is not lying on arm or hand

- Top arm supported by pillow

- Back supported by supportive device

- Top knee flexed

- Supportive device between legs with top knee flexed; knee and ankle supported

11. Return bed to lowest position. Remove privacy measures.
Lowering the bed provides for resident's safety.

12. Place call light within resident's reach.
Allows resident to communicate with staff as necessary.

13. Wash your hands.
Provides for infection prevention.

14. Report any changes in resident to the nurse.
Provides nurse with information to assess resident.

15. Document procedure using facility guidelines.
If you do not document the care, legally it did not happen.

Some residents' spinal columns must be kept in alignment. To turn these residents in bed, they have to be logrolled. **Logrolling** means moving a resident as a unit, without disturbing the alignment of the body. The head, back, and legs must be kept in a straight line. This is necessary in cases of neck or back problems, spinal cord injuries, or after back or hip surgeries. It is safer for two people to perform this procedure together. A draw sheet assists with moving.

Logrolling a resident

Equipment: draw sheet, coworker

1. Identify yourself by name. Identify the resident by name.
Resident has right to know identity of his or her caregiver. Addressing resident by name shows respect and establishes correct identification.

2. Wash your hands.
   Provides for infection prevention.

3. Explain procedure to resident. Speak clearly, slowly, and directly. Maintain face-to-face contact whenever possible.
   Promotes understanding and independence.

4. Provide for resident's privacy with curtain, screen, or door.
   Maintains resident's right to privacy and dignity.

5. Adjust bed to a safe level, usually waist high. Lock bed wheels.
   Prevents injury to you and to resident.

6. Lower the head of bed.
   When bed is flat, resident can be moved without working against gravity.

7. Both people stand on the same side of the bed. One person stands at the resident's head and shoulders. The other stands near the resident's midsection.

8. Place the resident's arms across his chest. Place a pillow between the knees.

9. Stand with feet shoulder-width apart. Bend your knees.
   Reduces your risk of injury. Promotes good body mechanics.

10. Grasp the draw sheet on the far side (Fig. 6-57).

Fig. 6-57. Both workers grasp the draw sheet on the far side.

11. On the count of three, gently roll the resident toward you. Turn the resident as a unit (Fig. 6-58). Your bodies will block resident and help prevent him from rolling out of bed.
    Work together for your safety and the resident's.

Fig. 6-58. On the count of three, both workers should roll the resident toward them, turning him as a unit.

12. Reposition resident comfortably.
    Maintains alignment.

13. Return bed to lowest position.
    Lowering the bed provides for resident's safety.

14. Place call light within resident's reach.
    Allows resident to communicate with staff as necessary.

15. Wash your hands.
    Provides for infection prevention.

16. Report any changes in resident to the nurse.
    Provides nurse with information to assess resident.

17. Document procedure using facility guidelines.
    If you do not document the care, legally it did not happen.

Before a resident who has been lying down stands up, he should dangle. To **dangle** means to sit up on the side of the bed with the legs hanging over the side. This helps residents regain balance. It allows blood pressure to stabilize.

Assisting resident to sit up on side of bed: dangling

1. Identify yourself by name. Identify the resident by name.
   Resident has right to know identity of his or her caregiver. Addressing resident by name shows respect and establishes correct identification.

2. Wash your hands.
   Provides for infection prevention.

3. Explain procedure to resident. Speak clearly, slowly, and directly. Maintain face-to-face contact whenever possible.
   Promotes understanding and independence.

4. Provide for resident's privacy with curtain, screen, or door.
   Maintains resident's right to privacy and dignity.

5. Adjust bed height to lowest position. Lock bed wheels.
   Allows resident's feet to touch floor when sitting. Reduces chance of injury if resident falls.

6. Raise the head of bed to sitting position.
   Resident can move without working against gravity.

7. Stand with feet shoulder-width apart. Bend your knees.
   Reduces your risk of injury. Promotes proper body mechanics.

8. Place one arm under the resident's shoulder blades. Place the other arm under the resident's thighs (Fig. 6-59).
   Placing your arm under the resident's neck may cause injury.

Fig. 6-59. *One arm should be under the resident's shoulder blades and the other arm should be under the thighs.*

9. On the count of three, slowly turn resident into sitting position with legs dangling over side of bed (Fig. 6-60).
   Communicating helps resident help you.

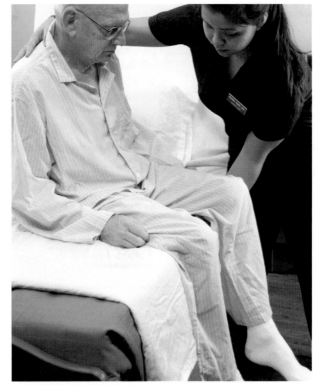

Fig. 6-60. *The weight of the resident's legs hanging down from the bed helps the resident sit up.*

10. Ask resident to hold onto edge of mattress with both hands. Assist resident to put on nonskid shoes or slippers.
    Prevents sliding on floor and protects resident's feet from contamination.

11. Have resident dangle as long as ordered. The care plan may direct you to allow the resident to dangle for several minutes and then return him to lying down, or it may direct you to allow the resident to dangle in preparation for walking or a transfer. Follow the care plan. Do not leave the resident alone. If the resident is dizzy for more than a minute, have him lie down again and report to the nurse.
    Change of position may cause dizziness due to a drop in blood pressure.

12. Take vital signs as ordered (Chapter 7).

13. Remove slippers or shoes.

14. Gently assist resident back into bed. Place one arm around resident's shoulders. Place the other arm under resident's knees. Slowly swing resident's legs onto bed.

15. Leave bed in lowest position. Remove privacy measures.
    Lowering the bed provides for resident's safety.

16. Place call light within resident's reach.
    Allows resident to communicate with staff as necessary.

17. Wash your hands.
    Provides for infection prevention.

18. Report any changes in resident to the nurse.
    Provides nurse with information to assess resident.

19. Document procedure using facility guidelines.
    If you do not document the care, legally it did not happen.

Transferring a resident means that an NA is moving him from one place to another. Transfers can move residents from a bed to a chair or wheelchair, from a wheelchair to a shower or toilet, and so on.

Safety is one of the most important things to consider during transfers. **Ergonomics** is the science of designing equipment, areas, and work tasks to make them safer and to suit the worker's abilities. OSHA states that manual lifting and transferring of residents should be reduced and eliminated when possible. Manual lifting, transferring, and repositioning of residents may increase risks of injury.

To reduce injuries, many facilities have adopted *no-lift*, *zero-lift*, or *lift-free* policies. These policies set strict guidelines for lifting and transferring of residents. Lift-free policies vary. Some facilities allow no lifting at all and require that equipment always be used when lifting and moving residents. The more restrictions placed on lifting, the less chance there is of injury. NAs must follow facility policies on lifting and use equipment properly. They should ask for help and always get help when they need it.

A **transfer belt** is a safety device used to assist staff in transferring residents who are weak, unsteady, or uncoordinated. It is called a **gait belt** when it is used to help residents walk. The belt is made of canvas or other heavy material. It has a buckle and sometimes has handles. It fits around the resident's waist outside the clothing. It should never be placed on bare skin. The belt gives NAs something firm to hold on to when helping with transfers. The NA should grasp the belt securely on both sides, with hands in an upward position. Transfer belts cannot be used if a resident has fragile bones or recent fractures.

A slide or transfer board may be used to help transfer residents who are unable to bear weight on their legs. Slide boards can be used for almost any transfer that involves moving from one sitting position to another (Fig. 6-61). Slide boards should not be used against bare skin.

Fig. 6-61. *A slide board can help with bed-to-chair transfers.*

Guidelines: Wheelchairs

G Learn how each wheelchair works. Residents may use manual (require human power to move) or electric wheelchairs. Know how to apply and release the brake and how to work the armrests and footrests. Always lock a wheelchair before helping a resident into or out of it (Fig. 6-62). After a transfer, unlock the wheelchair.

G To unfold a standard wheelchair, tilt the chair slightly to raise the wheels on the opposite side. Press down on one or both seat rails until the chair opens and the seat is flat. To fold a standard wheelchair, lift up under the center edge of the seat.

Fig. 6-62. Always lock the wheelchair before a resident gets into or out of it.

G   To remove an armrest, release the arm lock by the armrest, and lift the arm from the center. To replace the armrest, simply reverse the procedure.

G   To move a footrest out of the way, press or pull the release lever. Swing the footrest out toward the side of the wheelchair. To remove the footrest, lift it off when it is toward the side of the wheelchair (Fig. 6-63). To replace a footrest, simply put it back in the side position. Then swing it back to the front position. It should lock into place.

Fig. 6-63. To remove a footrest, swing the footrest toward the side of the wheelchair and lift it off.

G   To lift or lower a footrest, support the leg or foot. Squeeze the lever and pull up or push down.

G   To transfer to or from a wheelchair, the resident must use the side of the body that can bear weight to support and lift the side that cannot bear weight. Residents who can bear no weight with their legs may use leg braces or overhead trapezes to support themselves.

G   Before any transfer, make sure the resident is wearing nonskid footwear that is securely fastened. This promotes residents' safety and reduces the risk of falls.

G   During wheelchair transfers, make sure the resident is safe and comfortable. Ask the resident how you can help. Some may only want you to bring the chair to the bedside. Others may want you to be more involved.

G   Keep the resident's body in proper alignment while in a wheelchair or chair. Special cushions and pillows can be used for support. The hips should be well-positioned back in the chair.

G   When a resident is in a wheelchair or any chair, he or she should be repositioned at least every hour. The reasons for doing this are as follows:

•   It promotes comfort.

•   It reduces pressure.

•   It increases circulation.

•   It exercises the joints.

•   It improves muscle tone.

Falls

If a resident starts to fall during a transfer, the NA should do the following:

•   Widen his stance.

•   Bring the resident's body close to him to break the fall.

•   Bend his knees and support the resident as he lowers the resident to the floor (Fig. 6-64). If needed, the NA can drop to the floor with the resident to avoid injury to himself or the resident.

The NA should not try to reverse or stop a fall. The NA or the resident can suffer worse injuries if he tries to stop, rather than break, a fall. If a resident has fallen, the NA should call for help. He should not try to get the resident up after the fall.

Fig. 6-64. *A nursing assistant should not try to reverse or stop a fall. Instead, he should bend his knees and support the resident as he lowers her to the floor.*

Transferring a resident from bed to wheelchair

Equipment: wheelchair, transfer belt, nonskid footwear, lap robe or folded blanket

1. Identify yourself by name. Identify the resident by name.
   Resident has right to know identity of his or her caregiver. Addressing resident by name shows respect and establishes correct identification.

2. Wash your hands.
   Provides for infection prevention.

3. Explain procedure to resident. Speak clearly, slowly, and directly. Maintain face-to-face contact whenever possible.
   Promotes understanding and independence.

4. Provide for resident's privacy with curtain, screen, or door. Check the area to be certain it is uncluttered and safe.
   Maintains resident's right to privacy and dignity. Keeping area free from clutter promotes safety.

5. Place wheelchair at the head of the bed, facing foot of the bed, or at the foot of bed, facing head of bed. The arm of the wheelchair should be almost touching the bed. It should be placed on resident's stronger, or unaffected, side.
   Unaffected side supports weight.

6. Remove both wheelchair footrests close to the bed.

7. Lock wheelchair wheels.
   Wheel locks prevent chair from moving.

8. Raise the head of the bed. Adjust bed level to lowest position. Lock bed wheels.
   Prevents injury to you and to resident.

9. Assist resident to sitting position with feet flat on the floor. Let resident sit for a few minutes to adjust to change in position.

10. Put nonskid footwear on resident and fasten securely.
    Promotes resident's safety. Reduces risk of falls.

11. Stand in front of resident. Stand with feet about shoulder-width apart. Bend your knees.
    Reduces your risk of injury. Promotes proper body mechanics.

12. Place the transfer belt around resident's waist over clothing (not on bare skin). Tighten the buckle until it is snug. Leave enough room to insert flat fingers/hand comfortably under the belt. Check to make sure that skin or skin folds (for example, breasts) are not caught under the belt. Grasp the belt securely on both sides, with hands in upward position.

13. Provide instructions to allow resident to help with transfer. Instructions may include: "When you start to stand, push with your hands against the bed." "Once standing, if you're able, you can take small steps in the direction of the chair." "Once standing, reach for the chair with your stronger hand."

14. With your legs, brace (support) resident's lower legs to prevent slipping (Fig. 6-65). This can be done by placing one or both of your knees in front of the resident's knees.

15. Count to three to alert resident. On three, with hands still grasping the transfer belt on both sides and moving upward, slowly help resident to stand.
    Communicating helps resident help you.

Fig. 6-65. *Brace the resident's lower legs to prevent slipping.*

16. Tell the resident to take small steps in the direction of the chair while turning his back toward it. If more help is needed, help the resident pivot (turn) to stand in front of wheelchair with back of resident's legs against wheelchair (Fig. 6-66).
Pivoting is safer than twisting.

Fig. 6-66. *Help him pivot to the front of the wheelchair.*

17. Ask the resident to put hands on wheelchair armrests if able. When the chair is touching the back of the resident's legs, help him lower himself into the chair.

18. Reposition resident so that his hips touch the back of the wheelchair seat.
Using full seat of chair is safest.

19. Attach footrests. Place the resident's feet on the footrests. Check that the resident is in proper alignment. Gently remove the transfer belt. Place a folded blanket over the resident's lap as appropriate.
Protects feet and ankles.

20. Remove privacy measures.

21. Place call light within resident's reach.
Allows resident to communicate with staff as necessary.

22. Wash your hands.
Provides for infection prevention.

23. Report any changes in resident to the nurse.
Provides nurse with information to assess resident.

24. Document procedure using facility guidelines.
If you do not document the care, legally it did not happen.

Mechanical Lifts

Facilities often have mechanical, or hydraulic, lifts available to transfer residents. This equipment helps prevent injury to staff and residents. NAs may assist residents with many types of transfers using a mechanical lift. Using these lifts requires special training. NAs should not use equipment they have not been trained to use, as this could cause injury. There are many different types of mechanical lifts (Fig. 6-67). NAs should always ask for help if there is anything they do not understand about lift equipment.

Fig. 6-67. There are different types of lifts that transfer completely dependent residents and residents who can bear some weight. (PHOTOS COURTESY OF VANCARE INC., 800-694-4525)

Guidelines: Mechanical or Hydraulic Lifts

G Be careful when moving a resident using a mechanical lift. Have another person help you when using these lifts if possible. Many facilities require two staff members to assist when using a mechanical lift.

G Keep the chair or wheelchair to which the resident is to be moved close to the bed so that the resident is only moved a short distance in the lift.

G Check that the valves are working on the lift before using it.

G Use the correct sling for the lift that is being used. Using an incorrect sling may result in serious injury or death. If you are unsure which sling to use, talk to the nurse.

G Check the sling and straps for any fraying or tears. Do not use the lift if there are tears or holes.

G Open the legs of the stand to the widest position before helping the resident into the lift.

G Once the resident is in the sling and the straps are connected, pump up the lift only to the point where the resident's body clears the bed or chair.

Transferring a resident using a mechanical lift

Equipment: wheelchair or chair, coworker, mechanical or hydraulic lift

This is a basic procedure for transferring using a mechanical lift. Ask someone to help you before starting.

1. Identify yourself by name. Identify the resident by name.
    Resident has right to know identity of his or her caregiver. Addressing resident by name shows respect and establishes correct identification.

2. Wash your hands.
    Provides for infection prevention.

3. Explain procedure to resident. Speak clearly, slowly, and directly. Maintain face-to-face contact whenever possible.
    Promotes understanding and independence.

4. Provide for resident's privacy with curtain, screen, or door.
    Maintains resident's right to privacy and dignity.

5. Lock bed wheels.
    Wheel locks prevent bed from moving.

6. Position wheelchair next to bed. Lock brakes.
    Wheel locks prevent chair from moving.

7. Help the resident turn to one side of the bed. Position the sling under the resident, with the edge next to the resident's back. Fanfold if necessary. Make the bottom of the sling even with the resident's knees. Help the resident roll back to the middle of the bed. Spread out the fanfolded edge of the sling.

8. Roll the mechanical lift to bedside. Make sure the base is opened to its widest point. Push the base of the lift under the bed.

9. Place the overhead bar directly over the resident.

10. With the resident lying on his back, attach one set of straps to each side of the sling. Attach one set of straps to the overhead bar. Have coworker support the resident at the head, shoulders, and knees while being lifted. The resident's arms should be folded across his chest (Fig. 6-68). If the device has S hooks, they should face away from resident. Make sure all straps are connected properly and are smooth and straight.

Fig. 6-68. *With the resident's arms folded across his chest, attach the straps to the sling.*

11. Following manufacturer's instructions, raise the resident two inches above the bed. Pause a moment for the resident to gain balance.

12. Have coworker help support and guide the resident's body. You can then roll the lift so that the resident is positioned over the chair or wheelchair.
Having another person help promotes safety during the transfer and lessens chance of injury.

13. Slowly lower the resident into the chair or wheelchair. Push down gently on the resident's knees to help the resident into a sitting, rather than reclining, position.

14. Undo the straps from the overhead bar to the sling. Remove sling or leave in place; follow facility policy.

15. Be sure the resident is seated comfortably and correctly in the chair or wheelchair. Remove privacy measures.

16. Place call light within resident's reach.
Allows resident to communicate with staff as necessary.

17. Wash your hands.
Provides for infection prevention.

18. Report any changes in resident to the nurse.
Provides nurse with information to assess resident.

19. Document procedure using facility guidelines.
If you do not document the care, legally it did not happen.

7

Basic Nursing Skills

1. Explain admission, transfer, and discharge of a resident

Moving always requires an adjustment, but as a person ages, it can be even harder. This is especially true if illness, disability, and mobility problems are present. Nursing assistants play an important role in helping residents make a successful transition to long-term care facilities. By giving emotional support such as listening and being kind, compassionate, and helpful, NAs can help residents feel better about their new homes.

Residents' Rights

New LGBT Residents

Entering a long-term care facility can be especially difficult for lesbian, gay, bisexual, or transgender (LGBT) residents. LGBT residents may fear that they will not be accepted by staff or other residents. They may worry that their partners will not receive the same welcome the spouse or partner of a heterosexual resident would receive. NAs must not judge residents, even if they believe that homosexuality is wrong. Every resident deserves professional, caring service from staff. The facility is the resident's home. NAs should make every effort to make all residents feel comfortable and welcome.

Admission is often the first time an NA meets a new resident. This is a time of first impressions. The NA should try to make sure the resident has a good impression of him and his facility. Because change is difficult, staff must communicate with new residents. NAs can explain what to expect during the process. They can answer any questions that are within their scope of practice.

If residents or their families have questions that NAs cannot answer, they should find the nurse. It is a good idea for NAs to ask new residents questions to find out their personal preferences and routines. NAs can also ask residents' families about personal preferences if residents are not able to respond.

Guidelines: Admission

G Prepare the room before the resident arrives. This helps her to feel expected and welcome. Make sure the bed is made and the room is tidy. Restock supplies that are low. Make sure there is an admission kit available if used. Admission kits often contain personal care items, such as a bath basin, an emesis basin, a water pitcher and drinking glass, toothpaste, soap, a comb, lotion, and tissues (Fig. 7-1). The kit may also contain a urine specimen cup, label, and transport bag.

G When a new resident arrives at the facility, note the time and her condition. Is she using a wheelchair, on a stretcher, or walking? Who is with her? Observe the new resident for level of consciousness and if she seems confused. Look for signs of nervousness. Note any tubes she has, such as IVs or catheters.

G Introduce yourself. State your position. Smile and be friendly. Always call the person by her formal name until she tells you what she wants to be called.

Fig. 7-1. An admission kit is usually placed in a resident's room before he or she is admitted. It may contain personal care items that the resident will need. (REPRINTED WITH PERMISSION OF BRIGGS CORPORATION, 800-247-2343, WWW.BRIGGSCORP.COM)

G Never rush the process or the new resident. She should not feel like she is an inconvenience. Make sure that the new resident feels welcome and wanted.

G Explain day-to-day life in the facility. Offer to take the resident and her family on a tour. Show the resident important areas. When showing the resident where the dining room is, review the posted dining schedules. During the tour, introduce the resident to other residents and staff members you see. Introduce the roommate if there is one.

G Handle personal items with care and respect. A resident has a legal right to have her personal items treated carefully. When setting up the room, place personal items where the resident wants them (Fig. 7-2).

Fig. 7-2. Handle personal items carefully, and set up the room as the resident prefers.

G Admission is a stressful time. Observe the resident, as there could be something important that was missed. Report to the nurse if you notice any of the following:

- Disconnected tubing

- Resident seems confused, combative, and/or unaware of surroundings

- Resident is having difficulty breathing, pain, or any other signs of distress

- Resident has bruises or wounds

- Resident has missed a meal during admission process

- Resident has valuables, medications, hearing aids, eyeglasses, or dentures

G Follow facility policy on any other tasks that are required during admission.

G New residents may have good days followed by not-so-good days. Let residents adapt to their new homes at their own pace. However, report signs of confusion or depression to the nurse.

Residents' Rights

Admission

OBRA requires that on admission, residents must be told of their legal rights. They must be provided with a written copy of these rights. This includes rights about their funds and the right to file a complaint with the state survey agency. Residents must also be provided with information about their rights related to advance directives.

Admitting a resident

Equipment: may include admission paperwork (checklist and inventory form), gloves, and vital signs equipment

1. Identify yourself by name. Identify the resident by name.
    Resident has right to know identity of his or her caregiver. Addressing resident by name shows respect and establishes correct identification.

2. Wash your hands.
    Provides for infection prevention.

3. Explain procedure to resident. Speak clearly, slowly, and directly. Maintain face-to-face contact whenever possible.
    Promotes understanding and independence.

4. Provide for resident's privacy with curtain, screen, or door (Fig. 7-3). If the family is present, ask them to step outside until the admission process is over. Show them where they can wait.
    Maintains resident's right to privacy and dignity.

Fig. 7-3. All residents have a legal right to privacy, and providing privacy is part of doing your job professionally. Your professional, respectful behavior can help put a new resident at ease.

5. If part of facility procedure, do these things:

    •   Measure the resident's height and weight.

    •   Measure the resident's baseline vital signs. Baseline signs are initial values that can then be compared to future measurements.

    •   Obtain a urine specimen if required.

    •   Complete the paperwork. Take an inventory of all the personal items.

    •   Help the resident put personal items away. Label personal items according to facility policy.

    •   Provide fresh water.

6. Show the resident the room and bathroom. Explain how to work the bed controls and the call light. Show the resident the telephone, lights, and television controls.
    Promotes resident's safety.

7. Introduce the resident to his roommate if there is one. Introduce other residents and staff.
    Makes resident feel more comfortable.

8. Make sure resident is comfortable. Bring the family back inside if they were outside.

9. Place call light within resident's reach.
    Allows resident to communicate with staff as necessary.

10. Wash your hands.
    Provides for infection prevention.

11. Document procedure using facility guidelines.
    If you do not document the care, legally it did not happen.

Residents may be transferred to a different area of the facility. In cases of acute illness, they may be transferred to a hospital. Change is difficult. This is especially true when a person has an illness or her condition gets worse. Staff should make the transfer as smooth as possible for the resident. A resident should be informed of the transfer as soon as possible so that she can begin to adjust to the idea. The nurse will tell the resident about the transfer and should explain how, where, when, and why the transfer will occur. Any questions the resident has should be answered.

NAs help residents pack their personal items before transferring. Residents often worry about losing their belongings. NAs can involve them in the packing process. For example, the NA can let the resident see the empty closet, drawer, etc.

Transferring a resident

Equipment: may include a wheelchair, cart for belongings, the medical record, all of the resident's personal care items and packed personal items

1. Identify yourself by name. Identify the resident by name.
    Resident has right to know identity of his or her caregiver. Addressing resident by name shows respect and establishes correct identification.

2. Wash your hands.
Provides for infection prevention.

3. Explain procedure to resident. Speak clearly, slowly, and directly. Maintain face-to-face contact whenever possible.
Promotes understanding and independence.

4. Collect items to be moved onto the cart. Take them to the new location. If the resident is going into the hospital, they may be placed in temporary storage.

5. Help the resident into the wheelchair (or onto a stretcher if one is used). Take him or her to proper area.

6. Introduce new residents and staff.
Makes resident feel more comfortable.

7. Help the resident to put personal items away.

8. Make sure that the resident is comfortable.

9. Place call light within resident's reach.
Allows resident to communicate with staff as necessary.

10. Wash your hands.
Provides for infection prevention.

11. Report any changes in resident to the nurse.
Provides nurse with information to assess resident.

12. Document procedure using facility guidelines.
If you do not document the care, legally it did not happen.

To discharge a resident from a facility, a doctor must give the discharge order. The nurse then completes instructions for the resident to follow after discharge. The nurse will review these instructions and information with the resident and her family and friends. Some of these areas may be discussed:

- Future doctor or physical, speech, and occupational therapy appointments
- Home care, skilled nursing care
- Medications

- Ambulation instructions
- Medical equipment needed
- Medical transportation
- Any restrictions on activities
- Special exercises to keep the resident functioning at the highest level
- Special nutrition or dietary requirements
- Community resources

NAs help by collecting the resident's belongings and packing them carefully. The NA should know what the resident's condition is at the time of discharge and find out if the resident will be using a wheelchair or stretcher.

The day of discharge is often a happy day for residents who are going home. However, some residents may feel uncertainty or fear about leaving the facility. They may be concerned that their health will suffer. NAs can help by being positive. They can remind residents that their doctors believe they are ready to leave. However, if a resident has specific questions about care, the NA should inform the nurse.

Residents' Rights

Transfers or Discharges
OBRA requires that residents have the right to receive advance notice before being transferred or discharged from a facility. The written notice must contain the specifics of where and why they are being transferred or discharged. It must be in a language residents can understand. Staff must provide proper preparation for the transfer or discharge.

Discharging a resident

Equipment: may include a wheelchair, cart for belongings, discharge paperwork, including the inventory list from admission, resident's care items

1. Identify yourself by name. Identify the resident by name.
Resident has right to know identity of his or her caregiver. Addressing resident by name shows respect and establishes correct identification.

2. Wash your hands.
Provides for infection prevention.

3. Explain procedure to resident. Speak clearly, slowly, and directly. Maintain face-to-face contact whenever possible.
Promotes understanding and independence.

4. Provide for resident's privacy with curtain, screen, or door.
Maintains resident's right to privacy and dignity.

5. Measure the resident's vital signs.

6. Compare the checklist to the items there. If all items are there, ask the resident to sign.

7. Put the personal items to be taken onto the cart and take them to pick-up area.

8. Help the resident dress and then into the wheelchair or onto the stretcher if used.

9. Help the resident to say his goodbyes to the staff and residents.

10. Take resident to the pick-up area. Help him into vehicle. You are responsible for the resident until he is safely in the vehicle and the door is closed.

11. Wash your hands.
Provides for infection prevention.

12. Document procedure using facility guidelines. Include the following:
    • The vital signs at discharge
    • Time of discharge
    • Method of transport
    • Who was with the resident
    • What items the resident took with her (inventory checklist)
    If you do not document the care, legally it did not happen.

2. Explain the importance of monitoring vital signs

Nursing assistants monitor, document, and report residents' **vital signs**. Vital signs are important. They show how well the vital organs of the body, such as the heart and lungs, are working. They consist of the following:

• Measuring the body temperature

• Counting the pulse

• Counting the rate of respirations

• Measuring the blood pressure

• Observing and reporting the level of pain

Watching for changes in vital signs is very important. Changes can indicate a resident's condition is worsening. An NA should always notify the nurse if

• The resident has a fever (temperature is above average for the resident or outside the normal range)

• The resident has a respiratory or pulse rate that is too rapid or too slow

• The resident's blood pressure changes

• The resident's pain is worse or is not relieved by pain management

Ranges for Adult Vital Signs

Temp. Site	Fahrenheit	Celsius
Mouth (oral)	97.6°–99.6°	36.5°–37.5°
Rectum (rectal)	98.6°–100.6°	37.0°–38.1°
Armpit (axilla)	96.6°–98.6°	36.0°–37.0°
Ear (tympanic)	96.6°–99.7°	35.8°–37.6°
Temporal Artery	97.2°–100.1°	36.2°–37.8°

Normal Pulse Rate: 60–100 beats per minute
Normal Respiratory Rate: 12–20 respirations per minute

Blood Pressure

Normal	Systolic 100–119 Diastolic 60–79
Low	Below 100/60
Prehypertensive	Systolic 120–139 Diastolic 80–89
High	140/90 or above

Temperature

Body temperature is normally very close to 98.6°F (Fahrenheit) or 37°C (Celsius). Body temperature is a balance between the heat created by the body and the heat lost to the environment. Many factors affect body temperature: age, illness, stress, environment, exercise, and the circadian rhythm can all cause changes in body temperature. The circadian rhythm is the 24-hour day-night cycle. Average temperature readings change throughout the day. People tend to have lower temperatures in the morning. Increases in body temperature may indicate an infection or disease.

There are different sites for measuring body temperature: the mouth (oral), the rectum (rectal), the armpit (axilla), the ear (tympanic), and the temporal artery (the artery under the skin of the forehead). The different sites require different thermometers. Types of thermometers are as follows:

- Mercury-free (Fig. 7-4)

- Digital (Fig. 7-5)

- Electronic (Fig. 7-6)

- Disposable (Fig. 7-7)

- Tympanic (Fig. 7-8)

- Temporal artery (Fig. 7-9)

Fig. 7-4. *A mercury-free oral thermometer and a mercury-free rectal thermometer. Oral thermometers are usually green or blue; rectal thermometers are usually red.* (PHOTOS COURTESY OF RG MEDICAL DIAGNOSTICS OF WIXOM, MI, RGMD.COM)

Fig. 7-5. *A digital thermometer.*

Fig. 7-6. *An electronic thermometer.* (PHOTO COURTESY OF WELCH ALLYN, WWW.WELCHALLYN.COM, 800-535-6663)

Fig. 7-7. *A disposable thermometer.*

Fig. 7-8. *A tympanic thermometer.*

Fig. 7-9. *A temporal artery thermometer.* (PHOTO COURTESY OF EXERGEN CORPORATION, 800-422-3006, WWW.EXERGEN.COM)

Numbers on the thermometer allow the temperature to be read after it registers. Most thermometers show the temperature in degrees Fahrenheit (F). Each long line represents one degree. Each short line represents two-tenths of a degree. Some thermometers show the temperature in degrees Celsius (C). The long lines represent one degree. The short lines represent one-tenth of a degree. Small arrows or highlighted numbers show the normal temperature: 98.6°F and 37°C (Fig. 7-10).

Fig. 7-10. This shows a normal temperature reading: 98.6°F and 37°C.

There is a range of normal temperatures. Some people's temperatures normally run low. Others will run slightly higher, even in good health. Normal temperature readings also vary by the method used to take the temperature. A rectal temperature is generally considered to be the most accurate. However, taking a rectal temperature on an uncooperative person, such as a resident with dementia, can be dangerous. An axillary temperature is considered the least accurate.

An NA should not take an oral temperature on a person who

- Is unconscious

- Has recently had facial or oral surgery

- Is younger than 5 years old

- Is confused or disoriented

- Is heavily sedated

- Is likely to have a seizure

- Is coughing

- Is using oxygen

- Has facial paralysis

- Has a nasogastric tube (a feeding tube that is inserted through the nose and goes into the stomach)

- Has sores, redness, swelling, or pain in the mouth

- Has an injury to the face or neck

Measuring and recording oral temperature

Do not take an oral temperature on a resident who has smoked, eaten or drunk fluids, chewed gum, or exercised in the last 10 to 20 minutes.

Equipment: clean mercury-free, digital, or electronic thermometer, gloves, disposable sheath/cover for thermometer, tissues, pen and paper

1. Identify yourself by name. Identify the resident by name.
   Resident has right to know identity of his or her caregiver. Addressing resident by name shows respect and establishes correct identification.

2. Wash your hands.
   Provides for infection prevention.

3. Explain procedure to resident. Speak clearly, slowly, and directly. Maintain face-to-face contact whenever possible.
   Promotes understanding and independence.

4. Provide for resident's privacy with curtain, screen, or door.
   Maintains resident's right to privacy and dignity.

5. Put on gloves.

6. **Mercury-free thermometer**: Hold the thermometer by the stem. Before inserting it in the resident's mouth, shake thermometer down to below the lowest number (at least below 96°F or 35°C). To shake the thermometer down, hold it at the end opposite the bulb with the thumb and two fingers. With a snapping motion of the wrist, shake the thermometer (Fig. 7-11). Stand away from furniture and walls while doing so.
   Holding the stem end prevents contamination of the bulb end. The thermometer reading must be below the resident's actual temperature.

Fig. 7-11. Shake thermometer down to below the lowest number before inserting in a resident's mouth.

Digital thermometer: Put on the disposable sheath. Turn on thermometer and wait until *ready* sign appears.

Electronic thermometer: Remove the probe from base unit. Put on probe cover.

7. **Mercury-free thermometer**: Put on disposable sheath if available. Insert bulb end of the thermometer into resident's mouth, under tongue and to one side (Fig. 7-12).
The thermometer measures heat from blood vessels under the tongue.

Fig. 7-12. Insert thermometer under the resident's tongue and to one side.

Digital thermometer: Insert the end of digital thermometer into resident's mouth, under tongue and to one side.

Electronic thermometer: Insert the end of electronic thermometer into resident's mouth, under tongue and to one side.

8. **For all thermometers:** Tell the resident to hold the thermometer in his mouth with lips closed. Assist as necessary. Resident should breathe through his nose. Ask the resident not to bite down or talk.
The lips hold the thermometer in position. If it is broken, injury to the mouth may occur. More time may be required if resident opens mouth to talk.

Mercury-free thermometer: Leave the thermometer in place for at least three minutes.

Digital thermometer: Leave in place until thermometer blinks or beeps.

Electronic thermometer: Leave in place until you hear a tone or see a flashing or steady light.

9. **Mercury-free thermometer**: Remove the thermometer. Wipe with a tissue from stem to bulb or remove sheath. Dispose of the tissue or sheath. Hold the thermometer at eye level. Rotate until line appears, rolling the thermometer between your thumb and forefinger. Read the temperature. Remember the temperature reading.

Digital thermometer: Remove the thermometer. Read temperature on display screen. Remember the temperature reading.

Electronic thermometer: Read the temperature on the display screen. Remember the temperature reading. Remove the probe.

10. **Mercury-free thermometer**: Clean thermometer with soap and water. Rinse with clean water and dry. Return it to case.

Digital thermometer: Using a tissue, remove and dispose of sheath. Replace the thermometer in case.

Electronic thermometer: Press the eject button to discard the cover. Return the probe to the holder.

11. Remove and discard gloves.

12. Wash your hands.
Provides for infection prevention.

13. Immediately record the temperature, date, time, and method used (oral).
Record temperature immediately so you won't forget. Care plans are made based on your report.

14. Place call light within resident's reach.
Allows resident to communicate with staff as necessary.

15. Report any changes in resident to the nurse.
Provides nurse with information to assess resident.

NAs must always explain what they will do before starting to measure a rectal temperature. The NA needs the resident's cooperation. She should ask the resident to hold still. She should reassure him that the task will only take a few minutes. The NA should hold onto the thermometer at all times while taking a rectal temperature.

Measuring and recording rectal temperature

Equipment: clean rectal mercury-free, digital, or electronic thermometer, lubricant, gloves, tissue, disposable sheath/cover, pen and paper

1. Identify yourself by name. Identify resident by name.
    Resident has right to know identity of his or her caregiver. Addressing resident by name shows respect and establishes correct identification.

2. Wash your hands.
    Provides for infection prevention.

3. Explain procedure to resident. Speak clearly, slowly, and directly. Maintain face-to-face contact whenever possible.
    Promotes understanding and independence.

4. Provide for resident's privacy with curtain, screen, or door.
    Maintains resident's right to privacy and dignity.

5. Adjust bed to a safe level, usually waist high. Lock bed wheels.
    Promotes safety.

6. Help the resident to left-lying (Sims') position (Fig. 7-13).

Fig. 7-13. The resident must be in the left-lying (Sims') position.

7. Fold back linens to expose only the rectal area.

8. Put on gloves.

9. **Mercury-free thermometer**: Hold thermometer by stem. Shake the thermometer down to below the lowest number. Put on disposable sheath.

    Digital thermometer: Put on the disposable sheath. Turn on thermometer and wait until *ready* sign appears.

Electronic thermometer: Remove the probe from base unit. Put on probe cover.

10. Apply a small amount of lubricant to tip of bulb or probe cover (or apply pre-lubricated cover).

11. Separate the buttocks. Gently insert thermometer into rectum 1/2 to 1 inch. Stop if you meet resistance. Do not force the thermometer in (Fig. 7-14).

Fig. 7-14. Gently insert a rectal thermometer one-half to one inch into the rectum.

12. Replace the sheet over buttocks. Hold on to the thermometer at all times.

13. **Mercury-free thermometer**: Hold thermometer in place for at least three minutes.

    Digital thermometer: Hold thermometer in place until thermometer blinks or beeps.

    Electronic thermometer: Leave in place until you hear a tone or see a flashing or steady light.

14. Gently remove the thermometer. Wipe with tissue from stem to bulb or remove sheath. Discard tissue or sheath.

15. Read the thermometer at eye level as you would for an oral temperature. Remember the temperature reading.

16. **Mercury-free thermometer**: Clean thermometer with soap and water. Rinse with clean water and dry. Return it to case.

Digital thermometer: Clean thermometer according to policy and replace it in the case.

Electronic thermometer: Press the eject button to discard cover. Return probe to holder.

17. Remove and discard gloves.

18. Wash your hands.
    Provides for infection prevention.

19. Assist the resident to a comfortable position.

20. Immediately record the temperature, date, time, and method used (rectal).
    Record temperature immediately so you won't forget. Care plans are made based on your report.

21. Place call light within resident's reach.
    Allows resident to communicate with staff as necessary.

22. Report any changes in resident to the nurse.
    Provides nurse with information to assess resident.

Tympanic thermometers can take fast, accurate temperature readings. The NA should tell the resident that she will be placing a thermometer in the ear canal. She should reassure the resident that this is painless. The short tip of the thermometer will only go into the ear ¼ to ½ inch.

Measuring and recording tympanic temperature

Equipment: tympanic thermometer, gloves, disposable probe sheath/cover, pen and paper

1. Identify yourself by name. Identify the resident by name.
   Resident has right to know identity of his or her caregiver. Addressing resident by name shows respect and establishes correct identification.

2. Wash your hands.
   Provides for infection prevention.

3. Explain procedure to resident. Speak clearly, slowly, and directly. Maintain face-to-face contact whenever possible.
   Promotes understanding and independence.

4. Provide for resident's privacy with curtain, screen, or door.
   Maintains resident's right to privacy and dignity.

5. Put on gloves.

6. Put a disposable sheath over earpiece of the thermometer.
   Protects equipment. Reduces risk of contamination.

7. Position the resident's head so that the ear is in front of you. Straighten the ear canal by gently pulling up and back on the outside edge of the ear (Fig. 7-15). Insert the covered probe into the ear canal. Press the button.

Fig. 7-15. *Straighten the ear canal by gently pulling up and back on the outside edge of the ear.*

8. Hold thermometer in place either for one second or until thermometer blinks or beeps.

9. Read temperature. Remember temperature reading.

10. Dispose of sheath. Return thermometer to storage or to the battery charger if thermometer is rechargeable.

11. Remove and discard gloves.

12. Wash your hands.
    Provides for infection prevention.

13. Immediately record temperature, date, time, and method used (tympanic).
    Record temperature immediately so you won't forget. Care plans are made based on your report.

14. Place call light within resident's reach.
    Allows resident to communicate with staff as necessary.

15. Report any changes in resident to the nurse.
    Provides nurse with information to assess resident.

Axillary temperatures are less reliable than temperatures taken at other sites. However, they can be safer if a resident is confused, disoriented, uncooperative, or has dementia.

Measuring and recording axillary temperature

Equipment: clean mercury-free, digital, or electronic thermometer, gloves, tissues, disposable sheath/cover, pen and paper

1. Identify yourself by name. Identify resident by name.
    Resident has right to know identity of his or her caregiver. Addressing resident by name shows respect and establishes correct identification.

2. Wash your hands.
    Provides for infection prevention.

3. Explain procedure to resident. Speak clearly, slowly, and directly. Maintain face-to-face contact whenever possible.
    Promotes understanding and independence.

4. Provide for resident's privacy with curtain, screen, or door.
    Maintains resident's right to privacy and dignity.

5. Put on gloves.

6. Remove resident's arm from sleeve of gown or shirt to allow skin contact with the end of the thermometer. Wipe axillary area with tissues before placing the thermometer.

7. **Mercury-free thermometer**: Hold the thermometer by the stem. Shake the thermometer down to below the lowest number.

    Digital thermometer: Put on the disposable sheath. Turn on thermometer and wait until *ready* sign appears.

    Electronic thermometer: Remove the probe from base unit. Put on probe cover.

8. Position thermometer (bulb end for mercury-free) in center of the armpit. Fold resident's arm over his chest.

9. **Mercury-free thermometer**: Hold the thermometer in place, with the arm close against the side, for 8 to 10 minutes (Fig. 7-16).

Digital thermometer: Leave in place until thermometer blinks or beeps.

Electronic thermometer: Leave in place until you hear a tone or see a flashing or steady light.

Fig. 7-16. *After inserting the thermometer, fold the resident's arm over his chest and hold it in place for 8 to 10 minutes.*

10. **Mercury-free thermometer**: Remove the thermometer. Wipe with a tissue from stem to bulb or remove sheath. Dispose of the tissue or sheath. Read the thermometer at eye level as you would for an oral temperature. Remember the temperature reading.

    Digital thermometer: Remove the thermometer. Read temperature on display screen. Remember the temperature reading.

    Electronic thermometer: Read the temperature on the display screen. Remember the temperature reading. Remove the probe.

11. **Mercury-free thermometer**: Clean thermometer with soap and water. Rinse with clean water and dry. Return it to case.

    Digital thermometer: Using a tissue, remove and dispose of sheath. Replace the thermometer in case.

    Electronic thermometer: Press the eject button to discard the cover. Return the probe to the holder.

12. Remove and discard gloves.

13. Wash your hands.
    Provides for infection prevention.

14. Put resident's arm back into sleeve of gown.

15. Immediately record the temperature, date, time and method used (axillary).
    Record temperature immediately so you won't forget. Care plans are made based on your report.

16. Place call light within resident's reach.
    Allows resident to communicate with staff as necessary.

17. Report any changes in resident to the nurse.
    Provides nurse with information to assess resident.

Pulse

The pulse is the number of heartbeats per minute. The beat that is felt at certain pulse points in the body represents the wave of blood moving through the artery. This is a result of the heart pumping. The most common site for checking the pulse is on the inside of the wrist, where the radial artery runs just beneath the skin. This is called the **radial pulse**. The **brachial pulse** is the pulse inside the elbow. It is about one to one-and-a-half inches above the elbow. The radial and brachial pulses are involved in taking blood pressure. Blood pressure is explained later in this chapter. Common pulse sites are shown in Fig. 7-17.

For adults, the normal pulse rate is 60 to 100 beats per minute. Small children have faster pulses, in the range of 100 to 120 beats per minute. A newborn baby's pulse may be as high as 120 to 140 beats per minute. Many things can affect the pulse rate. These include exercise, fear, anger, anxiety, heat, infection, medications, and pain. An unusually high or low rate may not indicate disease. However, sometimes the pulse rate can signal that illness exists. For example, a rapid pulse may result from fever, dehydration, or heart failure. A slow or weak pulse may indicate infection.

Fig. 7-17. *Common pulse sites.*

Respirations

Respiration is the process of breathing air into the lungs, or **inspiration**, and exhaling air out of the lungs, or **expiration**. Each respiration consists of an inspiration and an expiration. The chest rises during inspiration and falls during expiration.

The normal respiration rate for adults ranges from 12 to 20 breaths per minute. Infants and children have a faster respiratory rate. Infants normally breathe at a rate of 30 to 40 respirations per minute. People may breathe more quickly if they know they are being observed. Because of this, respirations should be counted immediately after taking the pulse. The NA should keep her fingers on the resident's wrist or on the stethoscope over the heart. She should not make it obvious that she is watching the resident's breathing.

Measuring and recording radial pulse and counting and recording respirations

Equipment: watch with a second hand, pen and paper

1. Identify yourself by name. Identify the resident by name.
   Resident has right to know identity of his or her caregiver. Addressing resident by name shows respect and establishes correct identification.

2. Wash your hands.
    Provides for infection prevention.

3. Explain procedure to resident. Speak clearly, slowly, and directly. Maintain face-to-face contact whenever possible.
    Promotes understanding and independence.

4. Provide for resident's privacy with curtain, screen, or door.
    Maintains resident's right to privacy and dignity.

5. Place fingertips on thumb side of resident's wrist. Locate radial pulse (Fig. 7-18).

Fig. 7-18. Measure the radial pulse by placing fingertips on the thumb side of the wrist.

6. Count beats for one full minute.

7. Keep your fingertips on the resident's wrist. Count respirations for one full minute. Observe for the pattern and character of the resident's breathing. Normal breathing is smooth and quiet. If you see signs of troubled, shallow, or noisy breathing, such as wheezing, report it.
    Count will be more accurate if resident does not know you are counting his respirations.

8. Wash your hands.
    Provides for infection prevention.

9. Record pulse rate, date, time, and method used (radial). Record the respiratory rate and the pattern or character of breathing.
    Record pulse and respiration rate immediately so you won't forget. Care plans are made based on your report.

10. Place call light within resident's reach.
    Allows resident to communicate with staff as necessary.

11. Report any changes in resident to the nurse. Report to the nurse if the pulse is less than 60 beats per minute, over 100 beats per minute, if the rhythm is irregular, or if breathing is irregular.
    Provides nurse with information to assess resident.

Blood Pressure

Blood pressure is an important measure of health. Blood pressure is measured in millimeters of mercury (mmHg). The measurement shows how well the heart is working. There are two parts of blood pressure: the systolic measurement and the diastolic measurement.

In the **systolic** phase, the heart is at work. It contracts and pushes blood from the left ventricle of the heart. The reading shows the pressure on the walls of the arteries as blood is pumped through the body. The normal range for systolic blood pressure is 100 to 119 mmHg.

The second measurement reflects the **diastolic** phase. This is when the heart relaxes. The diastolic measurement is always lower than the systolic measurement. It shows the pressure in the arteries when the heart is at rest. The normal range for adults is 60 to 79 mmHg.

If blood pressure is between 120/80 mmHg and 139/89 mmHg, it is called prehypertension. This means that the person does not have high blood pressure now but is likely to develop it in the future.

People with high blood pressure, or hypertension, have elevated systolic and/or diastolic blood pressures. A blood pressure level of 140/90 mmHg or higher is considered high. Recent studies indicate, however, that blood pressure may measure as high as 150/90 in people over 60 without making it necessary to treat it with medication. There is still some disagreement among doctors about this issue. A measurement of 140/90 or higher is still considered hypertension.

Many factors can increase blood pressure. These include aging, exercise, physical or emotional stress, pain, medications, and the volume of blood in circulation.

Blood pressure is measured with a stethoscope and a blood pressure cuff, or sphygmomanometer (Fig. 7-19). There may be a digital sphygmomanometer available. The systolic and diastolic pressure readings and pulse are displayed digitally. The use of a stethoscope is not required with a digital sphygmomanometer.

Fig. 7-19. The top photo shows an aneroid sphygmomanometer. The bottom photo shows a type of digital sphygmomanometer that measures other vital signs as well.

When taking blood pressure, the first sound heard is the systolic pressure (top number). When the sound changes to a soft muffled thump or disappears, this is the diastolic pressure (bottom number). Blood pressure is

recorded as a fraction. The systolic reading is on top and the diastolic reading is on the bottom (for example: 120/80).

Blood pressure should not be measured on an arm that has an IV, a dialysis shunt, or any medical equipment. A side that has a cast, recent trauma, paralysis from a stroke, burn(s), or breast surgery (mastectomy) should be avoided.

It is important to use a cuff that is the correct size when measuring blood pressure. Available sizes include standard, pediatric, and large.

Measuring and recording blood pressure (one-step method)

Equipment: sphygmomanometer (blood pressure cuff), stethoscope, alcohol wipes, pen and paper

1. Identify yourself by name. Identify the resident by name.
    Resident has right to know identity of his or her caregiver. Addressing resident by name shows respect and establishes correct identification.

2. Wash your hands.
    Provides for infection prevention.

3. Explain procedure to the resident. Speak clearly, slowly, and directly. Maintain face-to-face contact whenever possible.
    Promotes understanding and independence.

4. Provide for resident's privacy with curtain, screen, or door.
    Maintains resident's right to privacy and dignity.

5. Before using stethoscope, wipe diaphragm and earpieces with alcohol wipes.
    Reduces pathogens, prevents ear infections, and prevents spread of infection.

6. Ask the resident to roll up his sleeve so that the upper arm is exposed. Do not measure blood pressure over clothing.

7. Position resident's arm with palm up. The arm should be level with the heart.
    A false low reading is possible if arm is above heart level.

8. With the valve open, squeeze the cuff. Make sure it is completely deflated.

9. Place blood pressure cuff snugly on resident's upper arm. The center of the cuff with sensor/arrow is placed over the brachial artery (1-1½ inches above the elbow, toward inside of elbow) (Fig. 7-20).
Cuff must be proper size and put on arm correctly so amount of pressure on artery is correct. If not, reading will be falsely high or low.

Fig. 7-20. *Place the center of the cuff over the brachial artery.*

10. Locate brachial pulse with fingertips.

11. Place earpieces of stethoscope in your ears.

12. Place diaphragm of stethoscope over brachial artery.

13. Close the valve (clockwise) until it stops. Do not over-tighten it (Fig. 7-21).
Tight valves are too hard to release.

Fig. 7-21. *Close the valve, but do not over-tighten it.*

14. Inflate cuff to between 160 mmHg to 180 mmHg. If a beat is heard immediately upon cuff deflation, completely deflate cuff. Reinflate cuff to no more than 200 mmHg.

15. Open the valve slightly with thumb and index finger. Deflate cuff slowly.
Releasing the valve slowly allows you to hear beats accurately.

16. Watch gauge. Listen for sound of the pulse.

17. Remember the reading at which the first pulse sound is heard. This is the systolic pressure.

18. Continue listening for a change or muffling of pulse sound. The point of a change or the point at which the sound disappears is the diastolic pressure. Remember this reading.

19. Open the valve. Deflate cuff completely. Remove cuff.
An inflated cuff left on resident's arm can cause numbness and tingling. If you must take blood pressure again, completely deflate cuff and wait 30 seconds. Never partially deflate a cuff and then pump it up again. Blood vessels will be damaged and reading will be falsely high or low.

20. Wash your hands.
Provides for infection prevention.

21. Record both the systolic and diastolic pressures. Record the numbers like a fraction, with the systolic reading on top and the diastolic reading on the bottom (for example: 120/80). Note which arm was used. Use *RA* for right arm and *LA* for left arm.
Record readings immediately so you won't forget. Care plans are made based on your report.

22. Wipe diaphragm and earpieces of stethoscope with alcohol wipes. Store equipment.

23. Place call light within resident's reach.
Allows resident to communicate with staff as necessary.

24. Wash your hands.
Provides for infection prevention.

25. Report any changes in resident to the nurse.
Provides nurse with information to assess resident.

In addition to other vital sign measurements, some NAs may be asked to obtain a pulse oximeter reading. A pulse oximeter is a device that uses a light to determine the amount of oxygen in the blood. A pulse oximeter also measures a person's pulse rate (Fig. 7-22).

Fig. 7-22. *A pulse oximeter sensor is usually clipped on a person's finger to measure the amount of oxygen in the blood, as well as pulse rate.*

A pulse oximeter may be used when residents have had surgery, are on oxygen, are in intensive care, or have cardiac or respiratory problems. When asked to obtain this reading, the NA should report the oxygen percentage to the nurse. The nurse will determine if the level is adequate for the resident.

Pain Management

Pain is often referred to as the fifth vital sign because it is as important to monitor as the other vital signs. NAs must observe and report residents' pain carefully. Pain is uncomfortable. It can quickly drain energy and hope. It is also a personal experience. This means it is different for each person. NAs spend the most time with residents. They play an important role in pain monitoring and prevention. Care plans are made based on NAs' reports.

Pain is **not** a normal part of aging. Sustained pain may lead to withdrawal, depression, and isolation. NAs must treat residents' complaints of pain seriously. They should listen to what residents are saying about the way they feel. They should take action to help them. If a resident complains of pain, the NA should ask these questions and then immediately report the information to the nurse:

- Where is the pain?

- When did the pain start?

- Is the pain mild, moderate, or severe? To help find out, the NA can ask the resident to rate the pain on a scale of 0 to 5 or 0 to 10, with 5 or 10 being the worst pain (Fig. 7-23).

Fig. 7-23. *The Wong-Baker FACES Pain Rating Scale is one type of pain scale. The NA can point to each face and ask the resident to choose the face that best describes his pain.* (FROM HOCKENBERRY MJ, WILSON D, WINKELSTEIN ML: WONG'S ESSENTIALS OF PEDIATRIC NURSING, ED. 7, ST. LOUIS, 2005, P. 1259. USED WITH PERMISSION. COPYRIGHT MOSBY.)

- Can you describe the pain? The NA should use the resident's words when reporting to the nurse.

- What were you doing before the pain started?

- How long does the pain last, and how often does it occur?

- What makes the pain better? What makes the pain worse?

Residents may have concerns about their pain. These concerns may make them hesitant to report their pain. Barriers to managing pain include the following:

- Fear of addiction to pain medication

- Feeling that pain is a normal part of aging

- Worrying about constipation and fatigue from pain medication

- Feeling that caregivers are too busy to deal with their pain

- Feeling that too much pain medication will cause death

NAs should be patient and caring when helping residents who are in pain. If residents are worried about the effects of pain medication or have questions about it, the NA should tell the nurse. Some people do not feel comfortable saying that they are in pain. A person's culture affects how he or she responds to pain. Some cultures believe that it is best not to react to pain. Other cultures believe in expressing pain freely. The NA should watch for body language or other messages that show that residents may be in pain.

Observing and Reporting: Pain

Report any of these to the nurse:

O/R Increased pulse, respirations, blood pressure

O/R Sweating

O/R Nausea

O/R Vomiting

O/R Tightening the jaw

O/R Squeezing eyes shut

O/R Holding or guarding a body part

O/R Frowning

O/R Grinding teeth

O/R Increased restlessness

O/R Agitation or tension

O/R Change in behavior

O/R Crying

O/R Sighing

O/R Groaning

O/R Breathing heavily

O/R Rocking

O/R Pacing

O/R Repetitive movements

O/R Difficulty moving or walking

To help reduce pain, the NA should

- Report complaints of pain or unrelieved pain promptly to the nurse.

- Gently position the body in proper alignment. Use pillows for support. Help in changes of position if the resident wishes.

- Give back rubs.

- Ask if the resident would like to take a warm bath or shower.

- Help the resident to the bathroom or commode or offer the bedpan or urinal.

- Encourage slow, deep breathing.

- Provide a calm and quiet environment. Soft music may distract the resident.

- Be patient, caring, gentle, and responsive.

3. Explain how to measure weight and height

NAs measure residents' weight and height as part of regular care. Height is checked less often than weight. Weight changes can be signs of illness. NAs must report **any** weight loss or gain, no matter how small. Weight will be measured using pounds or kilograms. A pound is a unit of weight equal to 16 ounces. A kilogram is a unit of mass equal to 1000 grams; one kilogram equals 2.2 pounds.

Measuring and recording weight of an ambulatory resident

Equipment: standing/upright scale, pen and paper

1. Identify yourself by name. Identify the resident by name.
   Resident has right to know identity of his or her caregiver. Addressing resident by name shows respect and establishes correct identification.

2. Wash your hands.
   Provides for infection prevention.

3. Explain procedure to resident. Speak clearly, slowly, and directly. Maintain face-to-face contact whenever possible.
   Promotes understanding and independence.

4. Provide for resident's privacy with curtain, screen, or door.
Maintains resident's right to privacy and dignity.

5. Make sure resident is wearing nonskid shoes that are fastened before walking to scale.

6. Start with scale balanced at zero before weighing the resident.
Scale must be balanced on zero for weight to be accurate.

7. Help resident to step onto the center of the scale. Be sure she is not holding, touching, or leaning against anything.
This interferes with weight measurement.

8. Determine resident's weight. Balance the scale by making the balance bar level. Move the small and large weight indicators until the bar balances. Read the two numbers shown (on the small and large weight indicators) when the bar is balanced. Add these two numbers together. This is the resident's weight (Fig. 7-24).

Fig. 7-24. *Move the small and large weight indicators until the bar balances. The weight shown in the illustration is 169 pounds.*

9. Help resident to safely step off scale before recording weight.
Protects against falls.

10. Wash your hands.
Provides for infection prevention.

11. Record the resident's weight.
Record weight immediately so you won't forget. Care plans are made based on your report.

12. Place call light within resident's reach.
Allows resident to communicate with staff as necessary.

13. Report any changes in resident to the nurse.
Provides nurse with information to assess resident.

Some residents will not be able to get out of wheelchairs easily. These residents may be weighed on a wheelchair scale. With this scale, wheelchairs are rolled directly onto the scale (Fig. 7-25). On some wheelchair scales, the NA will need to subtract the weight of the wheelchair from a resident's weight. If the wheelchair weight is not listed on the chair, the NA should weigh the empty wheelchair first. The footrests should be attached if they will be attached when the resident is in the chair. Then he should subtract the wheelchair's weight from the total.

Fig. 7-25. *Wheelchairs can be rolled directly onto wheelchair scales to determine weight.* (PHOTO COURTESY OF DETECTO, WWW.DETECTO.COM, 800-641-2008)

When residents are not able to get out of bed, they are weighed on special bed scales (Fig. 7-26). Before using a bed scale, the NA should know how to use it properly and safely.

Fig. 7-26. *A type of bed scale.* (PHOTO COURTESY OF DETECTO, WWW.DETECTO.COM, 800-641-2008)

For measuring height, the rod measures in inches and fractions of inches. The NA should record the total number of inches. If the NA has to convert inches into feet, there are 12 inches in one foot.

Measuring and recording height of a resident

For residents who can get out of bed, you will measure height using a standing scale.

Equipment: standing scale, pen, and paper

1. Identify yourself by name. Identify the resident by name.
   Resident has right to know identity of his or her caregiver. Addressing resident by name shows respect and establishes correct identification.

2. Wash your hands.
   Provides for infection prevention.

3. Explain procedure to resident. Speak clearly, slowly, and directly. Maintain face-to-face contact whenever possible.
   Promotes understanding and independence.

4. Provide for resident's privacy with curtain, screen, or door.
   Maintains resident's right to privacy and dignity.

5. Make sure resident is wearing nonskid shoes that are securely fastened before walking to scale.

6. Help resident to step onto scale, facing away from the scale.

7. Ask resident to stand straight if possible. Help as needed.
   Ensures accurate reading.

8. Pull up measuring rod from back of scale. Gently lower measuring rod until it rests flat on resident's head (Fig. 7-27).

9. Determine the resident's height.

10. Help resident off scale before recording height. Make sure measuring rod does not hit resident in the head.

Fig. 7-27. *To determine height on a standing scale, gently lower the measuring rod until it rests flat on the resident's head.*

11. Wash your hands.
    Provides for infection prevention.

12. Record the resident's height.
    Record height immediately so you won't forget. Care plans are made based on your report.

13. Place call light within resident's reach.
    Allows resident to communicate with staff as necessary.

14. Report any changes in resident to the nurse.
    Provides nurse with information to assess resident.

Some residents will be unable to get out of bed. Height is sometimes measured by using a tape measure and making two pencil marks on the sheet that is underneath the resident. The NA makes a mark at the top of the resident's head and one at his heel and measures the distance between the marks (Figs. 7-28 and 7-29). Height of a bedridden resident can also be measured using other methods. NAs should follow the procedures used at their facilities.

Basic Nursing Skills

Fig. 7-28. *Height can be measured in bed using a tape measure.*

Fig. 7-29. *One way that height of a bedridden resident can be measured is by making marks on the sheet at the resident's head and heel. Then the distance between the marks is measured.*

4. Explain restraints and how to promote a restraint-free environment

A **restraint** is a physical or chemical way to restrict voluntary movement or behavior. Examples of physical restraints are vest and jacket restraints, belt restraints, wrist/ankle restraints, and mitt restraints. Raised side rails on beds and geriatric chairs with tray tables attached are also physical restraints (Figs. 7-30 and 7-31). Chemical restraints are medications given to control a person's behavior.

Fig. 7-30. *Raised side rails are considered restraints because they restrict movement.*

Fig. 7-31. *While the tray table is attached or locked, a geriatric chair, or geri-chair, is considered a restraint.*

In the past, restraints were commonly used for these reasons:

- To prevent confused people from wandering
- To prevent falls
- To keep people from injuring themselves or others
- To prevent people from pulling out tubing needed for treatment

Restraint use was sometimes abused by caregivers. Residents were injured. This led to new laws restricting the use of restraints. Today, long-term care facilities are prohibited from using restraints unless they are medically necessary. They are only used as a last resort. They are only used after other measures have been tried. If a restraint is needed, a doctor must order it. Very specific guidelines apply to carrying out a restraint order. This includes frequent monitoring of the resident. NAs cannot use physical restraints unless a doctor has ordered it in the care plan and they have been trained in the restraint's use. It is against the law for staff to apply a restraint for convenience or to discipline a resident. NAs can check with their supervisor for policies regarding restraints.

There are many serious problems that occur with restraint use. They include the following:

- Pressure ulcers
- Pneumonia

- Risk of suffocation (suffocation is the stoppage of breathing from a lack of oxygen or excess of carbon dioxide in the body; it may result in unconsciousness or death)

- Reduced blood circulation

- Stress on the heart

- Incontinence

- Constipation

- Weakened muscles and bones

- Muscle atrophy (weakening or wasting away of the muscle)

- Loss of bone mass

- Poor appetite and malnutrition

- Depression and/or withdrawal

- Sleep disorders

- Loss of dignity

- Loss of independence

- Stress and anxiety

- Increased agitation (anxiety, restlessness)

- Loss of self-esteem

- Severe injury

- Death

Restraint usage has significantly decreased in facilities. State and federal agencies encourage facilities to take steps to create restraint-free environments. **Restraint-free care** means that restraints are not kept or used for any reason. Creative ideas that help avoid the need for restraints are being used instead. **Restraint alternatives** are any intervention used in the place of a restraint or that reduces the need for a restraint. Examples of restraint alternatives include the following:

- Improve safety measures to prevent accidents and falls. Improve lighting.

- Make sure call lights are within reach. Respond to call lights promptly.

- Ambulate the resident when he is restless. The doctor or nurse may add exercise into the care plan.

- Provide activities for those who wander at night.

- Encourage activities and independence. Escort the resident to social activities. Increase visits and social interaction.

- Give frequent help with toileting. Help with cleaning immediately after an episode of incontinence.

- Offer food or drink. Offer reading materials.

- Distract or redirect interest. Give the resident a repetitive task.

- Decrease the noise level. Listen to soothing music. Offer massage or use relaxation techniques.

- Reduce pain levels through medication. The resident should be monitored closely. Complaints of pain should be reported immediately.

- Provide familiar caregivers. Increase the number of caregivers with family and volunteers.

- Use a team approach to meeting needs. Offer training to teach gentle approaches to difficult people.

There are also several types of pads, belts, special chairs, and alarms that can be used instead of restraints. If a resident is ordered to have an alarm on his bed or chair, the NA should make sure it is there and is turned on.

OBRA sets specific rules for restraint use. Restraints can only be applied with a doctor's order. An NA cannot use a restraint unless the charge nurse has approved its use and the NA has been trained to use it properly. If a restraint has been ordered, the NA must place the call light where the resident can easily access it. She should answer call lights immediately. A restrained resident must be monitored constantly. He must be checked often, following facility policy. At regular, ordered intervals, the following must be done:

- Release the restraint (or discontinue use).

- Reassure the resident.

- Offer help with toileting. Check for episodes of incontinence. Provide incontinence care.

- Offer fluids and food.

- Check the skin for signs of irritation. Report any red, purple, blue, gray, or pale skin or any discolored areas to the nurse immediately.

- Check for swelling of the body part and report any swelling immediately.

- Reposition the resident.

- Ambulate the resident if he is able.

If any problems occur with the restraint, especially injury, the NA should notify the nurse and complete an incident report as soon as possible.

5. Define *fluid balance* and explain intake and output (I&O)

To maintain health, the body must take in a certain amount of fluid each day. Fluid comes in the form of liquids that a person drinks. It is also found in semi-liquid foods like gelatin, soup, ice cream, pudding, and yogurt. Generally, a healthy person needs about 64 ounces (oz) of fluid each day. The fluid a person consumes is called **intake**, or **input**. All fluid taken in each day cannot stay in the body. It must be eliminated as **output**. Output includes urine, feces (including diarrhea), and vomitus. It also includes perspiration and moisture in the air that a person exhales, and wound drainage.

Fluid balance is maintaining equal input and output, or taking in and eliminating equal amounts of fluids. Most people do this naturally. But some residents must have their intake and output, or I&O, monitored and recorded. To do this, the NA will need to measure and document

all fluids the resident takes by mouth, as well as all urine and vomitus produced. This is recorded on an Intake/Output (I&O) sheet (Fig. 7-32).

Fig. 7-32. *This is one type of intake/output record.*
(REPRINTED WITH PERMISSION OF BRIGGS CORPORATION, 800-247-2343, WWW.BRIGGSCORP.COM)

Conversions

One milliliter (mL) is a unit of measure equal to one cubic centimeter (cc). Follow your facility's policies on whether to document using mL or cc.

1 oz = 30 mL or 30 cc

2 oz = 60 mL

3 oz = 90 mL

4 oz = 120 mL

5 oz = 150 mL

6 oz = 180 mL

7 oz = 210 mL

8 oz = 240 mL

¼ cup = 2 oz = 60 mL

½ cup = 4 oz = 120 mL

1 cup = 8 oz = 240 mL

Measuring and recording urinary output

Equipment: I&O sheet, graduate (measuring container), gloves

1. Wash your hands.
   Provides for infection prevention.

2. Put on gloves before handling bedpan/urinal.

3. Pour the contents of the bedpan or urinal into graduate. Do not spill or splash any of the urine.

4. Place graduate on flat surface. Measure the amount of urine at eye level. Keep container level (Fig. 7-33). Remember the amount.
   A flat surface helps get an accurate reading.

Fig. 7-33. *Keep container on a flat surface while measuring output.*

5. After measuring urine, empty graduate into toilet. Do not splash urine.
   Reduces risk of contamination.

6. Rinse graduate. Pour rinse water into toilet.

7. Rinse bedpan/urinal. Pour rinse water into toilet. Flush the toilet.

8. Place graduate and bedpan/urinal in area for cleaning or clean and store according to facility policy.

9. Remove and discard gloves.

10. Wash hands before recording output.
    Provides for infection prevention.

11. Document the time and amount of urine in output column on sheet. For example: 1545 hours, 200 mL urine.
    Record amount immediately so you won't forget. Care plans are made based on your report. If you do not document the care, legally it did not happen.

12. Report any changes in resident to the nurse.
    Provides nurse with information to assess resident.

Collecting Specimens

NAs may need to collect a specimen from a resident. A **specimen** is a sample that is used for analysis in order to try to make a diagnosis. Different types of specimens are used for different tests. Different types of specimens that NAs may be asked to collect include the following:

- Urine (routine, clean-catch/mid-stream, or 24-hour)

- Stool (feces)

- Sputum (mucus coughed up from the lungs)

A **routine urine specimen** is collected anytime the resident **voids**, or urinates. The resident will void into a bedpan, urinal, commode, or hat. A **hat** is a plastic collection container sometimes put into a toilet to collect and measure urine or stool (Fig. 7-34). Some residents will be able to collect their own specimens. Others will need an NA's help. The seal must be intact on specimen containers before they are used. This helps avoid specimen contamination. All specimens must be labeled with the resident's first and last name, date of birth, room number, and the date and time the specimen was collected.

Fig. 7-34. *A hat is a container that is placed under the toilet seat to collect and measure urine or stool. Hats should be labeled. They must be cleaned after each use.*

Specimens

Body wastes and elimination needs are very private matters for most people. Residents may be embarrassed by having another person handle their body wastes. NAs should be sensitive to this. They should empathize with residents. An NA should be professional when collecting specimens. If she feels that this is an unpleasant task, she should not make it known. She should not make faces or frown. She should not use words that let the resident know she feels uncomfortable. Remaining professional when collecting specimens can help put residents at ease.

Collecting a routine urine specimen

Equipment: urine specimen container with completed label (labeled with resident's name, date of birth, room number, date, and time) and lid, specimen bag, 2 pairs of gloves, bedpan or urinal (if resident cannot use portable commode or toilet), hat for toilet (if resident uses portable commode or toilet), plastic bag, toilet paper, disposable wipes, paper towels, supplies for perineal care, lab slip

1. Identify yourself by name. Identify the resident by name.
    Resident has right to know identity of his or her caregiver. Addressing resident by name shows respect and establishes correct identification.

2. Wash your hands.
    Provides for infection prevention.

3. Explain procedure to the resident. Speak clearly, slowly, and directly. Maintain face-to-face contact whenever possible.
    Promotes understanding and independence.

4. Provide for resident's privacy with curtain, screen, or door.
    Maintains resident's right to privacy and dignity.

5. Put on gloves.
    Prevents you from coming into contact with body fluids.

6. Fit hat to toilet or commode, or provide resident with bedpan or urinal.

7. Ask resident to void into hat, urinal, or bedpan. Ask the resident not to put toilet paper in with the sample. Provide a plastic bag to discard toilet paper separately.
    Paper ruins the sample.

8. Place toilet paper and disposable wipes within resident's reach. Ask resident to clean his hands with a wipe when finished if he is able.

9. Remove and discard gloves. Wash your hands.

10. Place the call light within resident's reach. Ask resident to signal when done. Leave the room and close the door.
    Promotes resident's privacy and dignity.

11. When called, return and put on clean gloves. Give perineal care if help is needed.

12. Take bedpan, urinal, or hat to the bathroom.

13. Pour urine into the specimen container. Specimen container should be at least half full.

14. Cover the urine container with its lid. Do not touch the inside of container. Wipe off the outside with a paper towel. Apply label.
    Prevents contamination.

15. Place the container in a clean specimen bag (Fig. 7-35).
    Provides for safe transport.

Fig. 7-35. *Specimens must always be labeled with the resident's name, date of birth, room number, the date, and time, before being taken to the lab. A specimen may need to be placed in a clean specimen bag before transporting it.*

16. Discard extra urine in the toilet. Turn the faucet on with a paper towel. Rinse the bedpan, urinal, or hat with cold water and empty it into the toilet. Flush the toilet. Place equipment in proper area for cleaning or clean it according to facility policy.

17. Remove and discard gloves.

18. Wash your hands.
    Provides for infection prevention.

19. Place call light within resident's reach.
    Allows resident to communicate with staff as necessary.

20. Report any changes in resident to the nurse.
    Provides nurse with information to assess resident.

21. Take specimen and lab slip to proper area. Document procedure using facility guidelines. Note amount and characteristics of urine.
    If you do not document the care, legally it did not happen.

The **clean-catch specimen**, or mid-stream specimen (CCMS), does not include the first and

last urine in the sample. Its purpose is to determine the presence of bacteria in the urine.

Collecting a clean-catch (mid-stream) urine specimen

Equipment: specimen kit with container with completed label (labeled with resident's name, date of birth, room number, date, and time) and lid, specimen bag, cleaning solution, gloves, bedpan or urinal (if resident cannot use portable commode or toilet), plastic bag, toilet paper, disposable wipes, paper towels, towels, supplies for perineal care, lab slip

1. Identify yourself by name. Identify the resident by name.
   Resident has right to know identity of his or her caregiver. Addressing resident by name shows respect and establishes correct identification.

2. Wash your hands.
   Provides for infection prevention.

3. Explain procedure to resident. Speak clearly, slowly, and directly. Maintain face-to-face contact whenever possible.
   Promotes understanding and independence.

4. Provide for resident's privacy with curtain, screen, or door.
   Maintains resident's right to privacy and dignity.

5. Put on gloves.
   Prevents you from coming into contact with body fluids.

6. Open the specimen kit. Do not touch the inside of the container or inside of lid.
   Prevents contamination.

7. If the resident cannot clean his or her perineal area, you will do it. Use the wipes and cleaning solution to do this. Use a clean area of the wipe or clean wipe for each stroke. See bed bath procedure in Chapter 6 for a reminder on how to give perineal care.
   Improper cleaning can infect urinary tract and contaminate the sample.

8. Ask the resident to urinate a small amount into the bedpan, urinal, or toilet, and to stop before urination is complete.

9. Place the container under the urine stream. Have the resident start urinating again. Fill the container at least half full. Ask the resident to stop urinating and remove the container. Have the resident finish urinating in bedpan, urinal, or toilet.

10. After urination, provide a plastic bag so resident can discard toilet paper. Give perineal care if help is needed. Ask resident to clean his hands with a wipe if he is able.

11. Cover the urine container with its lid. Do not touch the inside of the container. Wipe off the outside with a paper towel. Apply label.

12. Place the container in a clean specimen bag.
    Provides for safe transport.

13. Discard extra urine in toilet. Turn the faucet on with a paper towel. Rinse the bedpan or urinal with cold water and empty it into the toilet. Flush the toilet. Place equipment in proper area for cleaning or clean it according to facility policy.

14. Remove and discard gloves.

15. Wash your hands.
    Promotes infection prevention.

16. Place call light within resident's reach.
    Allows resident to communicate with staff as necessary.

17. Report any changes in resident to the nurse.
    Provides nurse with information to assess resident.

18. Take specimen and lab slip to proper area. Document procedure using facility guidelines. Note amount and characteristics of urine.
    If you do not document the care, legally it did not happen.

The NA should ask the resident to let her know when he can have a bowel movement. She should be ready to collect the specimen.

Collecting a stool specimen

Equipment: specimen container with completed label (labeled with resident's name, date of birth, room number, date, and time) and lid, specimen bag, 2 pairs of gloves, 2 tongue blades, bedpan (if resident cannot use portable commode or toilet), hat for toilet (if resident uses portable commode or toilet), plastic bag, toilet paper, disposable wipes, paper towels, supplies for perineal care, lab slip

1. Identify yourself by name. Identify the resident by name.
   Resident has right to know identity of his or her caregiver. Addressing resident by name shows respect and establishes correct identification.

2. Wash your hands.
   Provides for infection prevention.

3. Explain procedure to resident. Speak clearly, slowly, and directly. Maintain face-to-face contact whenever possible.
   Promotes understanding and independence.

4. Provide for resident's privacy with curtain, screen, or door.
   Maintains resident's right to privacy and dignity.

5. Put on gloves.
   Prevents you from coming into contact with body fluids.

6. Fit hat to toilet or commode, or provide resident with bedpan.

7. Ask the resident not to urinate when he is ready to move bowels. Ask him not to put toilet paper in with the sample. Provide a plastic bag to discard toilet paper separately.
   Urine and paper ruin the sample.

8. Place toilet paper and disposable wipes within resident's reach. Ask resident to clean his hands with a wipe when finished if he is able.

9. Remove and discard gloves. Wash your hands.
   Promotes infection prevention.

10. Place the call light within resident's reach. Ask resident to signal when done. Leave the room and close the door.
Promotes resident's privacy and dignity.

11. When called, return and put on clean gloves. Give perineal care if help is needed.

12. Using the two tongue blades, take about two tablespoons of stool and put it in the container. Without touching the inside of the container, cover it tightly. Apply label and place container in a clean specimen bag.
Prevents contamination.

13. Wrap tongue blades in toilet paper. Put them in plastic bag with used toilet paper. Discard bag in proper container.

14. Empty the bedpan or container into the toilet. Turn the faucet on with a paper towel. Rinse the bedpan with cold water and empty it into the toilet. Flush the toilet. Place equipment in proper area for cleaning or clean it according to facility policy.

15. Remove and discard gloves.

16. Wash your hands.
Provides for infection prevention.

17. Place call light within resident's reach.
Allows resident to communicate with staff as necessary.

18. Report any changes in resident to the nurse.
Provides nurse with information to assess resident.

19. Take specimen and lab slip to proper area. Document procedure using facility guidelines. Note amount and characteristics of stool.
If you do not document the care, legally it did not happen.

Sputum specimens are collected to check for respiratory problems or illness. Early morning is the best time to collect sputum. The resident should cough up the sputum and spit it directly into the specimen container. Gloves must be worn when collecting sputum (or any specimen). A mask may be required as well.

6. Explain care guidelines for urinary catheters, oxygen therapy, and IV therapy

A **catheter** is a thin tube inserted into the body that is used to drain fluids or inject fluids. A **urinary catheter** is used to drain urine from the bladder. A **straight catheter** does not remain inside the person. It is removed immediately after urine is drained. An **indwelling catheter** (also called a *Foley catheter*) remains inside the bladder for a period of time (Fig. 7-36). The urine drains into a bag. Nursing assistants do not insert, remove, or irrigate catheters. NAs may be asked to provide daily care for the catheter, cleaning the area around the urethral opening, and emptying the drainage bag.

a)   b)

Fig. 7-36. *An illustration of a) an indwelling catheter (female) and b) an indwelling catheter (male).*

An external catheter, or **condom catheter** (also called a *Texas catheter*), has an attachment on the end that fits onto the penis. The attachment is fastened with special tape. Urine drains through the catheter into the tubing, then into the drainage bag. The external catheter is changed daily or as needed.

Guidelines: Urinary Catheters

G   Make sure that the drainage bag is always lower than the hips or bladder. Urine must never flow from the bag or tubing back into the bladder. This can cause infection.

G   Keep the drainage bag off the floor.

G   Keep the tubing as straight as possible. It should not be kinked.

G   Keep the genital area clean to prevent infection. Because the catheter goes all the way into the bladder, bacteria can enter the bladder more easily. Daily care of the genital area (perineal care) is especially important.

Observing and Reporting: Urinary Catheters

Report any of these to the nurse:

O/R   Blood in the urine or urine that looks unusual in any way

O/R   Catheter bag does not fill after several hours

O/R   Catheter bag fills suddenly

O/R   Catheter is not in place

O/R   Urine leaks from the catheter

O/R   Resident reports pain or pressure

O/R   Odor is present

Providing catheter care

Equipment: bath blanket, protective pads, bath basin with warm water, soap, bath thermometer, 2-4 washcloths or disposable wipes, towel, gloves

1. Identify yourself by name. Identify the resident by name.
   Resident has right to know identity of his or her caregiver. Addressing resident by name shows respect and establishes correct identification.

2. Wash your hands.
   Provides for infection prevention.

3. Explain procedure to resident. Speak clearly, slowly, and directly. Maintain face-to-face contact whenever possible.
   Promotes understanding and independence.

4. Provide for resident's privacy with curtain, screen, or door.
   Maintains resident's right to privacy and dignity.

5. Adjust bed to a safe level, usually waist high. Lock bed wheels.
   Prevents injury to you and to resident.

6. Lower head of bed. Position resident lying flat on her back.

7. Remove or fold back top bedding. Keep resident covered with bath blanket.
   Promotes resident's privacy.

8. Test water temperature with thermometer or on the inside of your wrist to ensure it is safe. Water temperature should be no higher than 105°F. Have resident check water temperature. Adjust if necessary.
   Resident's sense of touch may be different than yours; therefore, resident is best able to identify a comfortable water temperature.

9. Put on gloves.
   Prevents you from coming into contact with body fluids.

10. Ask the resident to flex her knees and raise her buttocks off the bed by pushing against the mattress with her feet. Place clean protective pad under her buttocks.
    Keeps linen from getting wet.

11. Expose only the area necessary to clean the catheter. Avoid overexposing resident.
    Promotes resident's privacy.

12. Place towel or pad under catheter tubing before washing.
    Helps keep linen from getting wet.

13. Wet washcloth in basin. Apply soap to washcloth. Clean area around meatus. Use a clean area of the washcloth for each stroke.

14. Hold catheter near meatus. Avoid tugging the catheter.

15. Clean at least four inches of catheter nearest meatus. Move in only one direction, away from the meatus. Use a clean area of the cloth for each stroke.
    Prevents infection.

16. Dip a clean washcloth in the water. Rinse area around meatus, using a clean area of washcloth for each stroke.

17. Dip a clean washcloth in the water. Rinse at least four inches of catheter nearest the meatus. Move in only one direction, away from meatus (Fig. 7-37). Use a clean area of the cloth for each stroke.

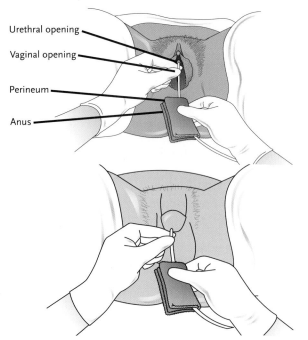

Urethral opening

Vaginal opening

Perineum

Anus

Fig. 7-37. *Hold the catheter near the meatus to avoid tugging the catheter. Moving in only one direction, away from meatus, helps prevent infection. Use a clean area of the washcloth for each stroke.*

18. With towel, dry at least four inches of catheter nearest meatus. Move in only one direction, away from meatus.

19. Remove pad from under resident. Remove towel or pad from under catheter tubing. Replace top covers. Remove bath blanket.

20. Dispose of linen in proper containers.

21. Empty basin into the toilet and flush. Place basin in proper area for cleaning or clean and store it according to facility policy.

22. Remove and discard gloves.

23. Wash your hands.
    Provides for infection prevention.

24. Return bed to lowest position.
    Lowering the bed provides for safety.

25. Place call light within resident's reach.
    Allows resident to communicate with staff as needed.

26. Report any changes in resident to the nurse.
    Provides nurse with information to assess resident.

27. Document procedure using facility guidelines.
    If you do not document the care, legally it did not happen.

Emptying the catheter drainage bag

Equipment: graduate (measuring container), alcohol wipes, paper towels, gloves

1. Identify yourself by name. Identify the resident by name.
   Resident has right to know identity of his or her caregiver. Addressing resident by name shows respect and establishes correct identification.

2. Wash your hands.
   Provides for infection prevention.

3. Explain procedure to resident. Speak clearly, slowly, and directly. Maintain face-to-face contact whenever possible.
   Promotes understanding and independence.

4. Provide for resident's privacy with curtain, screen, or door.
   Maintains resident's right to privacy and dignity.

5. Put on gloves.

6. Place paper towel on the floor under the drainage bag. Place graduate on the paper towel.

7. Open the drain or spout on the bag so that the urine flows out of the bag and into the graduate (Fig. 7-38). Do not let spout or clamp touch the graduate.

8. When urine has drained, close spout. Using alcohol wipes, clean the drain spout. Replace the drain in its holder on the bag.

Fig. 7-38. *Keep the spout and clamp from touching the graduate while draining urine.*

9. Go into the bathroom. Place graduate on a flat surface and measure at eye level. Note the amount and the appearance of the urine. Empty into toilet and flush toilet.

10. Clean and store graduate. Discard paper towels.

11. Remove and discard gloves.

12. Wash your hands.
    Provides for infection prevention.

13. Document procedure using facility guidelines. Note amount and characteristics of urine.
    If you do not document the care, legally it did not happen.

Oxygen therapy is the administration of oxygen to increase the supply of oxygen to the lungs. This increases oxygen to the body tissues. Oxygen therapy is used to treat breathing problems. It is prescribed by a doctor. Nursing assistants never stop, adjust, or administer oxygen.

Oxygen can be delivered in various ways. It may be piped into a resident's room through a central system. It may come in large tanks or in small, portable tanks. It may be produced by an oxygen concentrator. An oxygen concentrator is a box-like device that changes air in the room into air with more oxygen.

Some residents receive oxygen through a nasal cannula. A nasal cannula is a piece of plastic tubing that fits around the face and is secured by a strap that goes over the ears and around the back of the head (Fig. 7-39). The face piece has two short prongs made of tubing. These prongs fit inside the nose, pointing downward, and oxygen is delivered through them. A nurse or respiratory therapist fits the cannula.

Fig. 7-39. *Residents can still talk and eat while wearing a nasal cannula.*

Residents who do not need concentrated oxygen all the time may use a face mask when they need oxygen (Fig. 7-40). The face mask fits over the nose and mouth. It is secured by a strap that goes over the ears and around the back of the head.

Fig. 7-40. *Residents who need oxygen occasionally may use a face mask. The mask must be removed for the resident to eat or drink anything.*

Combustion means the process of burning. Oxygen is a very dangerous fire hazard because it supports combustion (makes other things burn). Working around oxygen requires special safety precautions.

Guidelines: Working Safely Around Oxygen

G Post *No Smoking* and *Oxygen in Use* signs. Never allow smoking where oxygen is used or stored.

G Remove all fire hazards from the room or area. Fire hazards include electrical equipment, such as electric razors and hair dryers. Other fire hazards are cigarettes, matches, and flammable liquids. **Flammable** means easily ignited and capable of burning quickly. Alcohol and nail polish remover are examples of flammable liquids. Notify the nurse if a resident does not want a fire hazard removed.

G Do not burn candles, light matches, or use lighters around oxygen. Any type of open flame that is present around oxygen is a dangerous fire hazard.

G Do not use an extension cord with an oxygen concentrator.

G Do not place electrical cords or oxygen tubing under rugs or furniture.

G Avoid using fabrics such as nylon and wool that can cause static electricity discharges.

G Report if the nasal cannula or face mask causes skin irritation. Check the nasal area and behind the ears for signs of irritation.

G Do not use any petroleum-based products, such as Vaseline or Chapstick, on the resident or on any part of the cannula or mask.

G Learn how to turn off oxygen in case of fire. Never adjust the oxygen setting or dose.

Intravenous therapy, often called **IV therapy**, is the delivery of medication, nutrition, or fluids through a person's vein. When a doctor prescribes IV therapy, a nurse inserts a needle or tube into a vein. This gives direct access to the bloodstream. Medication, nutrition, or fluids either drip from a bag suspended on a pole or are pumped by a portable pump through a tube and into the vein. Some residents with chronic conditions may have a permanent opening for IV lines, called a *port*. It has been surgically created to allow easy access for IV fluids. Nursing assistants never insert or remove IV lines. They are not responsible for care of the IV site. Their only responsibility for IV care is to report and document any observations of changes or problems with the IV.

Observing and Reporting: IV Therapy

Report any of the following to the nurse:

O/R The tube/needle falls out or is removed

O/R The tubing disconnects

O/R The dressing around the IV site is loose or not intact

O/R Blood is in the tubing or around the IV site

O/R The site is swollen or discolored

O/R The resident complains of pain

O/R The bag is broken or the level of fluid does not seem to decrease

O/R The IV fluid is not dripping or is leaking

O/R The IV fluid is nearly gone

O/R The pump beeps, indicating a problem

O/R The pump is dropped

NAs should document their observations and the care given. They should not get the IV site wet or lower the bag below the IV site. They should not disconnect the IV from the pump or turn off the alarm. NAs should not measure blood pressure on an arm with an IV line. Having an IV line in place makes some care procedures more difficult. The IV tubing must not pull or catch on anything, such as clothing. Special gowns with sleeves that snap and unsnap are available to lessen the risk of pulling out IV lines.

7. Discuss a resident's unit and related care

A resident's unit is the room or area where the resident lives. It contains furniture and personal items. The unit is the resident's home. It must be treated with respect. NAs must always knock and wait for permission before entering. Residents' units must be kept neat and clean. Providing a clean, safe, and orderly environment is an essential part of the NA's job.

Standard equipment often found in each resident's unit includes the following:

*   Electric or manual bed

*   Bedside stand

*   Urinal/bedpan and covers

*   Wash basin

*   Emesis basin

*   Soap dish and soap

*   Bath blanket

*   Toilet paper

*   Personal hygiene items

*   Overbed table

*   Chair

*   Call light

*   Privacy screen or curtain

Small items are usually stored in bedside stands. The water pitcher and cup are often placed on top of the bedside stand. A telephone, radio, and other items, such as photos, may also be placed there.

The overbed table may be used for meals or personal care. It is a clean area. It must be kept clean and free of clutter. Bedpans, urinals, soiled linen, and other contaminated items should not be placed on overbed tables.

The intercom system is the most common call system. When the resident presses the button, a light will be seen and/or a bell will be heard at the nurses' station. The call light allows the resident to contact staff when necessary. NAs must always place the call light within the resident's reach and answer all call lights immediately.

Residents' Rights

Privacy Curtains

All residents in a facility have the legal right to personal privacy. This means that they must always be protected from public view when receiving care. Each bed usually has a privacy curtain that extends all the way around the bed. Curtains keep others from seeing a resident undressed or while having care procedures done. To protect the resident's privacy, NAs must keep this curtain closed when giving care (Fig. 7-41). Although curtains and screens block vision, they do not block sound. NAs should keep their voices low. They should not discuss a resident's care near others. Closing the door, when possible, gives more complete privacy.

Fig. 7-41. Nursing assistants should pull the privacy curtain around the bed before giving care.

There are many types of equipment in a care facility. NAs must know how to use and care for all equipment properly. This helps prevent infection and injury. NAs should ask for help when needed. They should not try to use equipment that they do not know how to use.

Guidelines: Resident's Unit

G   Clean the overbed table after use. Place it within the resident's reach before leaving.

G   Keep the call light within the resident's reach. Check to see that it is within reach before you leave the room.

G   Keep equipment clean and in good condition. If any equipment appears damaged, report it to the nurse and/or file the proper paperwork to get it repaired. Do not use broken or damaged equipment.

G   OBRA requires that long-term care facilities have comfortable and safe environments by maintaining a temperature range of 71–81°F. Older people may feel cold often. Layer clothing and bed covers for warmth. Keep residents away from drafty areas. If residents control the heat and air conditioning in their rooms, do not change it for your comfort.

G   Remove meal trays right after meals. Check to make sure that there are no crumbs in the bed. Straighten bed linens as needed. Change linens if they become wet, soiled, or wrinkled.

G   Restock supplies. Make sure the resident has fresh drinking water and a clean cup within reach. Check that the resident is able to lift the pitcher and the cup. Make sure that tissues, paper towels, toilet paper, soap, and other supplies that are used daily are stocked before you leave.

G   If trash needs to be emptied or the bathroom needs to be cleaned, notify the housekeeping department. Trash should be emptied at least daily. Remove the trash when you leave the room if housekeeping staff is not available.

G   Report signs of insects or pests right away.

G   Do not move resident's belongings. Do not discard any personal items. Respect the resident's things.

G   Clean equipment and return it to storage or take it to the proper area for cleaning. Tidy the area.

8. Explain the importance of sleep and perform proper bedmaking

Sleep is a natural period of rest for the mind and body. As a person sleeps, the mind and body's energy is restored. During sleep, vital functions are performed. These include repairing and renewing cells, processing information, and organizing memory. Sleep is essential to a person's health and well-being.

A lack of sleep causes many problems. These include decreased mental function, reduced reaction time, and irritability. Sleep deprivation also decreases immune system function.

Many elderly persons, especially those who are living away from their homes, have sleep problems. Many things can affect sleep, such as fear, anxiety, stress, noise, diet, medications, and illness. Sharing a room with another person can disturb sleep.

Observing and Reporting: Sleep Issues

When a resident complains that he or she is not sleeping well, observe and report the following:

O/R   Sleeping too much during the day

O/R   Eating or drinking items that contain caffeine late in the day

O/R   Wearing night clothes during the day

O/R   Eating heavy meals late at night

O/R   Refusing to take medication ordered for sleep

O/R   Taking new medications

O/R   Having TV, radio, computer, or light on late at night

O/R   Having pain

Some residents spend much or all of their time in bed. Careful bedmaking is essential for comfort, cleanliness, and health. Linens should always be changed after personal care, such as bed baths. They should also be changed any time bedding or sheets are damp, soiled, or in need of straightening. Bed linens should be changed often for these reasons:

•   Sheets that are damp, wrinkled, or bunched up are uncomfortable. They may keep the resident from sleeping well.

- Microorganisms thrive in moist, warm places. Bedding that is damp or unclean may cause infection and disease.

- Residents who spend long hours in bed are at risk for pressure ulcers. Sheets that do not lie flat increase this risk by cutting off circulation.

Guidelines: Bedmaking

G Keep linens wrinkle-free and tidy. Change linen whenever wet, damp, wrinkled, or dirty.

G Wash your hands before handling clean linen (Fig. 7-42).

Fig. 7-42. Make sure you have washed your hands before gathering clean linen.

G Place clean linen on a clean surface, such as a chair or bedside stand. Do not place clean linen on the floor or on a contaminated area.

G Don (put on) gloves before removing bed linen from the bed.

G Look for personal items, such as dentures, hearing aids, jewelry, and glasses, before removing linens.

G When removing linen, fold or roll linen so that the dirtiest area is inside. Rolling puts the dirtiest surface of the linen inward. This lessens contamination.

G Do not shake linen or clothes. It may spread airborne contaminants.

G Bag soiled linen at the point of origin. Do not take it to other residents' rooms.

G Sort soiled linen away from resident care areas.

G Place wet linen in leakproof bags.

G Wear gloves when handling soiled linen. Hold soiled linen away from your body. Place it in the proper container or area immediately. If dirty linen touches your uniform, your uniform becomes contaminated.

G Change disposable bed protectors whenever they become soiled or wet. Dispose of them properly. Put a clean bed protector on the bed when you change linen.

If a resident cannot get out of bed, an NA must change the linens with the resident in bed. An **occupied bed** is a bed made while the resident is in the bed. When making the bed, the NA should use a wide stance and bend her knees. Bending from the waist should be avoided, especially when tucking sheets under the mattress. The height of the bed should be raised to make the job easier and safer.

Mattresses can be heavy. It is easier to make an empty bed than one with a resident in it. An **unoccupied bed** is a bed made while no resident is in the bed. If the resident can be moved, the NA's job will be easier.

Making an occupied bed

Equipment: clean linen—mattress pad, fitted or flat bottom sheet, waterproof bed protector (if needed), cotton draw sheet, flat top sheet, blanket(s), bath blanket, pillowcase(s), gloves

1. Identify yourself by name. Identify the resident by name.
   Resident has right to know identity of his or her caregiver. Addressing resident by name shows respect and establishes correct identification.

2. Wash your hands.
   Provides for infection prevention.

3. Explain procedure to resident. Speak clearly, slowly, and directly. Maintain face-to-face contact whenever possible.
   Promotes understanding and independence.

4. Provide for resident's privacy with curtain, screen, or door.
Maintains resident's right to privacy and dignity.

5. Place clean linen on clean surface within reach (e.g., bedside stand, overbed table, or chair).
Prevents contamination of linen.

6. Adjust bed to a safe level, usually waist high. Lower head of bed. Lock bed wheels.
When bed is flat, resident can be moved without working against gravity. Adjusting bed level and locking wheels prevents injury to you and resident.

7. Put on gloves.
Prevents you from coming into contact with body fluids.

8. Loosen top linen from the end of the bed on working side.

9. Unfold bath blanket over the top sheet to cover the resident. Remove top sheet. Keep the resident covered at all times with the bath blanket.

10. You will make the bed one side at a time. Raise side rail (if bed has them) on far side of bed. After raising side rail, go to other side of bed. Help resident to turn onto her side, moving away from you, toward the raised side rail (Fig. 7-43).

Fig. 7-43. Turn resident onto her side, toward raised side rail.

11. Loosen bottom soiled linen, mattress pad, and protector, if present, on the working side.

12. Roll bottom soiled linen toward resident, soiled side inside. Tuck it snugly against the resident's back.
Rolling puts dirtiest surface of linen inward, lessening contamination. The closer the linen is rolled to resident, the easier it is to remove from the other side.

13. Place the mattress pad (if used) on the bed, attaching elastic corners on working side.

14. Place and tuck in clean bottom linen. Finish with bottom sheet free of wrinkles. Make hospital corners to keep bottom sheet wrinkle-free (Fig. 7-44).
Hospital corners prevent a resident's feet from being restricted by or tangled in linen when getting in and out of bed.

Fig. 7-44. Hospital corners help keep the flat sheet smooth under the resident. They help prevent a resident's feet from being restricted by or tangled in linen when getting in and out of bed.

15. Smooth the bottom sheet out toward the resident. Be sure there are no wrinkles in the mattress pad. Roll the extra material toward the resident. Tuck it under the resident's body (Fig. 7-45).

Fig. 7-45. Tuck extra material under the resident's body.

16. If using a waterproof bed protector, unfold it and center it on the bed. Tuck the side near you under the mattress. Smooth it out toward the resident. Tuck as you did with the sheet.

17. If using a draw sheet, place it on the bed. Tuck in on your side, smooth, and tuck as you did with the other bedding.

18. Raise side rail nearest you. Go to the other side of the bed. Lower side rail on that side. Help resident turn onto clean bottom sheet (Fig. 7-46). Protect the resident from any soiled matter on the old linens.

Fig. 7-46. While helping resident turn onto clean linen, try to avoid contact with soiled matter on dirty linen.

19. Loosen the soiled linen. Check for any personal items. Roll linen from head to foot of the bed. Avoid contact with your skin or clothes. Place it in a hamper or bag. Never put it on the floor or furniture. Never shake it. Soiled linens are full of microorganisms

that should not be spread to other parts of the room.
Always work from cleanest (head of bed) to dirtiest (foot of bed) area to prevent spread of infection. Rolling puts dirtiest surface of linen inward, lessening contamination.

20. Pull the clean linen through as quickly as possible. Start with the mattress pad and wrap around corners. Pull and tuck in clean bottom linen just like the other side. Pull and tuck in waterproof bed protector and draw sheet if used. Finish with bottom sheet free of wrinkles.

21. Ask resident to turn onto her back. Help as needed. Keep resident covered and comfortable, with a pillow under her head. Raise the side rail.

22. Unfold the top sheet. Place it over the resident and center it. Ask the resident to hold the top sheet. Slip the bath blanket or old sheet out from underneath. Put it in the hamper or bag.

23. Place a blanket over the top sheet. Match the top edges. Tuck the bottom edges of top sheet and blanket under the bottom of the mattress. Make hospital corners on each side. Loosen the top linens over the resident's feet. At the top of the bed, fold the top sheet over the blanket about six inches.
Loosening the top linens over the feet prevents pressure on the feet, which can cause pressure ulcers.

24. Remove the pillow. Do not hold it near your face. Remove the soiled pillowcase by turning it inside out. Place it in the hamper or bag.

25. Remove and discard gloves. Wash your hands.
Provides for infection prevention.

26. With one hand, grasp the clean pillowcase at the closed end. Turn it inside out over your arm. Next, using the same hand that has the pillowcase over it, grasp one narrow edge of the pillow. Pull the pillowcase over it with

your free hand (Fig. 7-47). Do the same for any other pillows. Place them under resident's head with open end away from door.

Fig. 7-47. *After the pillowcase is turned inside out over your arm, grasp one end of the pillow. Pull the pillowcase over the pillow.*

27. Make resident comfortable.

28. Return bed to lowest position. Leave side rails in the ordered positions.
    Lowering the bed provides for safety.

29. Place call light within resident's reach.
    Allows resident to communicate with staff as necessary.

30. Take laundry bag or hamper to proper area.

31. Wash your hands.
    Provides for infection prevention.

32. Report any changes in resident to the nurse.
    Provides nurse with information to assess resident.

33. Document procedure using facility guidelines.
    If you do not document the care, legally it did not happen.

Making an unoccupied bed

Equipment: clean linen—mattress pad, fitted or flat bottom sheet, waterproof bed protector if needed, blanket(s), cotton draw sheet, flat top sheet, pillowcase(s), gloves

1. Wash your hands.
   Provides for infection prevention.

2. Place clean linen on clean surface within reach (e.g., bedside stand, overbed table, or chair).
   Prevents contamination of linen.

3. Adjust bed to a safe level, usually waist high. Put bed in flattest position. Lock bed wheels.
   Allows you to make a neat, wrinkle-free bed.

4. Put on gloves.
   Prevents you from coming into contact with body fluids.

5. Loosen soiled linen. Roll soiled linen (soiled side inside) from head to foot of bed. Avoid contact with your skin or clothes. Place it in a hamper or bag. Do not put it on the floor or furniture. Remove pillows and pillowcases and place pillowcases in hamper or bag.
   Always work from cleanest (head of bed) to dirtiest (foot of bed) area to prevent spread of infection. Rolling puts dirtiest surface of linen inward, lessening risk of contamination.

6. Remove and discard gloves. Wash your hands.
   Provides for infection prevention.

7. Remake the bed. Start with the mattress pad and wrap around corners. Place bottom sheet, tucking under mattress. Make hospital corners to keep the bottom sheet wrinkle-free. Put on waterproof bed protector and draw sheet, if used, smooth, and tuck under sides of bed.

8. Place top sheet and blanket over bed. Center these, tuck under end of bed, and make hospital corners. Fold down the top sheet over the blanket about six inches. Fold both top sheet and blanket down so resident can easily get into bed. If resident will not be returning to bed immediately, leave bedding up.

9. Put on clean pillowcases. Replace pillows.

10. Return bed to lowest position.

11. Take laundry bag or hamper to proper area.

12. Wash your hands.
    Provides for infection prevention.

13. Document procedure using facility
guidelines.
*If you do not document the care, legally it did not
happen.*

A **closed bed** is a bed completely made with the
bedspread and blankets in place. It is made for
residents who will be out of bed most of the day.
It is also made when a resident is discharged. A
closed bed is turned into an **open bed** by folding the linen down to the foot of the bed. An
open bed is a bed that is ready to receive a resident who has been out of bed all day or who is
being admitted to the facility.

9. Discuss dressings and bandages

Sterile dressings cover open or draining wounds.
A nurse changes these dressings. Non-sterile
dressings are applied to dry, closed wounds that
have less chance of infection. Nursing assistants
may be able to change non-sterile dressings.
State regulations vary, so NAs should follow state
and facility policies.

Changing a dry dressing using non-sterile technique

*Equipment: package of square gauze dressings, ad-
hesive tape, scissors, 2 pairs of gloves*

1. Identify yourself by name. Identify the resident by name.
*Resident has right to know identity of his or her care-
giver. Addressing resident by name shows respect and
establishes correct identification.*

2. Wash your hands.
Provides for infection prevention.

3. Explain procedure to resident. Speak clearly,
slowly, and directly. Maintain face-to-face contact whenever possible.
Promotes understanding and independence.

4. Provide for resident's privacy with curtain,
screen, or door.
Maintains resident's right to privacy and dignity.

5. Cut pieces of tape long enough to secure
the dressing. Hang tape on the edge of a
table within reach. Open the four-inch gauze
square package without touching the gauze.
Place the opened package on a flat surface.

6. Put on gloves.
*Protects you from coming into contact with body
fluids.*

7. Remove soiled dressing by gently peeling
tape toward the wound. Lift dressing off the
wound. Do not drag it over the wound. Observe dressing for any odor or drainage. Notice the color and size of the wound. Dispose
of used dressing in proper container.
*Avoids disturbing wound healing. Reduces risk of
contamination.*

8. Remove and discard gloves. Wash your
hands.
Provides for infection prevention.

9. Put on new gloves. Touching only outer
edges of new four-inch gauze, remove it from
package. Apply it to wound. Tape gauze in
place. Secure firmly (Fig. 7-48).
Keeps gauze as clean as possible.

Fig. 7-48. *Tape gauze in place to secure the dressing. Do
not completely cover all areas of the dressing with tape.*

10. Discard supplies.

11. Remove and discard gloves.

12. Wash your hands.
Provides for infection prevention.

13. Place call light within resident's reach.
*Allows resident to communicate with staff as
necessary.*

14. Report any changes in resident to the nurse.
Provides nurse with information to assess resident.

15. Document procedure according to facility guidelines.

If you do not document the care, legally it did not happen.

Elastic bandages (sometimes called *ACE bandages* or *ACE wraps*) are used to hold dressings in place, secure splints, and support and protect body parts. In addition, these bandages may decrease swelling that occurs from an injury (Fig. 7-49).

Fig. 7-49. *This is one type of elastic bandage.*

NAs may be required to help with elastic bandages. Duties may include the following:

• Bringing the bandage to the resident

• Positioning the resident to apply the bandage

• Washing and storing the bandage

• Documenting observations about the bandage

Some states allow NAs to apply and remove elastic bandages. They should follow their facility's policies and the care plan regarding elastic bandages.

Guidelines: Elastic Bandages

G Keep the area to be wrapped clean and dry.

G Apply bandage snugly enough to control bleeding and prevent movement of dressings. Make sure that the body part is not wrapped too tightly, which can decrease circulation.

G Wrap the bandage upwards and evenly, in a figure-eight pattern, so that no part of the wrapped area is pinched.

G Do not tie the bandage because this cuts off circulation to the body part; the end is held in place with special clips, tape, or fasteners.

G Remove the bandage as often as indicated in the care plan.

G Check the bandage often. It can become wrinkled or loose, which causes it to lose effectiveness. It can also become bunched up, which causes pressure and possible discomfort.

G Check on the resident 15 minutes after the bandage is applied to check for signs of poor circulation. Signs and symptoms of poor circulation include the following:

• Swelling

• Bluish, or cyanotic, skin

• Shiny, tight skin

• Skin that is cold to touch

• Sores

• Numbness

• Tingling

• Pain or discomfort

Loosen the bandage if you note any signs of poor circulation, and notify the nurse immediately.

8
Nutrition and Hydration

1. Identify the six basic nutrients and explain MyPlate

Proper nutrition is very important. **Nutrition** is how the body uses food to maintain health. Bodies need a well-balanced diet with nutrients and plenty of fluids. This helps the body grow new cells, maintain normal body function, and have energy. Proper nutrition in early life helps ensure good health later in life. For the ill or elderly, a well-balanced diet helps maintain muscle and skin tissues and prevent pressure ulcers. A healthy diet promotes healing. It also helps a person cope with stress.

A **nutrient** is a substance that is necessary for growth and life. Nutrients provide energy, promote growth and health, and help regulate metabolism. Metabolism is the process by which nutrients are broken down to be used by the body for energy and other needs. The body needs the following six nutrients for growth and development:

1. **Water**: Water is the most essential nutrient for life. One-half to two-thirds of the body's weight is water. A person needs about 64 ounces, or eight 8-ounce glasses, of water or other fluids per day. Without it, a person can only live a few days. Water assists in the digestion and absorption of food. It helps with waste elimination. Through perspiration, water also helps maintain normal body temperature. Keeping enough fluid in the body is necessary for good health.

The fluids a person drinks—water, juice, soda, coffee, tea, and milk—provide most of the water the body uses. Some foods are also sources of water, including soup, celery, lettuce, and apples.

2. **Carbohydrates**: Carbohydrates supply the body with energy and extra protein. They help the body use fat efficiently. Carbohydrates also provide fiber, which is necessary for bowel elimination. Carbohydrates can be divided into two basic types: complex and simple carbohydrates. Complex carbohydrates are found in bread, cereal, potatoes, rice, pasta, vegetables, and fruits (Fig. 8-1). Simple carbohydrates are found in sugars, sweets, syrups, and jellies. Simple carbohydrates do not have the same nutritional value that complex carbohydrates do.

Fig. 8-1. *Some sources of complex carbohydrates.*

3. **Protein**: Proteins are part of every body cell. They are needed for tissue growth and repair. Proteins also supply energy for the body. Excess proteins are excreted by the kidneys or stored as body fat. Sources of protein include seafood, poultry, meat, eggs, milk, cheese, nuts, nut but-

ters, peas, beans or legumes, and soy products (tofu, tempeh, some veggie burgers) (Fig. 8-2). Whole grain cereals, pastas, rice, and breads contain some proteins, too.

Fig. 8-2. Some sources of protein.

4. **Fats**: Fat helps the body store energy. In addition, fats add flavor to food. Fats also help the body absorb certain vitamins. Excess fat in the diet is stored as fat in the body.

Examples of fats are butter, margarine, salad dressings, oils, and animal fats in meats, dairy products, fowl, and fish (Fig. 8-3). Monounsaturated vegetable fats (including olive oil and canola oil) and polyunsaturated vegetable fats (including corn and safflower oils) are healthier fats. Saturated fats, including animal fats like butter, lard, bacon, and other fatty meats, are not as healthy. They should be limited.

Fig. 8-3. Some sources of fat.

5. **Vitamins**: Vitamins are substances needed by the body to function. The body cannot make most vitamins. They can only be obtained from certain foods. Vitamins A, D, E, and K are fat-soluble vitamins. This means they are carried and stored in body fat. Vitamins B and C are water-soluble vitamins. They are broken down by water in the body and used by the body, but cannot be stored. Excess B and C vitamins are eliminated in urine and feces.

6. **Minerals**: Minerals maintain body functions. Minerals help build bones, make hormones, and help in blood formation. They provide energy and control body processes. Zinc, iron, calcium, and magnesium are examples of minerals. Minerals are found in many foods.

Most foods have several nutrients. However, no one food has all the nutrients needed for a healthy body. This is why it is important to eat a daily diet that is well-balanced. There is not one single dietary plan that is right for everyone. People have different nutritional needs depending upon their age, gender, and activity level.

In 2011, the U.S. Department of Agriculture (USDA) developed MyPlate to help people build a healthy plate at meal times (Fig. 8-4). The MyPlate icon emphasizes vegetables, fruits, grains, protein, and low-fat dairy products.

Fig. 8-4. The U.S. Department of Agriculture developed the MyPlate icon and web address (ChooseMyPlate.gov) to help promote healthy eating practices.

MyPlate gives suggestions and tools for making healthy choices. It does not provide specific messages about what a person should eat. The MyPlate icon includes the following food groups:

Vegetables and fruits: A person should make half his plate fruits and vegetables. Vegetables include all fresh, frozen, canned, and dried vegetables, and vegetable juices. There are five subgroups within the vegetable group, organized by their nutritional content. These are dark green vegetables, red and orange vegetables, dry beans and peas, starchy vegetables, and other vegetables. A variety of vegetables from these subgroups should be eaten every day. Dark green, red, and orange vegetables have the best nutritional content (Fig. 8-5).

Fig. 8-5. Eating a variety of vegetables every day, especially dark green, red, and orange vegetables, helps promote good health.

Vegetables are low in fat and calories and have no cholesterol (although sauces and seasonings may add fat, calories, and cholesterol). They are good sources of dietary fiber, potassium, vitamin A, vitamin E, and vitamin C.

Fruits include all fresh, frozen, canned, and dried fruits, and 100% fruit juices. Most choices should be whole, cut-up, or pureed fruit, rather than juice, for the additional dietary fiber provided. Fruit can be added as a main dish, side dish, or as a dessert.

Fruits, like vegetables, are naturally low in fat, sodium, and calories and have no cholesterol. They are important sources of dietary fiber and many nutrients, including folic acid, potassium, and vitamin C. Foods containing dietary fiber help provide a feeling of fullness with fewer calories. Folic acid helps the body form red blood cells. Vitamin C is important for growth and repair of body tissues.

Grains: A person should make half his grain intake whole grains. There are many different grains. Some common ones are wheat, rice, oats, cornmeal, and barley. Foods made from grains include bread, pasta, oatmeal, breakfast cereals, tortillas, and grits. Grains can be divided into two groups: whole grains and refined grains. Whole grains contain bran and germ, as well as the endosperm. Refined grains retain only the endosperm. The endosperm is the tissue within flowering plants. It surrounds and nourishes the plant embryo. Examples of whole grains include brown rice, wild rice, bulgur, whole-grain corn, whole oats, whole wheat, and whole rye. Foods rich in fiber reduce the risk of heart disease and other diseases and may reduce constipation.

Protein: MyPlate guidelines emphasize the importance of eating a variety of protein foods every week. Meat, poultry, seafood, and eggs are animal sources of proteins. Beans, peas, soy products, nuts, and seeds are plant sources of proteins. Seafood should be eaten twice a week in place of meat or poultry. Seafood that is higher in oils and low in mercury, such as salmon or trout, is a better choice (Fig. 8-6). Lean meats and poultry, as well as eggs and egg whites, can be eaten on a regular basis. A person should eat plant-based protein foods more often. Beans and peas, soy products (tofu, tempeh, some veggie burgers), nuts, and seeds are low in saturated fat and high in fiber. Some nuts and seeds (flax, walnuts) are excellent sources of essential fatty acids. These acids may reduce the risk of heart disease. Sunflower seeds and almonds are good sources of vitamin E.

Fig. 8-6. Fish, like this salmon, contains healthy oils and is a good source of protein.

Dairy: All milk products and foods made from milk that retain their calcium content, such as yogurt and cheese, are part of the dairy category. Most dairy group choices should be fat-free or low-fat (1%). Fat-free or low-fat milk or yogurt should be chosen more often than cheese. Milk and yogurt contain less sodium than most cheeses.

Milk provides nutrients that are vital for the health and maintenance of the body. These nutrients include calcium, potassium, vitamin D, and protein. Fat-free or low-fat milk provides these nutrients without the extra calories and saturated fat. Soy products enriched with calcium are an alternative to dairy foods.

The following guidelines provide additional tips for making healthy food choices:

Guidelines: Healthy Food Choices

G   Balance calories. Calorie balance is the relationship between the calories obtained from food and fluids consumed and the calories used during normal body functions and physical activity. Proper calorie intake varies from person to person. To find the proper calorie intake, the USDA suggests visiting ChooseMyPlate.gov.

G   Enjoy your food, but eat less. Eating too fast or eating without paying attention to your food can lead to overeating. Know when you feel hungry and when you are full. Notice what you are eating. Stop eating when you feel satisfied.

G   Avoid oversized portions. Choose smaller-sized portions when eating. Portion out food before you eat it. Use smaller bowls and plates for meals. When eating out, split food with others or take part of your meal home.

G   Eat these foods more often: vegetables, fruits, whole grains, and fat-free or 1% milk and low-fat dairy products. These foods have better nutrients for health.

G   Eat these foods less often: foods high in solid fats, added sugars, and salt. These foods include fatty meats, like bacon and hot dogs, cheese, fried foods, ice cream, and cookies.

G   Compare sodium in foods. Read product labels to determine if they contain salt or sodium. Foods high in sodium include the following:

- Cured meats, including ham, bacon, lunch meat, and sausage

- Salty or smoked fish, including herring, sardines, anchovies, and smoked salmon

- Processed cheese and some other cheeses

- Salted foods, including nuts, pretzels, potato chips, and dips

- Vegetables preserved in brine, such as pickles, sauerkraut, and olives

- Sauces with high concentrations of salt, including steak and soy sauces, ketchup, and mayonnaise

- Commercially-prepared foods such as breads, canned soups and vegetables, and certain breakfast cereals

Select canned foods that are labeled *sodium-free, very low sodium, low-sodium,* or *reduced sodium.*

G   Drink water instead of sugary drinks. Drinking water or unsweetened beverages reduces sugar and calorie intake. Sweetened beverages, such as soda, fruit punch, and sports drinks, are a major source of sugar and calories in diets.

2. Describe factors that influence food preferences

Culture, ethnicity, income, education, religion, and geography all affect ideas about nutrition. Food preferences may be formed by what a person ate as a child, by what tastes good, or by personal beliefs about what should be eaten (Fig. 8-7). Some people choose not to eat any animals or animal products, such as steak, chicken, butter, or eggs. These people are vegetarians or vegans, depending on what they eat.

Fig. 8-7. Food likes and dislikes are influenced by what a person ate as a child.

The region or culture a person grows up in often affects his food preference. People from the southwestern United States may like spicy food. Southern cooking may include fried foods, like fried chicken or fried okra. Ethnic groups often share common foods. These may be eaten at certain times of the year or all the time. Religious beliefs affect diet, too. Some Muslim and Jewish people do not eat any pork. Mormons may not drink alcohol, coffee, or tea.

Food preferences may change while a resident is living at a facility. Just as anyone may decide that he likes some foods for a time and then changes his mind, so may residents. Whatever residents' food preferences may be, NAs should respect them. It is never appropriate to make fun of personal preferences. If an NA notices that certain food is not being eaten—no matter how small the amount—she should report it to the nurse.

Residents' Rights

Food Choices

Residents have the legal right to make choices about their food. They can choose what kind of food they want to eat. They can refuse the food and drink being offered. NAs must honor a resident's personal beliefs and preferences about selecting and avoiding specific foods. Although residents have the right to refuse, it is best to ask questions when they do.

For example, if a resident refuses dinner, the NA can ask if there is something wrong with the food. The resident may say he is Jewish and cannot eat a pork chop because it is not kosher. NAs should respond to requests for different food in a pleasant way. The NA can explain that she will report to the nurse and will get him another meal as quickly as possible. She can take the tray to the dietitian or dietary department so that an alternative may be offered.

3. Explain special diets

A doctor sometimes places residents who are ill on special diets. These diets are known as **therapeutic**, **modified**, or **special diets**. Certain nutrients or fluids may need to be restricted or removed. Some medications may interact with certain foods, which then must be eliminated. Doctors may order special diets for residents who do not eat enough. Diets are also used for weight control and food allergies.

Several types of modified diets are available. Some residents may be on a combination of special diets. The care plan should specify any special diet the resident is on (Fig. 8-8). Examples of special diets are listed below:

NUTRITION	Diet Order: Low fat			
✓	Meal Preparation			
	Assist with Feeding			
✓	Limit/Encourage Fluids			
	Grocery Shopping			
	Wash Clothes			

Fig. 8-8. The care plan specifies special diets or dietary restrictions.

Low-Sodium Diet: Residents with high blood pressure, heart disease, kidney disease, or fluid retention may be placed on a low-sodium diet. Many foods have sodium, but people are most familiar with it as an ingredient in table salt. Salt is restricted first in a low-sodium diet because it is high in sodium. For residents on a low-sodium diet, salt will not be used. Salt shakers or packets will not be on the diet tray. Common abbreviations for this diet are *Low Na*, which means low sodium, or *NAS*, which stands for *No Added Salt*.

Nutrition and Hydration

Fluid-Restricted Diet: The fluid taken into the body through food and fluids must equal the fluid that leaves the body through perspiration, stool, urine, and expiration. This is fluid balance. When fluid intake is greater than fluid output, body tissue becomes swollen with fluid. People with severe heart disease or kidney disease may have trouble processing fluid. To prevent further damage, doctors may restrict fluid intake. For residents on fluid restriction, the NA will measure and document exact amounts of fluid intake and report excesses to the nurse. Additional fluids or foods that count as fluids, such as ice cream, puddings, gelatin, etc., should not be offered. If the resident complains of thirst or requests fluids, the NA should tell the nurse. A common abbreviation for this diet is *RF*, which stands for *Restrict Fluids*.

Low-Protein Diet: People who have kidney disease may be on low-protein diets. Protein is restricted because it breaks down into compounds that may further damage the kidneys. The extent of the restrictions depends on the stage of the disease and if the resident is on dialysis. Vegetables and starches, such as breads and pasta, are encouraged.

Low-Fat/Low-Cholesterol Diet: People who have high levels of cholesterol in their blood are at risk for heart attacks and heart disease. People with gallbladder disease, diseases that interfere with fat digestion, and liver disease are also placed on a low-fat/low-cholesterol diet. This diet permits skim milk, low-fat cottage cheese, fish, white meat of turkey and chicken, fresh fruits and vegetables, and vegetable fats (especially monounsaturated fats such as olive and canola oils) (Fig. 8-9). People who have gallbladder disease or other digestive problems may be placed on a diet that restricts all fats. A common abbreviation for this diet is *Low-Fat/Low-Chol*.

Modified Calorie Diet: Some residents may need to reduce calories to lose weight or prevent weight gain. Other residents may need to increase calories because of malnutrition, surgery,

illness, or fever. Common abbreviations for this diet are *Low-Cal* or *High-Cal*.

Fig. 8-9. Vegetables are an important part of a low-fat/low-cholesterol diet.

Diabetic Diet: Calories and carbohydrates are carefully controlled in the diets of residents who have diabetes. Protein and fats are also regulated. The foods and the amounts are determined by nutritional and energy needs. A dietitian and the resident will make up a meal plan. It will include all the right types and amounts of food for each day. The meal plan may use a carbohydrate-counting approach (often called *carb counting*). After the proper amount of carbohydrates is determined by the dietitian, they need to be counted in each meal or snack. Meal planning can also be done by using the exchange system. In this system, similar foods can be substituted for one another to make up a menu. Looking at the exchange list, the resident makes food choices while controlling his diet.

To keep their blood glucose levels near normal, diabetic residents must eat the right amount of the right type of food at the right time. They must eat all that is served. NAs should encourage them to do so. NAs should not offer other foods without the nurse's approval. If a resident will not eat what is directed or is not following the diet, the NA should tell the nurse.

Diabetics should avoid foods that are high in sugar. Sugary foods can cause problems with insulin balance. A meal tray for a resident with diabetes may have artificial sweetener, low-calorie jelly, and/or low-calorie maple syrup. Artificial sweeteners may be used in coffee or tea, rather than sugar. The American Diabetes Association's (ADA) website, diabetes.org, has more information.

Vegetarian Diet: Health issues may cause a person to require a vegetarian diet. A person may also choose to eat a vegetarian diet for religious reasons, or due to a dislike of meat, a compassion for animals, a belief in non-violence, or financial issues. Different types of vegetarian diets are

- A lacto-ovo vegetarian diet excludes all meats, fish, and poultry, but allows eggs and dairy products.
- A lacto-vegetarian diet eliminates poultry, meats, fish, and eggs, but allows dairy products.
- An ovo-vegetarian diet omits all meats, fish, poultry, and dairy products, but allows eggs.
- A vegan diet eliminates poultry, meats, fish, eggs, and dairy products, along with all foods that are derived from animals.

Diets may also be modified in consistency:

Liquid Diet: A liquid diet is usually ordered for a short time due to a medical condition or before or after a test or surgery. It is ordered when a resident needs to keep the intestinal tract free of food. A liquid diet consists of foods that are in a liquid state at body temperature. Liquid diets are usually ordered as *clear* or *full*. A clear liquid diet includes clear juices, broth, gelatin, and popsicles. A full liquid diet includes all the liquids served on a clear liquid diet, with the addition of cream soups, milk, and ice cream.

Soft Diet and Mechanical Soft Diet: The soft diet is soft in texture and consists of soft or chopped foods that are easier to chew and swallow. Foods that are hard to chew and swallow, such as raw fruits and vegetables and some meats, will be restricted. High-fiber foods, fried foods, and spicy foods may also be limited. Doctors order this diet for residents who have trouble chewing and swallowing due to dental problems or other medical conditions. It is also ordered for people who are going from a liquid diet to a regular diet.

The mechanical soft diet consists of chopped or blended foods that are easier to chew and swallow. Foods are prepared with blenders, food processors, meat grinders, or cutting utensils. Unlike the soft diet, the mechanical soft diet does not limit spices, fat, and fiber. Only the texture of foods is changed. This diet is used for people recovering from surgery or who have trouble chewing and swallowing.

Pureed Diet: To **puree** a food means to blend or grind it into a thick paste of baby food consistency. The food should be thick enough to hold its form in the mouth. This diet does not require a person to chew his food. A pureed diet is often used for people who have trouble chewing and/or swallowing more textured foods.

Nutritional Supplements

Illness often causes residents to need extra nutrients, as well as additional calories. Sometimes a resident will be advised by his doctor or dietitian to add a high-nutrition supplement to the regular or modified diet. Usually this is done to encourage weight gain or the intake of proteins, vitamins, or minerals. Nutritional supplements may come in a powdered or liquid form. Supplements may be pre-mixed and ready to drink. Powdered supplements need to be mixed with a liquid before being taken. NAs may not be allowed to prepare supplements and/or hand them to residents. They should follow facility policy.

NAs can help by encouraging residents to drink their supplements. A resident who is ill, tired, or in pain may not have much of an appetite. It may take a long time for him to drink a large glass of a thick liquid. The NA should be patient. If a resident does not want to drink the supplement, the NA should not insist that he do so. However, she should report this to the nurse.

4. Describe how to assist residents in maintaining fluid balance

Most residents should be encouraged to drink at least 64 ounces of water or other fluids a day. Water is an essential nutrient for life. Proper fluid intake is important. It helps prevent constipation and urinary incontinence. Without enough fluid, urine becomes concentrated. More concentrated urine creates a higher risk for infection. Proper fluid intake also helps to dilute wastes and flush out the urinary system. It may even help prevent confusion.

The sense of thirst can lessen as people age. Infection, fever, diarrhea, and some medications will also increase the need for fluid intake. NAs should remind residents to drink fluids often (Fig. 8-10). Some residents will drink more fluids if they are offered them in smaller amounts, rather than in one large glassful. Some residents will have an order to force fluids or restrict fluids because of medical conditions. **Force fluids (FF)** means that the resident should be encouraged to drink more fluids. **Restrict fluids (RF)** means the resident is allowed to drink, but must limit the daily amount to a level set by the doctor. When a resident has a restrict fluids order, the NA should not give the resident any extra fluids or a water pitcher unless the nurse approves it.

Fig. 8-10. *Drinking enough water and other fluids promotes health. NAs should encourage residents to drink fluids often.*

The abbreviation **NPO** stands for *nothing by mouth*. This means that a resident is not allowed to have anything to eat or drink. Some residents have such a severe problem with swallowing that it is unsafe to give them anything by mouth. These types of residents will receive nutrition through a feeding tube or intravenously. Some residents may not be able to eat and drink for a short time before a medical test or surgery. NAs

need to know this abbreviation. They should never offer any food or drink, even water, to a resident with this order.

Dehydration occurs when a person does not have enough fluid in the body. Dehydration is a serious condition. It is a major problem among the elderly. People can become dehydrated if they do not drink enough or if they have diarrhea or are vomiting. Preventing dehydration is very important.

Guidelines: Preventing Dehydration

G   Report observations and warning signs to the nurse immediately.

G   Encourage residents to drink every time you see them.

G   Offer fresh water or other fluids often. Offer drinks that the resident enjoys. Some may not like water and prefer other types of beverages, such as juice, soda, tea, or milk. Some residents do not want ice in their drinks. Honor personal preferences. Report to the nurse if the resident tells you he does not like the fluids being served.

G   Ice chips, frozen flavored ice sticks, and gelatin are also liquids. Offer them often. Do not offer ice chips or sticks if a resident has a swallowing problem.

G   If appropriate, offer sips of liquid between bites of food at meals and snacks.

G   Make sure pitcher and cup are near enough and light enough for the resident to lift.

G   Offer assistance if resident cannot drink without help. Use adaptive cups as needed.

G   Record fluid intake and output.

Observing and Reporting: Dehydration

Report any of these to the nurse:

O/R   Resident drinks less than six 8-ounce glasses of liquid per day

O/R Resident drinks little or no fluids at meals

O/R Resident needs help drinking from a cup or glass

O/R Resident has trouble swallowing liquids

O/R Resident has frequent vomiting, diarrhea, or fever

O/R Resident is easily confused or tired

Report any of these signs and symptoms:

O/R Dry mouth

O/R Cracked lips

O/R Sunken eyes

O/R Dark urine

O/R Strong-smelling urine

O/R Weight loss

O/R Complaints of abdominal pain

Serving fresh water

Equipment: water pitcher, ice scoop, glass, straw, gloves

1. Identify yourself by name. Identify the resident by name.
   Resident has right to know identity of his or her caregiver. Addressing resident by name shows respect and establishes correct identification.

2. Wash your hands.
   Provides for infection prevention.

3. Put on gloves.
   Promotes infection prevention.

4. Scoop ice into water pitcher. Add fresh water.

5. Use and store ice scoop properly. Do not allow ice to touch your hand and fall back into container. Place scoop in proper receptacle after each use.
   Avoids contamination of ice.

6. Take pitcher to resident.

7. Pour glass of water for resident. Leave pitcher and glass at the bedside.
   Encourages resident to maintain hydration.

8. Make sure that pitcher and glass are light enough for resident to lift. Leave a straw if the resident desires it and does not have swallowing problems.
   Demonstrates understanding of resident's abilities and/or limitations. Prevents dehydration.

9. Place call light within resident's reach.
   Allows resident to communicate with staff as necessary.

10. Remove and discard gloves.

11. Wash your hands.
    Provides for infection prevention.

Fluid overload occurs when the body cannot handle the fluid consumed. This often affects people with heart or kidney disease.

Observing and Reporting: Fluid Overload

Report any of these to the nurse:

O/R Swelling/edema of extremities (ankles, feet, fingers, hands); **edema** is swelling caused by excess fluid in body tissues.

O/R Weight gain (daily weight gain of one to two pounds)

O/R Decreased urine output

O/R Shortness of breath

O/R Increased heart rate

O/R Anxiety

O/R Skin that appears tight, smooth, or shiny

5. List ways to identify and prevent unintended weight loss

Unintended weight loss is a serious problem for the elderly. Weight loss can mean that the resident has a serious medical condition. It can lead to skin breakdown. This leads to pressure ulcers. It is very important for NAs to report any weight loss, no matter how small. If a resident has diabetes, COPD, cancer, HIV, or other diseases, he is at a greater risk for malnutrition. (Chapter 4 has more information.)

Guidelines: Preventing Unintended Weight Loss

G Report observations and warning signs to the nurse.

G Food should look, taste, and smell good. The resident may have a poor sense of taste and smell.

G Encourage residents to eat. Talk about food being served in a positive tone of voice. Use positive words (Fig. 8-11).

Fig. 8-11. Be friendly and positive while helping residents with eating. This helps promote appetite and prevent weight loss.

G Honor residents' food likes and dislikes.

G Offer different kinds of foods and beverages.

G Help residents who have trouble feeding themselves.

G Season foods to residents' preferences.

G Allow time for residents to finish eating.

G Tell the nurse if residents have trouble using utensils.

G Record meal/snack intake.

G Give oral care before and after meals if the resident requests it.

G Position residents sitting upright for eating.

G If resident has had a loss of appetite and/or seems sad, ask about it.

Observing and Reporting: Unintended Weight Loss

Report any of these to the nurse:

O/R Resident needs help eating or drinking

O/R Resident eats less than 70% of meals served

O/R Resident has mouth pain

O/R Resident has dentures that do not fit

O/R Resident has difficulty chewing or swallowing

O/R Resident coughs or chokes while eating

O/R Resident is sad, has crying spells, or withdraws from others

O/R Resident is confused, wanders, or paces

6. Identify ways to promote appetites at mealtime

Mealtimes are often the times of day that residents look forward to the most. Meals are important for getting proper nourishment. They are also times for socializing, which has a positive effect on eating. Socializing can help prevent weight loss, dehydration, and malnutrition. It can also prevent loneliness and boredom.

Promoting healthy eating is an important part of a nursing assistant's job. Mealtime should be pleasant and enjoyable.

Guidelines: Promoting Appetites

G Assist residents with grooming and hygiene tasks before dining as needed.

G Give oral care before eating if requested.

G Offer a trip to the bathroom or help with toileting before eating.

G Help residents wash hands before eating.

G Encourage the use of dentures, eyeglasses, and hearing aids. If these are damaged, notify the nurse.

G   Check the environment. The temperature should be comfortable. Address any odors. Keep noise level low. Do not shout or raise your voice. Do not bang plates or cups.

G   Seat residents next to their friends or people with like interests. Encourage conversation.

G   Properly position residents for eating. Usually the proper position is upright, at a 90-degree angle. This helps prevent swallowing problems. If residents use a wheelchair, make sure they are sitting at a table that is the right height. Most facilities have adjustable tables for wheelchairs. Residents who use geri-chairs—reclining chairs on wheels—should be upright, not reclined, while eating.

G   Serve food promptly to maintain the correct temperature. Keep food covered until ready to serve.

G   Plates and trays should look appetizing. If they do not, inform your supervisor.

G   Give the resident the proper eating tools. Use assistive utensils if needed (Fig. 8-12).

Fig. 8-12. *These are examples of assistive, or adaptive, devices that can help with eating.* (PHOTOS COURTESY OF NORTH COAST MEDICAL, INC., 800-821-9319, WWW.NCMEDICAL.COM)

G   Be cheerful, positive, and helpful. Make conversation if the resident wishes to talk.

G   Honor requests regarding food. Residents have the legal right to ask for and receive different food. They can also ask for additional food.

7. Demonstrate how to assist with eating

Residents will need different levels of help with eating. Some residents will not need any help.

Other residents will only need help setting up. They may need someone to open cartons and cut and season their food. Once that is done, they can feed themselves. The NA should check with these residents from time to time to see if they need anything else.

Other residents will be completely unable to feed themselves. It will be the NA's job to feed them. Residents who must be fed are often embarrassed and depressed about their dependence on another person. NAs should be sensitive to this and give privacy while residents are eating. Residents should not be rushed while eating.

NAs should only give assistance as specified, when necessary, or when residents request it. They should encourage residents to do what they can. For example, if a resident can hold and use a napkin, she should. If she can hold and eat finger foods, they should be offered. There are devices that help residents eat more independently (see Fig. 8-12). More adaptive devices are shown in Chapter 9.

Guidelines: Assisting a Resident with Eating

G   Before you begin serving or helping residents, wash your hands.

G   It is very important to identify residents before serving a meal tray. Feeding a resident the wrong food can cause serious problems, even death. Verify that you have the right resident. Check the diet card against the name listed outside the door (if available). Ask the resident to state his name. Check that the diet on the tray is correct and matches the diet card.

G   Sit at a resident's eye level. Resident should be sitting upright, at a 90-degree angle. Make eye contact with the resident.

G   If the resident wishes, allow time for prayer.

G   Never treat the resident like a child. This is embarrassing and disrespectful. It is hard for many people to accept help with feeding. Be supportive and encouraging.

G Test the temperature of the food by putting your hand over the dish to sense the heat. Do not touch food to test its temperature. If you think the food is too hot, do not blow on it to cool it. Offer other food to give it time to cool.

G Cut foods and pour liquids as needed. Season foods to the resident's preference.

G Identify the foods and fluids that are in front of the resident. Call pureed foods by the correct name. For example, ask, "Would you like green beans?" rather than referring to it as "some green stuff."

G Ask the resident which food he wants to eat first. Allow him to make the choice, even if he wants to eat dessert first.

G Do not mix foods unless the resident requests it.

G Do not rush the meal. Allow time for the resident to chew and swallow each bite. Be relaxed.

G Be social and friendly. Make simple conversation if the resident wishes to do so. Use appropriate topics, such as the news, weather, the resident's life, things the resident enjoys, and food preferences. Say positive things about the food being served, such as, "This smells really good," and, "This looks really fresh."

G Give the resident your full attention while he is eating. Do not talk to other staff members while helping a resident eat.

G Alternate food and drink. Alternating cold and hot foods or bland foods and sweets can help increase appetite.

G If the resident wants a different food from what is being served, inform the dietitian so that an alternative may be offered.

Residents' Rights

Clothing Protectors

Residents have the right to refuse to wear a clothing protector. The NA can offer a clothing protector, but should not insist that a resident wear one. She should respect the resident's wishes. A clothing protector should not be referred to as a *bib*. This promotes residents' dignity and avoids treating them like children.

Feeding a resident

Equipment: meal, eating utensils, clothing protector, washcloths or wipes

1. Identify yourself by name. Identify the resident by name.
    Resident has right to know identity of his or her caregiver. Addressing resident by name shows respect and establishes correct identification.

2. Wash your hands.
    Provides for infection prevention.

3. Explain procedure to resident. Speak clearly, slowly, and directly. Maintain face-to-face contact whenever possible.
    Promotes understanding and independence.

4. Look at the diet card or menu. Ask resident to state her name. Verify that resident has received the right tray.
    Tray should only contain foods, fluids, and condiments permitted on the diet.

5. Raise the head of the bed. Make sure resident is in an upright sitting position (at a 90-degree angle).
    Promotes ease of swallowing. Prevents aspiration of food and beverage.

6. Adjust bed height to where you will be able to sit at resident's eye level. Lock bed wheels.

7. Place meal tray where it can be easily seen by the resident, such as on the overbed table.

8. Help resident to clean her hands with hand wipes if resident cannot do it herself.
    Promotes good hygiene and infection prevention.

9. Help resident to put on clothing protector if desired.
Protects resident's clothing from food and beverage spills.

10. Sit facing resident at the resident's eye level (Fig. 8-13). Sit on the stronger side if the resident has one-sided weakness.
Promotes good communication. Lets resident know that he or she will not be rushed while eating.

Fig. 8-13. *The resident should be sitting upright, and the NA should be sitting at her eye level.*

11. Tell the resident what foods are on the plate. Ask resident what she would like to eat first.
Resident has legal right to make decisions.

12. Check the temperature of the food. Using utensils, offer the food in bite-sized pieces. Tell the resident the content of each bite of food offered (Fig. 8-14). Alternate types of food, allowing for resident's preferences. Do not feed all of one type before offering another type. Make sure resident's mouth is empty before next bite or sip. Report any swallowing problems to the nurse immediately.
Small pieces are easier to chew and lessen the risk of choking. If the mouth is empty before offering more food, it lessens the risk of choking.

Fig. 8-14. *Offer the food in bite-sized pieces. Tell resident the content of each bite of food.*

13. Offer sips of beverage to the resident throughout the meal. If you are holding the cup, touch it to the resident's lips before you tip it. Give small, frequent sips.
Promotes ease of swallowing.

14. Talk with the resident during the meal (Fig. 8-15). Do not rush the resident.
Makes mealtime more enjoyable.

Fig. 8-15. *Socializing during mealtime makes eating more enjoyable. It may help promote a healthy appetite.*

15. Use washcloth or wipes to wipe food from resident's mouth and hands as needed during the meal (Fig. 8-16). Wipe mouth and hands at the end of the meal.
Maintains resident's dignity.

Fig. 8-16. *Wiping food from the mouth during the meal helps to maintain the resident's dignity.*

16. Remove clothing protector if used. Dispose of it in proper container.

17. Remove the food tray. Check for eyeglasses, dentures, or any personal items before removing tray. Place tray in proper area.

18. Make resident comfortable. Keep resident in the upright position for at least 30 minutes if ordered. Make sure bed is free from crumbs.
Food left on sheets can cause skin breakdown.

19. Return bed to lowest position. Remove privacy measures.
    Provides for safety.

20. Place call light within resident's reach.
    Allows resident to communicate with staff as necessary.

21. Wash your hands.
    Provides for infection prevention.

22. Report any changes in resident to the nurse.
    Provides nurse with information to assess resident.

23. Document procedure using facility guidelines.
    If you do not document the care, legally it did not happen.

Food trays and plates should also be observed after the meal. This helps to identify residents with poor appetites. It may also signal illness, a problem such as dentures that do not fit properly, or a change in food preferences.

All facilities keep track of how much food and liquid a resident consumes. Percentages are often used to document food intake, but the method can vary. The dietitian calculates the percentages for meals. The NA may be asked to document how much of the entire meal a resident ate. For example, if the resident ate the entire meal served, the NA would document that 100% was eaten. If the resident ate about half of the meal, the NA would document 50% eaten, and so on. NAs must document food intake accurately. They should follow their facility's policies.

8. Identify signs and symptoms of swallowing problems

Residents may have conditions that make eating or swallowing difficult. **Dysphagia** means difficulty in swallowing. A stroke, or CVA, can cause weakness on one side of the body and paralysis. Nerve and muscle damage from head and neck cancer, multiple sclerosis, Parkinson's or Alzheimer's disease may also be present. If a resident has trouble swallowing, soft foods and thickened liquids will be served. A special cup will help make swallowing easier.

NAs need to be able to recognize and report signs that a resident has a swallowing problem. Signs and symptoms of swallowing problems include the following:

* Coughing during or after meals

* Choking during meals

* Dribbling saliva, food, or fluid from the mouth

* Having food residue inside the mouth or cheeks during and after meals

* Gurgling during or after meals or losing voice

* Eating slowly

* Avoiding eating

* Spitting out pieces of food

* Swallowing several times per mouthful

* Clearing the throat frequently during and after meals

* Watering eyes when eating or drinking

* Food or fluid coming up into the nose

* Making a visible effort to swallow

* Breathing rapidly or with shorter breaths while eating or drinking

* Difficulty chewing food

* Difficulty swallowing medications

Residents with swallowing problems may be restricted to consuming only thickened liquids. Thickened liquids have a thickening powder or agent added to them. This improves the ability to control fluid in the mouth and throat. A doctor orders the necessary thickness after the resident has been evaluated by a speech-language pathologist.

Some beverages arrive already thickened and ready to drink. Other beverages must have the thickening agent added before serving. If thickening is ordered, it must be used with all liquids. This means that NAs should not offer regular liquids, such as water or other beverages, to residents who must have thickened liquids. There are three basic thickened consistencies:

1. **Nectar Thick**: This consistency is thicker than water. It is the thickness of a thick juice, such as a pear nectar or tomato juice. A resident can drink this from a cup.

2. **Honey Thick**: This consistency has the thickness of honey. It will pour very slowly. A resident will usually use a spoon to consume it.

3. **Pudding Thick**: With this consistency, the liquids have become semi-solid, much like pudding. A spoon should stand up straight in the glass when put into the middle of the drink. A resident must consume these liquids with a spoon.

Swallowing problems put residents at high risk for choking on food or drink. Inhaling food, fluid, or foreign material into the lungs is called **aspiration**. Aspiration can cause pneumonia or death. An NA should alert the nurse immediately if any problems occur while feeding.

Guidelines: Preventing Aspiration

G   Position residents in a straight, upright position when eating or drinking. Do not try to feed residents in a reclining position.

G   Offer small pieces of food or small spoonfuls of pureed food.

G   Feed residents slowly. Do not rush them.

G   Place food in the unaffected, or stronger, side of the mouth.

G   Make sure mouth is empty before offering another bite of food or sip of drink.

G   Keep residents in the upright position for at least 30 minutes after eating and drinking.

When the digestive system does not function properly, **hyperalimentation** or **total parenteral nutrition** (**TPN**) may be needed. With TPN, a solution of nutrients goes directly into the bloodstream. It bypasses the digestive system.

When a person is unable to swallow, he or she may be fed through a tube. A **nasogastric tube** is inserted into the nose and goes to the stomach. A tube can also be placed into the stomach through the abdominal wall. This is called a **percutaneous endoscopic gastrostomy** (**PEG**) **tube**. The surgically-created opening into the stomach that allows the insertion of a tube is called a **gastrostomy** (Fig. 8-17). Tube feedings are used when residents cannot swallow but can digest food. Conditions that may prevent swallowing include coma, cancer, stroke, refusal to eat, or extreme weakness. It is important to remember that residents have the legal right to refuse treatment. This includes the insertion of tubes.

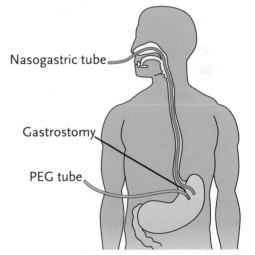

Fig. 8-17. Nasogastric tubes are inserted through the nose. PEG tubes are inserted through the abdominal wall into the stomach.

NAs never insert or remove tubes, do the feeding, or irrigate (clean) the tubes. They may assemble equipment and supplies and hand them to the nurse. NAs may position the resident in a sitting position for feeding. They may also discard or clean and store used equipment and supplies. In addition, NAs may observe, report, and document any changes in the resident or problems with the feeding.

Guidelines: Tube Feedings

G Wash your hands before assisting with any aspect of tube feedings.

G Make sure the tubing is not coiled or kinked or resting underneath the resident.

G Be aware if resident has an order for *nothing by mouth* or *NPO*.

G The tube is only inserted and removed by a doctor or nurse. If it comes out, report it immediately.

G A doctor will prescribe the type and amount of feeding. The feedings should be at room temperature and in liquid form.

G A resident with a feeding tube should always have the head of the bed elevated 30 degrees. However, during a feeding, the resident should remain in a sitting position with the head of the bed elevated at least 45 degrees. This helps prevent serious problems, such as aspiration. The elderly can develop pneumonia or even die from improper positioning during tube feedings. After the feeding, keep the resident upright for as long as ordered, at least 30 minutes.

G If the resident must remain in bed for long periods during feedings, give careful skin care. This helps to prevent pressure ulcers on the hips and sacral area.

Observing and Reporting: Tube Feedings

Report any of these to the nurse immediately:

O/R Redness or drainage around the opening

O/R Skin sores or bruises

O/R Cyanotic skin

O/R Resident complaints of pain or nausea

O/R Choking or coughing

O/R Vomiting

O/R Diarrhea

O/R Swollen abdomen

O/R Fever

O/R Tube falls out

O/R Problems with equipment

O/R Sound of feeding pump alarm

O/R Change of resident's inclined position

9. Describe how to assist residents with special needs

Residents with specific diseases or conditions, such as stroke, Parkinson's disease, Alzheimer's disease or other dementias, head trauma, blindness, or confusion may need special assistance when eating.

Guidelines: Dining Techniques

G Use assistive devices such as utensils with built-up handle grips, plate guards, and drinking cups. Assistive or adaptive devices for eating help people feed themselves. These devices are ordered for specific residents and should be included on the meal tray.

G Residents may benefit from physical and verbal cues. These promote independence. The hand-over-hand approach is an example of a physical cue. The resident lifts a utensil if he is able. You put your hand over his to help with eating. With your hand placed over the resident's hand, help the resident get food on the utensil. Steer the utensil from the plate to the mouth and back. Repeat this until the resident is finished.

G Verbal cues must be short and clear. The cues should prompt the resident to do something. Give verbal cues one at a time. Wait until the resident has finished one task before asking him to do another. The cues are repeated until the resident is finished eating. Examples of verbal cues include the following:

- "Pick up your spoon."
- "Put some carrots on your spoon."
- "Raise the spoon to your lips."
- "Open your mouth."
- "Place the spoon in your mouth."
- "Close your mouth."
- "Take the spoon out of your mouth."
- "Chew."
- "Swallow."
- "Drink some water."

G For visually-impaired residents, use the face of an imaginary clock to explain the position of what is in front of them (Fig. 8-18).

Fig. 8-18. Use the face of an imaginary clock to explain the position of food to visually-impaired residents.

G For residents who have had a stroke and have a paralyzed or weaker side, place food in the unaffected, or stronger, side of the mouth. Make sure food is swallowed before offering another bite.

G Place food in the resident's field of vision. The nurse will determine a resident's field of vision.

G For residents who have Parkinson's disease, tremors or shaking can make it difficult to eat. Help by using physical cues. Place food and drinks close so that the resident can easily reach them. Use assistive devices as needed.

G If a resident has poor sitting balance, seat him in a regular dining room chair with armrests, rather than in a wheelchair. Proper position in chair means hips are at a 90-degree angle, knees are flexed, and feet and arms are fully supported. Push the chair under the table. Place forearms on the table. If a resident tends to lean to one side, ask him to keep his elbows on the table.

G If a resident has poor neck control, a neck brace may be used to stabilize the head. Use assistive devices as needed. If resident is in a geri-chair, a wedge cushion behind the head and shoulders may be used.

G If the resident bites down on utensils, ask him to open his mouth. Do not pull the utensil out of the mouth. Wait until the jaw relaxes.

G If the resident pockets food in his cheeks, ask him to chew and swallow the food. Touch the side of his cheek. Ask him to use his tongue to get the food. Using your fingers on the cheek (near the lower jaw), gently push food toward teeth.

G If the resident holds food in his mouth, ask him to chew and swallow the food. You may need to trigger swallowing. To do this, gently press down on the tongue when taking the spoon out of the mouth. You can also try to gently press down on the top of his head with your hand. Make sure the resident has swallowed the food before offering more.

9

Rehabilitation and Restorative Care

1. Discuss rehabilitation and restorative care

When a resident loses some ability to function due to illness or injury, rehabilitation may be ordered. **Rehabilitation** is care that is managed by professionals. It helps to restore a person to his highest possible level of functioning. It involves helping residents move from illness, disability, and dependence toward health, ability, and independence. Rehabilitation involves all parts of the person's disability. This includes physical (e.g., eating, elimination) and psychosocial (e.g., independence, self-esteem) needs. Goals of a rehabilitation program include the following:

*   To help a resident regain function or recover from illness

*   To develop and promote a resident's independence

*   To help a resident to feel in control of his life

*   To help a resident accept or adapt to the limitations of a disability

Rehabilitation will be used for many residents, particularly those who have suffered a stroke, accident, or trauma. Restorative care usually follows rehabilitation. The goal of restorative care is to keep the resident at the level achieved by rehabilitative services. Both rehabilitation and restorative care take a team approach (Fig. 9-1).

Because nursing assistants spend many hours with these residents, they are a very important part of the team. NAs play a critical role in helping residents recover and regain independence.

Fig. 9-1. *A team of specialists, including doctors, nurses, physical therapists, and other kinds of therapists, helps residents with rehabilitation.*

Guidelines: Restorative Care

G Be patient. Progress may be slow. The more patient you are, the easier it will be for them to regain abilities and confidence.

G Be positive and supportive.

G Focus on small tasks and small accomplishments. Break tasks down into small steps. Take everything one step at a time.

G Recognize that setbacks occur. Progress occurs at different rates. Reassure residents that setbacks are normal.

G Be sensitive to the resident's needs. Some residents may need more encouragement than others. Some may be embarrassed by encouragement. Understand what motivates your residents.

G Encourage independence. Independence improves self-image and attitude. It also helps speed recovery.

G Involve residents in their care. Residents who feel involved may be more motivated to work hard in rehabilitation.

Observing and Reporting: Restorative Care

---

o/r Any increase or decrease in abilities

o/r Any change in attitude or motivation, positive or negative

o/r Any change in general health, such as changes in skin condition, appetite, energy level, or general appearance

o/r Signs of depression or mood changes

2. Describe the importance of promoting independence and list ways exercise improves health

Maintaining independence is vital during and after rehabilitation and restorative services. When an active and independent person is dependent, physical and mental problems may result. The body becomes less mobile. The mind is less focused. Studies show that the more active a person is, the better the mind and body work.

Inactivity and immobility can result in many problems, including the following:

- Loss of self-esteem
- Depression
- Pneumonia
- Urinary tract infection
- Constipation
- Blood clots
- Dulling of the senses
- Muscle atrophy
- Contractures

- Increased risk for pressure ulcers
- Problems with independence and self-esteem

The staff's job is to keep residents as active as possible—whether they are bedbound or are able to walk (ambulate). Regular ambulation and exercise help improve these things:

- Quality and health of the skin
- Circulation
- Strength
- Sleep and relaxation
- Mood
- Self-esteem
- Appetite
- Elimination
- Blood flow
- Oxygen level

Promoting social interaction and thinking abilities is important too. Most facilities have activities geared to residents' ages and abilities. Social involvement should be encouraged. When possible, NAs should join in activities with residents. This promotes independence. It also gives NAs a chance to observe residents' abilities.

3. Discuss ambulation and describe assistive devices and equipment

Ambulation is walking. A resident who is **ambulatory** is one who can get out of bed and walk. Many older residents are ambulatory, but need help to walk safely. Several tools, including gait belts, canes, walkers, and crutches, help with ambulation. NAs should check the care plan before helping a resident ambulate. The NA should discuss the resident's abilities, limitations, and disabilities with the nurse. It is important that the NA communicate what she would like to do and allow the resident to do what he can.

Assisting a resident to ambulate

Equipment: gait belt, nonskid shoes

1. Identify yourself by name. Identify the resident by name.
   Resident has right to know identity of his or her caregiver. Addressing resident by name shows respect and establishes correct identification.

2. Wash your hands.
   Provides for infection prevention.

3. Explain procedure to resident. Speak clearly, slowly, and directly. Maintain face-to-face contact whenever possible.
   Promotes understanding and independence.

4. Provide for resident's privacy with curtain, screen, or door.
   Maintains resident's right to privacy and dignity.

5. Adjust bed to lowest position so that the feet are flat on the floor. Lock bed wheels.
   Prevents injury and promotes stability.

6. Before ambulating, put nonskid footwear on resident and securely fasten.
   Promotes resident's safety. Prevents falls.

7. Stand in front of and face the resident. Place your feet about shoulder-width apart.
   Promotes proper body mechanics.

8. Place gait belt around resident's waist over clothing (not on bare skin). Grasp belt securely on both sides.

9. If resident is unable to stand without help, brace (support) the resident's lower extremities. This can be done by placing one of your knees against the resident's knee (Fig. 9-2). It can also be done by placing both of your knees against both of the resident's knees (Fig. 9-3). Bend your knees.

10. Hold the resident close to your center of gravity. Provide instructions to allow resident to help with standing. Tell the resident to lean forward, push down on the bed with his hands, and stand on the count of three. On three, with hands still grasping the gait belt

on both sides and moving upward, slowly help resident to stand.

Fig. 9-2. *If resident has a weak knee, brace it against your knee.*

Fig. 9-3. *You can also use both knees to brace the resident's knees.*

11. Walk slightly behind and to one side of resident for the full ordered distance, while holding onto the gait belt (Fig. 9-4). If the resident has a weaker side, stand on the weaker side. Ask resident to look forward, not down at the floor, during ambulation.

12. After ambulation, help resident to the bed or chair. Remove gait belt. Check that the resident is in proper alignment.

13. Leave bed in lowest position.
    Provides for safety.

Fig. 9-4. *Walk behind and to one side while holding onto the gait belt when assisting with ambulation.*

14. Place call light within resident's reach.
    Allows resident to communicate with staff as necessary.

15. Wash your hands.
    Provides for infection prevention.

16. Report any changes in resident to nurse.
    Provides nurse with information to assess resident.

17. Document procedure using facility guidelines.
    If you do not document the care, legally it did not happen.

When helping a visually-impaired resident walk, the NA should let the person walk beside and slightly behind her, as he rests a hand on the NA's elbow. The NA should walk at a normal pace. She should let the resident know when they are about to turn a corner or when a step is approaching. The NA should state whether they will be stepping up or down.

Residents who have trouble walking may use canes, walkers, or crutches to help themselves. Canes help with balance. Residents using canes should be able to bear weight on both legs. If one leg is weaker, the cane should be held in the hand on the strong side.

Types of canes are the C cane, the functional grip cane, and the quad cane. The C cane is a straight cane with a curved handle at the top. It has a rubber-tipped bottom to prevent slipping. A C cane is used to improve balance. A functional grip cane is similar to the C cane, except that it has a straight grip handle, rather than a curved handle. The grip handle helps improve grip control. It provides more support than the C cane. A

quad cane has four rubber-tipped feet and a rectangular base. It is designed to bear more weight than the other canes (Fig. 9-5).

Fig. 9-5. *A quad cane has four rubber-tipped feet and can bear more weight than other canes.*

A walker is used when the resident can bear some weight on the legs. The walker gives stability for residents who are unsteady or lack balance. The metal frame may have rubber-tipped feet and/or wheels (Fig. 9-6). Crutches are used for residents who can bear no weight or limited weight on one leg. Some people use one crutch. Some use two.

Fig. 9-6. *The photo on the left shows a standard walker and the photo on the right shows a Hemi Walker, which is a walker that is designed for people who have difficulty using an arm or a hand.* (© INVACARE CORPORATION. USED WITH PERMISSION. WWW.INVACARE.COM)

Guidelines: Cane or Walker Use

G Be sure the walker or cane is in good condition. It must have rubber tips on the bottom. The tips should not be cracked. Walkers may have wheels. If so, roll the walker to make sure the wheels are moving properly.

G Be sure the resident is wearing securely fastened, nonskid shoes before ambulating.

G When using a cane, the resident should place it on his stronger side.

G When using a walker, have the resident place both hands on the walker. The walker should not be over-extended. It should be placed no more than six inches in front of the resident.

G Stay near the resident on the weaker side.

G Do not hang purses or clothing on the walker.

G If height of the cane or walker does not appear to be correct (too short, too tall, etc.), tell the nurse.

Assisting with ambulation for a resident using a cane, walker, or crutches

Equipment: gait belt, nonskid shoes, cane, walker, or crutches

1. Identify yourself by name. Identify the resident by name.
   Resident has right to know identity of his or her caregiver. Addressing resident by name shows respect and establishes correct identification.

2. Wash your hands.
   Provides for infection prevention.

3. Explain procedure to resident. Speak clearly, slowly, and directly. Maintain face-to-face contact whenever possible.
   Promotes understanding and independence.

4. Provide for resident's privacy with curtain, screen, or door.
   Maintains resident's right to privacy and dignity.

5. Adjust bed to lowest position so that the feet are flat on the floor. Lock bed wheels.
   Prevents injury and promotes stability.

6. Before ambulating, put nonskid footwear on resident and securely fasten.
   Promotes resident's safety. Prevents falls.

7. Stand in front of and face resident. Place your feet about shoulder-width apart.
   Promotes proper body mechanics.

8. Place gait belt around resident's waist over clothing (not on bare skin). Grasp belt securely on both sides.

9. If resident is unable to stand without help, brace (support) resident's lower extremities (see previous procedure). Bend your knees. Help the resident to stand as described in the previous procedure.

10. Help as needed with ambulation.

   a. **Cane**: Resident places cane about six inches, or a comfortable distance, in front of his stronger leg. He brings weaker leg even with cane. He then brings stronger leg forward slightly ahead of cane. Repeat.

   b. **Walker**: Resident picks up or rolls the walker. He places it about six inches, or a comfortable distance, in front of him. All four feet or wheels of the walker should be on the ground before resident steps forward to the walker. The walker should not be moved again until the resident has moved both feet forward and is steady. The resident should never put his feet ahead of the walker.
   Promotes stability and prevents falls.

   c. **Crutches**: Resident should be fitted for crutches and taught to use them correctly by a physical therapist or nurse. The resident may use crutches several different ways. It depends on what his weakness is. No matter how they are used, weight should be on the resident's hands and arms. Weight should not be on the underarm area.

11. Walk slightly behind and to one side of resident. Stay on the weaker side if resident has one. Hold the gait belt.
   Provides security.

12. Watch for obstacles in the resident's path. Ask the resident to look forward, not down at the floor, during ambulation.
   Promotes resident's safety. Prevents injury.

13. Encourage resident to rest if he is tired. When a person is tired, it increases the

chance of a fall. Let the resident set the pace. Discuss how far he plans to go based on the care plan.

14. After ambulation, remove gait belt. Help resident to the bed or chair. Check that the resident is in proper alignment.

15. Leave bed in lowest position.
    Provides for safety.

16. Place call light within resident's reach.
    Allows resident to communicate with staff as necessary.

17. Wash your hands.
    Provides for infection prevention.

18. Report any changes in resident to nurse.
    Provides nurse with information to assess resident.

19. Document procedure using facility guidelines.
    If you do not document the care, legally it did not happen.

Many devices are available to help people who are recovering from or adapting to a physical condition. **Assistive** or **adaptive devices** are equipment that helps residents perform their activities of daily living (ADLs). Each device is made to support a particular disability.

Personal care equipment includes long-handled brushes and combs. Plate guards prevent food from being pushed off the plate. They make it easier to scoop food onto utensils. Reachers can help put on underwear or pants. A sock aid can pull on socks. A long-handled shoehorn assists in putting shoes on without bending. Long-handled sponges help with bathing.

Supportive devices, such as canes, walkers, and crutches, are used to assist residents with ambulation. Safety devices, such as shower chairs and gait or transfer belts, help prevent accidents. Safety bars/grab bars are often installed in and near the tub and toilet to give the resident something to hold on to while changing position.

More examples of assistive devices are shown in Figure 9-7 below.

4. Explain guidelines for maintaining proper body alignment

Residents who are confined to bed need proper body alignment. This aids recovery and prevents injury to muscles and joints. These guidelines help residents maintain proper alignment and make progress when they can get out of bed:

Fig. 9-7. *Many assistive items are available to help residents adapt to physical changes.* (PHOTOS COURTESY OF NORTH COAST MEDICAL, INC. WWW.NCMEDICAL.COM, 800-821-9319)

Guidelines: Alignment and Positioning

G   Observe principles of alignment. Proper alignment is based on straight lines. The spine should be in a straight line. Pillows or rolled or folded blankets can support the small of the back and raise the knees or head in the supine position. They can support the head and one leg in the lateral position (Fig. 9-8).

Fig. 9-8. Pillows or rolled or folded blankets help provide extra support.

G   Keep body parts in natural positions. In a natural hand position, the fingers are slightly curled. Use a rolled washcloth, gauze bandage, or a rubber ball inside the palm to support the fingers in this position. Use bed cradles to keep covers from resting on feet in the supine position.

G   Prevent external rotation of hips. When legs and hips turn outward during bedrest, hip contractures can result. A rolled blanket or towel tucked alongside the hip and thigh can keep the leg from turning outward.

G   Change positions often to prevent muscle stiffness and pressure ulcers. This should be done at least every two hours. The position used will depend on the resident's condition and preference. Check the skin every time you reposition the resident.

G   Give back rubs as ordered for comfort and relaxation.

5. Describe care guidelines for prosthetic devices

Amputation is the surgical removal of some or all of a body part, usually a hand, arm, leg, or foot. Amputation may be the result of an injury or disease. After amputation, some people feel that the limb is still there. They may feel pain in the part that has been amputated. **Phantom sensation** is the term used when a person feels that the body part is still there. **Phantom limb pain** occurs when the person feels pain in a limb (or extremity) that has been amputated. It may last for a short time or for years. The pain or sensation is real. It should not be ignored.

A **prosthesis** is a device that replaces a body part that is missing or deformed because of an accident, injury, illness, or birth defect. It is used to improve a person's ability to function and/or to improve appearance. Examples of prostheses include the following:

*   Artificial limbs, such as artificial hands, arms, feet, and legs, are made to resemble the body part that they are replacing.

*   An artificial breast is made of a lightweight, soft, spongy material.

*   A hearing aid is a small, battery-operated device that amplifies sound for persons with hearing loss.

*   An artificial eye, or ocular prosthetic, replaces an eye that has been lost to disease or injury. An ocular prosthetic does not provide vision. It can, however, improve appearance.

*   Dentures are artificial teeth. They may be necessary when teeth have been damaged, lost, or must be removed.

Guidelines: Amputation and Prosthesis Care

G   Residents who have had a body part amputated must make many physical, psychological, social, and occupational adjustments due to disability. Be supportive.

G   Help residents with their ADLs.

G   Prostheses are specially-fitted, expensive pieces of equipment (some cost tens of thousands of dollars). Care for them as assigned. Handle them carefully.

G A therapist or nurse will demonstrate application of a prosthesis. Follow instructions to apply and remove the prosthesis. Follow the manufacturer's care directions.

G Keep a prosthesis and the skin under it dry and clean. The socket of the prosthesis must be cleaned at least daily. Follow the care plan and the nurse's instructions.

G If ordered, apply a stump sock before putting on the prosthesis.

G Observe the skin on stump. Watch for signs of skin breakdown caused by pressure and abrasion. Report any redness or open areas.

G Never try to fix a prosthesis. Report any problems to the nurse.

G Do not show negative feelings about the stump during care.

G Phantom limb pain is real pain. Treat it that way. Report complaints of pain to the nurse.

G If the resident has an artificial eye, review the care plan with the nurse. Always wash your hands and don gloves before handling an artificial eye. Never clean or soak the eye in rubbing alcohol. It will crack the plastic and destroy it. If the eye is to be removed and not reinserted, store it in water or saline solution. Make sure the container is labeled with the resident's name and room number. The resident may be able to remove, clean, and insert the eye himself. Know any instructions for assisting with care.

Information on care of hearing aids is in Chapter 2. Denture care is located in Chapter 6.

6. Describe how to assist with range of motion exercises

Range of motion (**ROM**) exercises put a joint through its full arc of motion. The goal of these exercises is to decrease or prevent contractures or atrophy, improve strength, and increase circulation. Active range of motion (AROM) exercises are done by a resident himself, without help.

The NA's role in AROM exercises is to encourage the resident. Active assisted range of motion (AAROM) exercises are done by the resident with some help and support from the NA. Passive range of motion (PROM) exercises are used when residents are not able to move on their own. A staff member performs these exercises without the resident's help.

ROM exercises are specific for each body area. They include these movements (Fig. 9-9):

Fig. 9-9. *The different range of motion body movements.*

- **Abduction**: moving a body part away from the midline of the body
- **Adduction**: moving a body part toward the midline of the body
- **Extension**: straightening a body part
- **Flexion**: bending a body part
- **Dorsiflexion**: bending backward
- **Rotation**: turning a joint
- **Pronation**: turning downward
- **Supination**: turning upward
- **Opposition**: touching the thumb to any other finger

NAs will not do ROM exercises without an order from a doctor, nurse, or physical therapist. The NA will repeat each exercise three to five times, once or twice a day, working on both sides of the body. When doing ROM exercises, the NA should begin at the resident's shoulders and work down the body. The upper extremities (arms) should be exercised before the lower extremities (legs). The NA should give support above and below the joint. The joints should be moved gently, slowly, and smoothly. The NA should stop the exercises if the resident complains of pain and report the pain to the nurse.

Assisting with passive range of motion exercises

1. Identify yourself by name. Identify the resident by name.
    Resident has right to know identity of his or her caregiver. Addressing resident by name shows respect and establishes correct identification.

2. Wash your hands.
    Provides for infection prevention.

3. Explain procedure to resident. Speak clearly, slowly, and directly. Maintain face-to-face contact whenever possible.
    Promotes understanding and independence.

4. Provide for resident's privacy with curtain, screen, or door.
    Maintains resident's right to privacy and dignity.

5. Adjust bed to a safe level, usually waist high. Lock bed wheels.
    Prevents injury to you and to resident.

6. Position the resident lying supine—flat on her back—on the bed. Use proper alignment.
    Reduces stress to joints.

7. While supporting the limbs, move all joints gently, slowly, and smoothly through the range of motion to the point of resistance. Repeat each exercise at least three times. Stop if any pain occurs.
    Rapid movement may cause injury. Pain is a warning sign for injury.

8. **Shoulder**: Support the resident's arm at the elbow and wrist while performing ROM for the shoulder. Place one hand under the elbow and the other hand under the wrist. Raise the straightened arm from the side position upward toward head to ear level. Return arm

down to side of the body (extension/flexion) (Fig. 9-10).

Fig. 9-10. Raise the straightened arm upward toward head to ear level and return it to the side of the body.

Move straightened arm away from side of body to shoulder level. Return arm to side of body (abduction/adduction) (Fig. 9-11).

Fig. 9-11. Move straightened arm away from side of body to shoulder level and return arm to side.

9. **Elbow**: Hold the resident's wrist with one hand and the elbow with the other hand. Bend the elbow so that the hand touches the shoulder on that same side (flexion). Straighten the arm (extension) (Fig. 9-12).

Fig. 9-12. Bend the elbow so that the hand touches the shoulder on the same side. Then straighten the arm.

Exercise the forearm by moving it so the palm is facing downward (pronation) and then the palm is facing upward (supination) (Fig. 9-13).

Fig. 9-13. *Exercise the forearm so that the palm is facing downward and then upward.*

10. **Wrist**: Hold the wrist with one hand. Use the fingers of the other hand to help move the joint through the motions. Bend the hand down (flexion); bend the hand backward (dorsiflexion) (Fig. 9-14).

Fig. 9-14. *While supporting the wrist, gently bend the hand down and then backward.*

Turn the hand in the direction of the thumb (radial flexion). Then turn the hand in the direction of the little finger (ulnar flexion) (Fig. 9-15).

Fig. 9-15. *Turn the hand in the direction of the thumb, then turn it in the direction of the little finger.*

11. **Thumb**: Move the thumb away from the index finger (abduction). Move the thumb back next to the index finger (adduction) (Fig. 9-16).

Fig. 9-16. *Move the thumb away from the index finger and then back to the index finger.*

Touch each fingertip with the thumb (opposition) (Fig. 9-17).

Fig. 9-17. *Touch each fingertip with the thumb.*

Bend thumb into the palm (flexion) and out to the side (extension) (Fig. 9-18).

Fig. 9-18. *Bend the thumb into the palm and then out to the side.*

12. **Fingers**: Make the hand into a fist (flexion). Gently straighten out the fist (extension) (Fig. 9-19).

Fig. 9-19. *Make the fingers into a fist and then gently straighten out the fist.*

Spread the fingers and the thumb far apart from each other (abduction). Bring the fingers back next to each other (adduction) (Fig. 9-20).

Fig. 9-20. *Spread the fingers and thumb far apart from each other and then bring them back next to each other.*

13. **Hip**: Support the leg by placing one hand under the knee and one under the ankle. Straighten the leg and raise it gently upward. Move the leg away from the other leg (abduction). Move the leg toward the other leg (adduction) (Fig. 9-21).

Fig. 9-21. *Straighten the leg and gently raise it. Move the leg away from the other leg and then back toward the other leg.*

Gently turn the leg inward (internal rotation), then turn the leg outward (external rotation) (Fig. 9-22).

Fig. 9-22. *Gently turn the leg inward and then outward.*

14. **Knee**: Support the leg under the knee and under the ankle while performing ROM for the knee. Bend the knee to the point of resistance (flexion). Return leg to resident's normal position (extension) (Fig. 9-23).

Fig. 9-23. *Gently bend the knee to the point of resistance and return the leg to its normal position.*

15. **Ankle**: Support the foot and ankle close to the bed while performing ROM for the ankle. Push/pull foot up toward the head (dorsiflexion). Push/pull foot down, with the toes pointed down (plantar flexion) (Fig. 9-24).

Fig. 9-24. Push the foot up toward the head and then push it back down.

Turn the inside of the foot inward toward the body (supination). Bend the sole of the foot so that it faces away from the body (pronation) (Fig. 9-25).

Fig. 9-25. Turn inside of foot inward, toward the body, and then bend it to face away from the body.

16. **Toes**: Curl and straighten the toes (flexion and extension) (Fig. 9-26).

Fig. 9-26. Curl and straighten the toes.

Gently spread the toes apart (abduction) (Fig. 9-27).

Fig. 9-27. Gently spread the toes apart.

17. Return resident to comfortable position. Return bed to lowest position.
    Promotes resident's safety.

18. Place call light within resident's reach.
    Allows resident to communicate with staff as necessary.

19. Wash your hands.
    Provides for infection prevention.

20. Report any changes in resident to nurse.
    Provides nurse with information to assess resident.

21. Document procedure using facility guidelines. Note any decrease in range of motion or any pain experienced by the resident. Notify the nurse or the physical therapist if you find increased stiffness or physical resistance. Resistance may be a sign that a contracture is developing.
    If you do not document the care, legally it did not happen.

7. List guidelines for assisting with bladder and bowel retraining

Injury, illness, or inactivity may cause a loss of normal bladder or bowel function. Residents may need help to re-establish a regular routine and normal function. Problems with elimination can be embarrassing or difficult to discuss. NAs should be sensitive to this. They should be professional when handling incontinence or working to re-establish routines.

Guidelines: Bladder or Bowel Retraining

G   Follow Standard Precautions. Wear gloves when handling body wastes.

G   Explain the training schedule to the resident. Follow the schedule carefully.

G   Keep a record of the resident's bladder and bowel habits. When you see a pattern of elimination, you can predict when the resident will need a bedpan or a trip to the bathroom.

G   Offer a bedpan or a trip to the bathroom before beginning long procedures.

G   Encourage residents to drink plenty of fluids. Do this even if urinary incontinence is a problem. About 30 minutes after fluids are taken, offer a trip to the bathroom or a bedpan or urinal.

G   Encourage the resident to eat foods that are high in fiber. Encourage residents to follow special diets as ordered.

G   Answer call lights promptly. Residents cannot wait long when the urge to go to the bathroom occurs. Leave call lights within reach.

G   Provide privacy for elimination—both in the bed and in the bathroom.

G   If a resident has trouble urinating, try running water in the sink. Have her lean forward slightly. This puts pressure on the bladder.

G   Do not rush the resident.

G   Help residents with careful perineal care. This helps prevent skin breakdown and promotes proper hygiene. Observe for skin changes.

G   Discard wastes according to facility policy.

G   Discard clothing protectors and incontinence briefs properly (Fig. 9-28). Double-bag these items if ordered. This stops odors from collecting.

G   Some facilities use washable bed pads or briefs. Follow Standard Precautions when handling these items.

Fig. 9-28. *A type of incontinence pad.*

G   Keep an accurate record of urination and bowel movements. This includes episodes of incontinence.

G   Praise successes or even attempts to control the bladder and bowels. However, do not talk to residents as if they are children. Keep your voice low. Do not draw attention to any aspect of retraining. Do not discuss accidents or retraining in public areas.

G   Never show frustration or anger toward residents who are incontinent. The problem is out of their control. Negative reactions will only make things worse. Be kind, supportive, and professional.

G   When the resident is incontinent or cannot use the toilet when asked, be positive. Never make the resident feel like a failure. Praise and encouragement are essential for a successful program. Some residents will always be incontinent. Be patient. Offer these residents extra care and attention. Skin breakdown may lead to pressure ulcers without proper care. Always report changes in skin.

Changing Incontinence Briefs

When changing an incontinence brief, the NA should make sure to assemble all needed items beforehand, including a protective pad, perineal care supplies, disposable wipes, gloves, and a clean brief. She should put on gloves before handling the brief. When removing the soiled brief, the NA should roll it inward, soiled side inside, without spilling its contents. Working from front to back, she should carefully remove all urine and/or feces from the skin. After cleaning the area thoroughly, she should blot it dry and apply the clean brief.

10
Caring for Yourself

The first nine chapters of this book introduce readers to the long-term care setting. They cover the knowledge, skills, and qualities a person needs to work as a nursing assistant. This final chapter is more personal. It addresses the reader directly. This chapter includes information on how to find and keep a job, as well as how to build good working relationships. It also includes helpful tips for managing stress and staying healthy.

1. Describe how to find a job

You may soon be looking for a job. Nursing assistants may be able to work in long-term care facilities, in assisted living facilities, in hospitals, in the home, and in other places. To find a job, you must first find potential employers. Then you must contact them to find out about job opportunities. To find employers, use the Internet, newspaper, or personal contacts (Fig. 10-1). You can also ask your instructor about potential employers.

Fig. 10-1. Using the Internet is a good way to find a job.

Once you have a list of potential employers, you need to contact them. Emailing or phoning first, unless they mention not to do so, is a good way to find out what jobs are available. Ask how to apply for a job with each potential employer.

When making an appointment, ask what information to bring with you. Make sure you have this information with you when you go. Some of these documents may be required:

*   Identification, including driver's license, social security card, birth certificate, passport, or other official form of identification

*   Proof of your legal status in this country and proof that you are legally able to work, even if you are a U.S. citizen. All employers must have files showing that all employees are legally allowed to work in this country. Do not be offended by this request.

*   High school diploma or equivalency, school transcripts, and diploma or certificate from your nursing assistant training course. Take your instructor's name, phone number, and email address with you as well.

*   References are people who can be contacted to recommend you as an employee. They include former employers and/or former teachers. Do not use relatives or friends as references. You can ask references to write letters for you beforehand. They can be addressed "To Whom It May Concern" and should explain how they know you and

describe your skills, qualities, and work habits. Take copies of these with you.

Some potential employers will ask you for a résumé. A résumé is a summary or listing of relevant job experience and education. When creating your résumé, keep it brief (one page is best) and clear. Include this information:

- Your contact details: name, address, telephone number, email address

- Your educational experience, starting with the most current first

- Your work experience, starting with the most current first

- Any special skills, such as knowledge of computer software, typing skills, or speaking other languages

- Any memberships in professional organizations

- Volunteer work

You may need to complete a job application. Write down the general information you will need. Take it with you, along with your résumé if you have one. This will save time and avoid mistakes. Include this information:

- Your address, phone number, and email address

- Your birth date

- Your social security number

- Name and address of the school or program where you were trained, the date you completed your training, and your certification number, as well as information about other certifications such as CPR and first aid

- Names, titles, addresses, phone numbers, and email addresses of former employers, and the dates you worked there

- Salary information from your former jobs

- Reasons why you left each of your former jobs

- Names, addresses, phone numbers, and email addresses of your references

- Days and hours you can work

- A brief statement of why you are changing jobs or why you want to work as a nursing assistant

Fill out the application carefully and neatly. Never lie. Before you write anything, read it all the way through once. If you are not sure what is being asked, find out before filling in that space. Fill in all of the blanks. Write *N/A* (not applicable) if the question does not apply to you.

By law, your employer must do a criminal background check on all new aides hired. You may be asked to sign a form granting permission to do this. Do not take it personally. It is a law intended to protect patients and residents.

To make the best impression at a job interview, be professional. Do the following:

- Shower or bathe. Use deodorant.

- Brush your teeth.

- Wear only simple makeup and jewelry or none at all.

- Clean and file your nails. Nails should be medium length or shorter. Do not wear artificial nails.

- Style clean hair simply.

- Shave or trim facial hair before the interview.

- Dress neatly and appropriately. Make sure clothing is clean, ironed, and has no holes in it. Do not wear jeans, shorts, or short dresses or skirts (no shorter than knee-length). Shoes should be clean and polished. Do not wear sneakers or flip-flops.

- Do not wear perfume or cologne. Many people dislike or are allergic to scents.

- Do not smoke beforehand. You will smell like smoke in the interview.

- Arrive 10 or 15 minutes early.

- Introduce yourself. Smile and shake hands (Fig. 10-2). Your handshake should be firm and confident.

- Answer questions clearly and completely.

- Make eye contact to show you are sincere.

- Avoid slang words or expressions.

- Do not eat, drink, chew gum, or smoke in an interview.

- Sit up or stand up straight. Look happy to be there.

- Do not bring friends or children with you.

- Relax and be confident. You have worked hard to get this far.

Fig. 10-2. Smile, shake hands confidently, and make eye contact when arriving at a job interview.

Be positive when answering questions. Emphasize what you enjoy or think you will enjoy about the job. Do not complain about any previous jobs you have had. Make it clear that you are hardworking and willing to work with all kinds of residents.

Usually interviewers will ask if you have any questions. Have some prepared. Write them down so you do not forget things you really want to know. Questions you may want to ask include

- What hours would I work? Is there any mandatory overtime I would need to work?

- What benefits does the job include? Is health insurance available? Would I get paid sick days or holidays?

- What is the average caseload for nursing assistants?

- What orientation or training is provided?

- How will I contact my supervisor when I need to do so?

- Are there any policies regarding ongoing education or advancement?

- How soon will you be making a decision about this position?

Later in the interview, you may want to ask about salary or wages if you have not already been given this information. Listen carefully to the answers to your questions. Take notes if needed. You will probably be told when you can expect to hear from the employer about the job. Do not expect to be offered a job at the interview. When the interview is over, stand up and shake hands again. Thank the employer for meeting with you.

Send a letter after every job interview to say thank you. Express your continued interest in the job. If you have not heard back from the employer within the time frame you discussed with your interviewer, call and ask if the job has been filled.

2. Describe a standard job description and explain how to manage time and assignments

A job description is an agreement between the employer and the employee. When you start a new job, you will receive a job description. It states the responsibilities and tasks of the job. It also describes the skills required for the job, to whom you must report, and the salary range.

The job description provides protection for both you and your employer. It protects you, the employee, from the facility changing duties without notifying you. It protects you from being fired based on something not related to your job description. The employer is protected if you ever were to claim you did not know certain duties were part of the job. The job description reduces misunderstandings. It can be used to document what was agreed upon if legal issues occur.

When taking care of residents, you must be able to manage your time well. There is a variety of tasks that must be done during your shift. Managing time properly helps you complete these tasks. Many of the following ideas for managing time on the job can be used to manage personal time as well:

Plan ahead. Planning is the single best way to manage time better. Sometimes it is hard even to find time to plan, but it is important to sit down and list everything that has to be done. Often just making the list will help you feel better and be able to focus. It is also helpful to take time to check to see if you have all the supplies needed for a procedure before you begin.

The nurse creates nursing assistants' work assignments based on the needs of residents and availability of staff. The assignments allow staff to work as a team. Your responsibilities in completing assignments include the following:

- Helping others when needed

- Never ignoring a resident who needs help

- Answering all call lights even when not assigned to a particular resident

- Notifying the nurse if you cannot complete an assignment

Prioritize. Identify the most important things to get done and do these first.

Make a schedule. Write out the hours of the day and fill in what needs to be done and when. This allows for a realistic schedule.

Combine activities. You can visit with residents while providing care, which combines two important tasks. Work more efficiently whenever possible.

Get help. It is a simple reality that it is not possible for you to do everything. Sometimes you will need help to ensure a resident's safety. Do not be afraid to ask for help.

3. Discuss how to manage and resolve conflict

Everyone experiences conflict at some point in his or her life. For example, families may argue at home, coworkers may disagree on the job, and so on. If conflict at work is not managed or resolved, it may affect the ability to function well. The work environment may suffer. When conflict occurs, there is a proper time and place to address it. You may need to talk to your supervisor for help. In general, follow these guidelines:

Guidelines: Resolving Conflict

G   Plan to discuss the issue at the right time. Do not start a conversation while you are helping residents. Wait until the supervisor has decided on the right time and place. Privacy is important. Shut the door. Limit distractions, such as TV and conversations.

G   Agree not to interrupt the person. Do not be rude or sarcastic, or name-call. Use active listening. Take turns speaking.

G   Do not get emotional. Some situations may be upsetting. However, you will be more effective in communicating if you can keep your emotions out of it.

G   Check your body language. Make sure it is not tense, unwelcoming, or threatening.

Maintain eye contact. Use a posture that says you are listening and interested. Lean forward slightly. Do not slouch.

G   Keep the focus on the issue at hand. When discussing conflict, state how you feel when a behavior occurs. Use "I" statements. First describe the actual behavior. Then use "feeling" words to describe how you feel. Let the person know how the problem is affecting you. For example, "When you are late to work, I feel upset because I end up doing your work along with my own."

G   People involved in the conflict may need to come up with possible solutions. Think of ways that the conflict can be resolved. A solution that does not satisfy everyone may be chosen by a supervisor. You may have to compromise. Be prepared to do this.

4. Describe employee evaluations and discuss appropriate responses to criticism

Handling criticism is hard for most people. Being able to accept and learn from criticism is important in all relationships. This includes work relationships. From time to time you will get evaluations from your employer. They contain ideas to help you improve your job performance. Here are some tips for handling criticism and using it to your benefit:

•   Listen to the message that is being sent. Do not get so upset that you cannot understand the message.

•   Hostile criticism and constructive criticism are not the same. Hostile criticism is angry and negative. Examples are, "You are useless!" or, "You are lazy and slow." Hostile criticism should not come from your employer or supervisor. You may hear hostile criticism from residents, family members, or others. The best response is something like, "I'm sorry you are so disappointed,"

and nothing more. Give the person a chance to calm down before trying to discuss their comments.

•   Constructive criticism is meant to help you improve. Constructive criticism may come from your employer, supervisor, or others. Examples are, "You really need to be more accurate in your charting," or, "You are late too often. You'll have to make more of an effort to be on time." Listening to and acting on constructive criticism can help you be more successful in your job. Pay attention to it (Fig. 10-3).

Fig. 10-3. *Ask for suggestions when receiving constructive criticism.*

•   If you are not sure how to avoid a mistake you have made, always ask for suggestions on improving your performance.

•   Apologize and move on. If you have made a mistake, apologize as needed (Fig. 10-4). This may be to a supervisor, a resident, or others. Learn from the incident and put it behind you. Do not dwell on it or hold a grudge. Responding professionally to criticism is important for success in any job.

I'm sorry I've been late several times this month. I know it's inconvenient for you. I am making more of an effort to be on time, and I expect not to be late again.

Fig. 10-4. *Be willing to apologize if you have made a mistake.*

An evaluation will also cover overall knowledge, conflict resolution, and team effort. Flexibility, friendliness, trustworthiness, and excellent customer service are very important. Evaluations are often the basis for salary increases. A good evaluation can help you advance within the facility. Being open to criticism and suggestions for improvement will help you be more successful.

If you decide to change jobs, be responsible. Always give your employer at least two weeks' written notice that you will be leaving. Otherwise, your facility may be understaffed. Both the residents and other staff will suffer. Future employers may talk with past supervisors. People who change jobs too often or who do not give notice before leaving are less likely to be hired.

5. Discuss certification and explain the state's registry

To meet the requirements set forth in the Omnibus Budget Reconciliation Act (OBRA), states must regulate nursing assistant training, evaluation, and certification. OBRA requires 75 hours as the minimum level of initial training and a 12-hour minimum for annual continuing education (called *in-services*). Many states' requirements exceed the minimum hours. It is a good idea to know your state's rules.

After completing an approved training program, NAs are given a competency evaluation (a certification exam or test) so that they can be certified to work in a state. This exam usually has both a written and skills evaluation. You must pass both parts in order to be certified to work as a nursing assistant.

OBRA also requires that each state keep a registry of nursing assistants. This registry is maintained by a state department. Often this is the state's Board of Nursing or Department of Health. The registry contains NAs' training information and results of certification exams. It also has any findings of abuse, neglect, or theft by nursing assistants. Employers are able to access this list to check if you have passed the certification exam. They can see if your certification is current. They are also able to see if you have been investigated for or found guilty of abuse or neglect.

Each state has different requirements for maintaining certification. Learn your state's requirements. Follow them exactly or you will not be able to keep working. Once you are certified, you can lose your certification if you fail to follow your state's rules. This can occur if you do not work in long-term care for a period of time or fail to get the required number of continuing education hours. You can also lose certification due to criminal activities, including abuse and neglect.

6. Describe continuing education

The federal government requires that nursing assistants have a 12-hour minimum of continuing education each year. Many states may require more. In-service continuing education courses help you keep your knowledge and skills fresh. Classes also give more information about certain conditions, challenges in working with residents, or regulation changes. You need to be up-to-date on the latest that is expected of you.

Your employer may be responsible for offering in-service courses. However, you are responsible for attending and completing them. You must do the following:

- Sign up for the course or find out where it is offered.

- Attend all class sessions.

- Pay attention and complete all the class requirements.

- Make the most of your in-service programs. Participate (Fig. 10-5).

Fig. 10-5. *Students should pay attention and participate during continuing education courses.*

- Keep original copies of all certificates and records of your successful attendance so you can prove you took the class.

7. Explain ways to manage stress

Stress is the state of being frightened, excited, confused, in danger, or irritated. It is often thought that only bad things cause stress. However, positive situations cause stress, too. For example, getting married or having a baby are usually positive situations. But both can bring enormous stress from the changes they bring to a person's life.

You may be thrilled when you get your new job. But starting work may also cause you stress. You may be afraid of making mistakes, excited about earning money or helping people, or confused about your new duties. Learning how to

recognize stress and what causes it is helpful. Then you can master a few simple methods for relaxing and learn to manage stress.

A **stressor** is something that causes stress. Anything can be a stressor. Some examples include the following:

- Divorce

- Marriage

- New baby

- Parenthood

- Children growing up

- Children leaving home

- Feeling unprepared for a task

- Starting a new job

- Problems at work

- New responsibilities at work

- Feeling unsupported at work (not enough guidance and resources)

- Losing a job

- Supervisors

- Coworkers

- Residents

- Illness

- Finances

Stress is not only an emotional response. It is also a physical response. When a person has stress, changes occur in the body. The endocrine system makes more of the hormone adrenaline. This can increase nervous system response, heart rate, respiratory rate, and blood pressure. This is why, in stressful situations, your heart beats fast, you breathe hard, and you may feel warm or perspire.

Each person has a different tolerance level for stress. What one person would find overwhelming might not bother another person. A person's tolerance for stress depends on his personality, life experiences, and physical health.

Guidelines: Managing Stress

To manage stress in your life, develop healthy dietary, exercise, and lifestyle habits:

G   Eat nutritious foods.

G   Exercise regularly (Fig. 10-6). You can exercise alone or with a partner.

Fig. 10-6. Regular exercise, such as walking, is one healthy way to decrease stress.

G   Get enough sleep.

G   Drink only in moderation.

G   Do not smoke.

G   Find time at least a few times a week to do something relaxing, such as reading a book or watching a movie.

Not managing stress can cause many problems. Some of these problems will affect how well you do your job. Signs that you are not managing stress include the following:

• Showing anger or being abusive to residents

• Arguing with your supervisor about assignments

• Having poor relationships with coworkers and residents

• Complaining about your job and your responsibilities

• Feeling work-related burnout (burnout is a state of mental or physical exhaustion caused by stress)

• Feeling tired even when you are rested

• Having trouble focusing on residents and procedures

Stress can seem overwhelming when you try to handle it yourself. Often just talking about stress can help you manage it better. Sometimes another person can offer helpful suggestions. You may think of new ways to handle stress just by talking it through with another person. Get help from one or more of these resources when managing stress:

• Your supervisor or another member of the care team for work-related stress

• Your family

• Your friends

• A support group

• Your place of worship

• Your doctor

• A local mental health agency

• Any phone hotline that deals with related problems (check the Internet)

It is not appropriate to talk to your residents or their family members to help you with your personal or job-related stress.

Developing a plan to manage stress can be helpful. The plan can include nice things you will do for yourself every day and things to do in stressful situations. Before making a plan, you first need to answer these questions:

• What are the sources of stress in my life?

• When do I most often feel stress?

• What effects of stress do I see in my life?

• What can I change to decrease my stress?

• What do I have to learn to cope with because I cannot change it?

When you have answered these questions, you will have a clearer picture of the challenges you face. Then you can come up with strategies for managing stress.

The Body Scan

Sometimes a relaxation exercise can help you feel refreshed and relaxed in only a short time. Below is a simple relaxation exercise. Try it out. See if it helps you feel more relaxed.

Close your eyes. Focus on your breathing and posture. Be sure you are comfortable. Starting at the balls of your feet, concentrate on your feet. Find any tension hidden in the feet. Try to relax and release the tension. Continue very slowly. Take a breath between each body part. Move up from the feet, focusing on and relaxing the legs, knees, thighs, hips, stomach, back, shoulders, neck, jaw, eyes, forehead, and scalp. Take a few very deep breaths. Open your eyes.

Look back over all you have learned in this program. Your work as a nursing assistant is very important. Every day may be different and challenging. In a hundred ways every week you will offer help that only a caring person like you can give.

Do not forget to value the work you have chosen to do (Fig. 10-7). It is important. Your work can mean the difference between living with independence and dignity and living without. The difference you make is sometimes life versus death. Look in the face of each of your residents. Know that you are doing important work. Look in a mirror when you get home. Be proud of how you make your living.

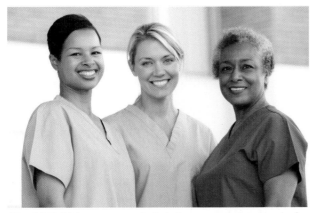

Fig. 10-7. *Value your work. It is important. Be proud of what you have chosen to do.*

Abbreviations

ā	before
ad lib	as desired
ADLs	activities of daily living
amb	ambulate, ambulatory
amt	amount
ap	apical
as tol	as tolerated
ax.	axillary (armpit)
BID, b.i.d.	two times a day
BM	bowel movement
BP, B/P	blood pressure
BPM	beats per minute
BRP	bathroom privileges
BSC	bedside commode
c̄	with
C	Centigrade
cath.	catheter
C. diff	*clostridium difficile*
CHF	congestive heart failure
c/o	complains of
COPD	chronic obstructive pulmonary disease
CPR	cardiopulmonary resuscitation
CVA	cerebrovascular accident, stroke
DAT	diet as tolerated
DNR	do not resuscitate
DOB	date of birth
DON	director of nursing
Dx, dx	diagnosis
F	Fahrenheit
FF	force fluids
ft	foot
H₂O	water
h, hr, hr.	hour
HBV	hepatitis B virus
HOB	head of bed
HS, hs	hours of sleep
ht	height
HTN	hypertension
hyper	above normal, too fast, rapid
hypo	low, less than normal
I&O	intake and output
inc	incontinent
isol	isolation
IV, I.V.	intravenous (within a vein)
lab	laboratory
lb.	pound
LTC	long-term care
meds	medications
mL	milliliter
mmHg	millimeters of mercury
MRSA	methicillin-resistant *Staphylococcus aureus*
N/A	not applicable
NKA	no known allergies
NPO	nothing by mouth
O₂	oxygen
OBRA	Omnibus Budget Reconciliation Act
OOB	out of bed
oz	ounce
p̄	after
peri care	perineal care
per os, PO	by mouth
PPE	personal protective equipment
p.r.n., prn	when necessary
q̄	every
q2h	every two hours
q3h	every three hours
q4h	every four hours
R	respirations, rectal
rehab	rehabilitation
RF	restrict fluids
ROM	range of motion
s̄	without
S&S, S/S	signs and symptoms
SOB	shortness of breath
spec.	specimen
stat	immediately
T., temp	temperature
TB	tuberculosis
TID, t.i.d.	three times a day
TPR	temperature, pulse, and respiration
UTI	urinary tract infection
VS, vs	vital signs
w/c, W/C	wheelchair
wt.	weight

Glossary

abdominal thrusts: method of attempting to remove an object from the airway of someone who is choking.

abduction: moving a body part away from the midline of the body.

abrasion: an injury that rubs off the surface of the skin.

abuse: purposeful mistreatment that causes physical, mental, or emotional pain or injury to someone.

active neglect: the purposeful failure to provide needed care, resulting in harm to a person.

activities of daily living (ADLs): daily personal care tasks such as bathing; caring for skin, nails, hair, and teeth; dressing; toileting; eating and drinking; walking; and transferring.

acute care: 24-hour skilled care for short-term illnesses or injuries; generally given in hospitals and ambulatory surgical centers.

adaptive devices: special equipment that helps a person who is ill or disabled to perform activities of daily living; also called *assistive devices*.

adduction: moving a body part toward the midline of the body.

adult day services: care for people who need some help during certain hours, but who do not live in the facility where care is given.

advance directives: legal documents that allow people to choose what medical care they wish to have if they are unable to make those decisions themselves.

affected side: a weakened side from a stroke or injury; also called *weaker* or *involved* side.

ageism: prejudice toward, stereotyping of, and/or discrimination against older persons or the elderly.

Alzheimer's disease: a progressive, incurable disease that causes tangled nerve fibers and protein deposits to form in the brain, eventually causing dementia.

ambulation: walking.

ambulatory: capable of walking.

amputation: the surgical removal of some or all of a body part, usually a hand, arm, leg, or foot.

angina pectoris: chest pain, pressure, or discomfort.

antimicrobial: an agent that destroys, resists, or prevents the development of pathogens.

anxiety: uneasiness or fear, often about a situation or condition.

apathy: a lack of interest.

aspiration: the inhalation of food, fluid or foreign material into the lungs.

assault: a threat to harm a person, resulting in the person feeling fearful that he or she will be harmed.

assisted living: residences for people who do not need skilled, 24-hour care, but do require some help with daily care.

assistive devices: special equipment that helps a person who is ill or disabled to perform activities of daily living; also called *adaptive devices*.

atrophy: the wasting away, decreasing in size, and weakening of muscles from lack of use.

autoimmune illness: an illness in which the body's immune system attacks normal tissue in the body.

battery: the intentional touching of a person without his or her consent.

bipolar disorder: a type of depression that causes a person to swing from periods of deep depression to periods of extreme activity; also called *manic-depressive illness*.

bloodborne pathogens: microorganisms found in human blood, body fluid, draining wounds, and mucous membranes that can cause infection and disease in humans.

body mechanics: the way the parts of the body work together when a person moves.

bony prominences: areas of the body where the bone lies close to the skin.

brachial pulse: the pulse located inside the elbow, about one to one-and-a-half inches above the elbow.

cardiopulmonary resuscitation (CPR): medical procedures used when a person's heart or lungs have stopped working.

care plan: a plan developed for each resident to achieve certain goals; it outlines the steps and tasks that the care team must perform.

catastrophic reaction: reacting to something in an unreasonable, exaggerated way.

catheter: a thin tube inserted into the body to drain or inject fluids.

causative agent: a pathogenic microorganism that causes disease.

Centers for Disease Control and Prevention (CDC): a government agency under the U.S. Department of Health and Human Services that issues information to protect the health of individuals and communities.

cerebrovascular accident (CVA): a condition that occurs when blood supply to a part of the brain is blocked or a blood vessel leaks or ruptures within the brain; also called *stroke*.

chain of command: the line of authority within a facility.

chain of infection: way of describing how disease is transmitted from one being to another.

charting: documenting important information and observations about residents.

Cheyne-Stokes: alternating periods of slow, irregular breathing and rapid, shallow breathing.

chronic: long-term or long-lasting.

cite: in a long-term care facility, to find a problem through a survey.

claustrophobia: the fear of being in a confined space.

clean: in health care, a condition in which objects are not contaminated with pathogens.

clean-catch specimen: a urine specimen that does not include the first and last urine voided; also called *mid-stream specimen*.

clichés: phrases that are used over and over again and do not really mean anything.

closed bed: a bed completely made with the bedspread and blankets in place.

***Clostridium difficile* (C. diff, C. difficile):** bacterial illness that can cause diarrhea and colitis.

cognition: the ability to think logically and clearly.

cognitive: related to thinking and learning.

cognitive impairment: loss of ability to think logically; concentration and memory are affected.

combative: violent or hostile behavior.

combustion: the process of burning.

communication: the process of exchanging information with others by sending and receiving messages.

compassionate: caring, concerned, considerate, empathetic, and understanding.

condom catheter: catheter that has an attachment on the end that fits onto the penis; also called *external* or *Texas catheter*.

confidentiality: the legal and ethical principle of keeping information private.

confusion: the inability to think clearly.

conscientious: guided by a sense of right and wrong; principled.

conscious: the state of being mentally alert and having awareness of surroundings, sensations, and thoughts.

constipation: the inability to eliminate stool, or the infrequent, difficult, and often painful elimination of a hard, dry stool.

constrict: to narrow.

contracture: the permanent and often painful shortening of a muscle or tendon, usually due to lack of activity.

cultural diversity: the different groups of people with varied backgrounds and experiences who live together in the world.

culture: a system of learned behaviors, practiced by a group of people, that is considered to be the tradition of that people and is passed on from one generation to the next.

culture change: a term given to the process of transforming services for elders so that they are based on the values and practices of the person receiving care; core values include choice, dignity, respect, self-determination, and purposeful living.

cyanotic: skin that is blue or gray.

dangle: to sit up with the legs hanging over the side of the bed in order to regain balance and stabilize blood pressure.

defense mechanisms: unconscious behaviors used to release tension or cope with stress.

dehydration: a serious condition that results from inadequate fluid in the body.

delirium: a state of severe confusion that occurs suddenly and is usually temporary.

delusions: false beliefs.

dementia: the serious loss of mental abilities, such as thinking, remembering, reasoning, and communicating.

dentures: artificial teeth.

developmental disabilities: disabilities that are present at birth or emerge during childhood that restrict physical or mental ability.

diabetes: a condition in which the pancreas produces too little insulin or does not properly use insulin.

diabetic ketoacidosis (DKA): a complication of diabetes that is caused by having too little insulin; also called *hyperglycemia*.

diagnoses: physicians' determinations of an illness.

diastolic: second measurement of blood pressure; phase when the heart relaxes or rests.

digestion: the process of preparing food physically and chemically so that it can be absorbed into the cells.

dilate: to widen.

direct contact: a way of transmitting pathogens through touching the infected person or his or her secretions.

dirty: in health care, a condition in which objects have been contaminated with pathogens.

disinfection: process that kills pathogens, but not all pathogens; it reduces the pathogen count to a level that is considered not infectious.

disorientation: confusion about person, place, or time.

disposable: only to be used once and then discarded.

disposable razor: type of razor that is discarded after one use; requires the use of shaving cream or soap.

diuretics: medications that reduce fluid volume in the body.

doff: to remove.

domestic violence: physical, sexual, or emotional abuse by spouses, intimate partners, or family members.

don: to put on.

do-not-resuscitate (DNR): a type of advance directive that instructs medical professionals not to perform CPR if a person's heartbeat or breathing stops.

dorsiflexion: bending backward.

draw sheet: an extra sheet placed on top of the bottom sheet; used for moving residents in bed.

durable power of attorney for health care: a signed, dated, and witnessed legal document that appoints someone else to make the medical decisions for a person in the event he or she becomes unable to do so.

dysphagia: difficulty swallowing.

dyspnea: difficulty breathing.

edema: swelling caused by excess fluid in body tissues.

electric razor: type of razor that runs on electricity; does not require the use of soap or shaving cream.

elimination: the process of expelling solid wastes (made up of the waste products of food) that are not absorbed into the cells.

elope: in medicine, when a person with Alzheimer's disease wanders away from a protected area and does not return.

embolism: an obstruction of a blood vessel, usually by a blood clot.

emesis: the act of vomiting, or ejecting stomach contents through the mouth and/or nose.

emotional lability: laughing or crying without any reason or when it is inappropriate.

empathy: identifying with the feelings of others.

enema: a specific amount of water, with or without an additive, that is introduced into the colon to stimulate the elimination of stool.

ergonomics: the science of designing equipment, areas, and work tasks to make them safer and to suit the worker's abilities.

ethics: the knowledge of right and wrong.

expiration: exhaling air out of the lungs.

expressive aphasia: trouble communicating thoughts through speech or writing.

extension: straightening a body part.

false imprisonment: unlawful restraint that affects a person's freedom of movement; includes both the threat of being physically restrained and actually being physically restrained.

fecal incontinence: the inability to control the bowels, leading to involuntary passage of stool.

financial abuse: the improper or illegal use of a person's money, possessions, property, or other assets.

first aid: emergency care given immediately to an injured person.

flammable: easily ignited and capable of burning quickly.

flexion: bending a body part.

fluid balance: taking in and eliminating equal amounts of fluid.

fluid overload: a condition that occurs when the body cannot handle the amount of fluid consumed.

foot drop: a weakness of muscles in the feet and ankles that causes problems with the ability to flex the ankles and walk normally.

force fluids (FF): a medical order to encourage a person to drink more fluids.

Fowler's: a semi-sitting body position in which a person's head and shoulders are elevated 45 to 60 degrees.

fracture: a broken bone.

fracture pan: a bedpan that is flatter than a regular bedpan.

full weight-bearing (FWB): a doctor's order stating that a person has the ability to support full body weight (100%) on both legs.

gait: manner of walking.

gait belt: a belt made of canvas or other heavy material used to help people who are weak, unsteady, or uncoordinated to stand, sit, or walk; also called *transfer belt*.

gastrostomy: a surgically-created opening into the stomach that allows insertion of a tube.

gestational diabetes: type of diabetes that appears in pregnant women who have never had diabetes before but who have high glucose levels during pregnancy.

glands: organs that produce and secrete chemicals called hormones.

glucose: natural sugar.

gonads: sex glands.

grief: deep distress or sorrow over a loss.

grooming: practices to care for oneself, such as caring for fingernails and hair.

hallucinations: seeing, hearing, smelling, tasting, or feeling things that are not there.

hand hygiene: washing hands with either plain or antiseptic soap and water and using alcohol-based hand rubs.

hat: in health care, a collection container that is sometimes inserted into a toilet to collect and measure urine or stool.

healthcare-associated infection (HAI): an infection acquired within a healthcare setting during the delivery of medical care.

Health Insurance Portability and Accountability Act (HIPAA): a federal law that requires health information be kept private and secure and that organizations must take special steps to protect this information.

hemiparesis: weakness on one side of the body.

hemiplegia: paralysis on one side of the body.

hepatitis: inflammation of the liver caused by certain viruses and other factors, such as alcohol abuse, some medications, and trauma.

hoarding: collecting and putting things away in a guarded way.

holistic care: a type of care that involves caring for the whole person—the mind as well as the body.

home health care: care that is provided in a person's home.

homeostasis: the condition in which all of the body's systems are working at their best.

hormones: chemical substances created by the body that control numerous body functions.

hospice care: holistic, compassionate care given to dying people and their families.

hygiene: practices to keep bodies clean and healthy.

hypertension (HTN): high blood pressure, measuring 140/90 or higher.

impairment: a loss of function or ability.

incident: an accident, problem, or unexpected event during the course of care that is not part of the normal routine in a healthcare facility.

incontinence: the inability to control the bladder or bowels.

indirect contact: a way of transmitting pathogens by touching something contaminated by the infected person.

indwelling catheter: a type of catheter that remains inside the bladder for a period of time; urine drains into a bag.

infection: the state resulting from pathogens invading the body and multiplying.

infection prevention: the set of methods practiced in healthcare facilities to prevent and control the spread of disease.

infectious: contagious.

inflammation: swelling.

informed consent: the process in which a person, with the help of a doctor, makes informed decisions about his or her health care.

input: the fluid a person consumes; also called *intake*.

inspiration: breathing in.

insulin: a hormone that converts glucose into energy for the body.

insulin reaction: complication of diabetes that can result from either too much insulin or too little food; also known as *hypoglycemia*.

intake: the fluid a person consumes; also called *input*.

intravenous (IV): into a vein.

intravenous (IV) therapy: the delivery of medication, nutrition, or fluids through a person's vein.

involuntary seclusion: the separation of a person from others against the person's will.

involved: term used to refer to the weaker, or affected, side of the body after a stroke or injury.

lateral: body position in which a person is lying on either side.

laws: rules set by the government to help people live peacefully together and to ensure order and safety.

length of stay: the number of days a person stays in a healthcare facility.

liability: a legal term that means someone can be held responsible for harming someone else.

living will: a document that outlines the medical care a person wants, or does not want, in case he or she becomes unable to make those decisions.

localized infection: an infection that is limited to a specific location in the body and has local symptoms.

logrolling: moving a person as a unit, without disturbing the alignment of the body.

long-term care (LTC): care given in long-term care facilities for people who need 24-hour, skilled care.

major depressive disorder: a type of depression that causes withdrawal, lack of energy, and loss of interest in activities, as well as other symptoms; also called *major depression*.

malpractice: injury to a person due to professional misconduct through negligence, carelessness, or lack of skill.

masturbation: to touch or rub sexual organs in order to give oneself or another person sexual pleasure.

Medicaid: a medical assistance program for people with low incomes, as well as for people with disabilities.

medical asepsis: refers to practices such as handwashing that reduce, remove, and control the spread of microorganisms.

Medicare: a federal health insurance program for people who are 65 or older, are disabled, or are ill and cannot work.

menopause: the end of menstruation.

mental health: the normal functioning of emotional and intellectual abilities.

mental illness: a disorder that affects a person's ability to function at a normal level in the family, home, or community.

metabolism: physical and chemical processes by which substances are produced or broken down into energy or products for use by the body.

microbe: a living thing or organism that is so small that it can be seen only under a microscope; also called *microorganism*.

microorganism (MO): a living thing or organism that is so small that it can be seen only under a microscope; also called *microbe*.

Minimum Data Set (MDS): a detailed form with guidelines for assessing residents in long-term care facilities; also details what to do if resident problems are identified.

mode of transmission: the method of describing how a pathogen travels.

modified diets: diets for people who have certain illnesses; also called *special* or *therapeutic diets.*

MRSA (methicillin-resistant *Staphylococcus aureus*): an infection caused by specific bacteria that have become resistant to many antibiotics.

mucous membranes: the membranes that line body cavities that open to the outside of the body, such as the linings of the mouth, nose, eyes, rectum, or genitals.

nasogastric tube: a feeding tube that is inserted into the nose and goes to the stomach.

neglect: the failure to provide needed care that results in physical, mental, or emotional harm to a person.

negligence: actions, or the failure to act or provide the proper care, that result in unintended injury to a person.

non-intact skin: skin that is broken by abrasions, cuts, rashes, acne, pimples, lesions, surgical incisions, or boils.

nonverbal communication: communicating without using words.

non-weight-bearing (NWB): a doctor's order stating that a person is unable to touch the floor or support any body weight on one or both legs.

NPO (nothing by mouth): medical order to withhold all food and fluids taken orally.

nutrient: a substance that is necessary for growth and life; it provides energy, promotes growth and health, and helps regulate metabolism.

nutrition: how the body uses food to maintain health.

objective information: information based on what a person sees, hears, touches, or smells; also called *signs.*

obsessive compulsive disorder (OCD): an anxiety disorder characterized by obsessive behavior or thoughts.

obstructed airway: a condition in which the tube through which air enters the lungs is blocked.

Occupational Safety and Health Administration (OSHA): a federal government agency that makes rules to protect workers from hazards on the job.

occupied bed: a bed made while a person is in the bed.

ombudsman: a legal advocate for residents in long-term care facilities; helps resolve disputes and settle conflicts.

Omnibus Budget Reconciliation Act (OBRA): law passed by the federal government that includes minimum standards for nursing assistant training, staffing requirements, resident assessment instructions, and information on rights for residents.

open bed: a bed made with linen folded down to the foot of the bed.

opposition: touching the thumb to any other finger.

oral care: care of the mouth, teeth, and gums.

orthosis: a device that helps support and align a limb and improve its functioning; also called *orthotic device.*

orthotic device: a device that helps support and align a limb and improve its functioning; also called *orthosis.*

osteoarthritis: common type of arthritis that usually affects the hips, knees, fingers, thumbs, and spine; also called *degenerative joint disease (DJD)* or *degenerative arthritis.*

osteoporosis: a disease that causes bones to become porous and brittle, causing them to break easily.

ostomy: a surgically-created opening from an area inside the body to the outside.

outpatient care: care given for less than 24 hours for people who have had treatment or surgery and need short-term skilled care.

output: all fluid that is eliminated from the body; includes fluid in urine, feces, vomitus, and perspiration, moisture that is exhaled in the air, and wound drainage.

oxygen therapy: the administration of oxygen to increase the supply of oxygen to the lungs.

pacing: walking back and forth in the same area.

palliative care: care that focuses on the comfort and dignity of the person, rather than on curing him or her.

panic disorder: a disorder in which a person has repeated episodes of intense fear that something bad will occur.

paraplegia: loss of function of lower body and legs.

partial bath: a bath given on days when a complete bath or shower is not done; includes washing the face, hands, underarms, and perineum.

partial weight-bearing (PWB): a doctor's order stating that a person is able to support some body weight on one or both legs.

passive neglect: the unintentional failure to provide needed care, resulting in physical, mental, or emotional harm to a person.

pathogens: microorganisms that are capable of causing infection and disease.

pediculosis: an infestation of lice.

percutaneous endoscopic gastrostomy (PEG) tube: a feeding tube placed through the abdominal wall into the stomach.

perineal care: care of the genitals and anal area.

perineum: the genital and anal area.

perseveration: the repetition of words, phrases, questions, or actions.

personal: relating to life outside one's job, such as family, friends, and home life.

personal protective equipment (PPE): equipment that helps protect employees from serious workplace injuries or illnesses resulting from contact with workplace hazards.

person-directed care: a type of care that places the emphasis on the person needing care and his or her individuality and capabilities.

phantom limb pain: pain in a limb (or extremity) that has been amputated.

phantom sensation: warmth, itching, or tingling in a body part that has been amputated.

phobia: an intense form of anxiety or fear.

physical abuse: any treatment, intentional or not, that causes harm to a person's body.

pillaging: taking things that belong to someone else.

policy: a course of action that should be taken every time a certain situation occurs.

portable commode: a chair with a toilet seat and a removable container underneath that is used for elimination; also called *bedside commode.*

portal of entry: any body opening on an uninfected person that allows pathogens to enter.

portal of exit: any body opening on an infected person that allows pathogens to leave.

positioning: the act of helping people into positions that promote comfort and health.

postmortem care: care of the body after death.

post-traumatic stress disorder (PTSD): an anxiety disorder caused by a traumatic experience.

posture: the way a person holds and positions his body.

pre-diabetes: a condition that occurs when a person's blood glucose levels are above normal but are not high enough for a diagnosis of type 2 diabetes.

pressure points: areas of the body that bear much of its weight.

pressure ulcer: a serious wound resulting from skin breakdown; also called *pressure sore*, *bed sore*, or *decubitus ulcer*.

procedure: a method, or way, of doing something.

professional: having to do with work or a job.

professionalism: how a person behaves when he is on the job; it includes how a person dresses, the words he uses, and the things he talks about.

pronation: turning downward.

prone: body position in which a person is lying on his stomach, or front side of the body.

prosthesis: a device that replaces a body part that is missing or deformed because of an accident, injury, illness, or birth defect; used to improve a person's ability to function and/or his appearance.

protected health information(PHI): a person's private health information, which includes name, address, telephone number, social security number, email address, and medical record number.

psychological abuse: emotional harm caused by threatening, scaring, humiliating, intimidating, isolating, or insulting a person, or by treating him as a child; also includes verbal abuse.

psychosocial needs: needs that involve social interaction, emotions, intellect, and spirituality.

psychotherapy: a method of treating mental illness that involves talking about one's problems with mental health professionals.

puree: to blend or grind food into a thick paste of baby food consistency.

quadriplegia: loss of function of legs, trunk, and arms.

radial pulse: the pulse located on the inside of the wrist, where the radial artery runs just beneath the skin.

range of motion (ROM): exercises that put a joint through its full arc of motion.

receptive aphasia: difficulty understanding spoken or written words.

rehabilitation: care that is given by specialists to help restore or improve function after an illness or injury.

reproduce: to create new human life.

reservoir: a place where a pathogen lives and grows.

Residents' Rights: numerous rights identified in the OBRA law that relate to how residents must be treated while living in a facility; they provide an ethical code of conduct for healthcare workers.

respiration: the process of breathing air into the lungs and exhaling air out of the lungs.

restraint: a physical or chemical way to restrict voluntary movement or behavior.

restraint alternatives: any intervention used in place of a restraint or that reduces the need for a restraint.

restraint-free care: an environment in which restraints are not kept or used for any reason.

restrict fluids (RF): a medical order to limit the amount of fluids a person drinks to the level set by the doctor.

rheumatoid arthritis: a type of arthritis in which joints become inflamed, red, swollen, and very painful, resulting in restricted movement and possible deformities.

rotation: turning a joint.

routine urine specimen: a urine specimen that can be collected any time a person voids.

safety razor: a type of razor that has a sharp blade with a special safety casing to help prevent cuts; requires the use of shaving cream or soap.

scalds: burns caused by hot liquids.

schizophrenia: a form of mental illness that affects a person's ability to think, communicate, make decisions, and understand reality.

scope of practice: defines the tasks that healthcare providers are legally allowed to do and how to do them correctly.

sexual abuse: the forcing of a person to perform or participate in sexual acts against his or her will; includes unwanted touching, exposing oneself, and the sharing of pornographic material.

sexual harassment: any unwelcome sexual advance or behavior that creates an intimidating, hostile, or offensive working environment.

sharps: needles or other sharp objects.

shearing: rubbing or friction that results from the skin moving one way and the bone underneath it remaining fixed or moving in the opposite direction.

shock: a condition that occurs when organs and tissues in the body do not receive an adequate blood supply.

Sims': body position in which a person is lying on his left side with the upper knee flexed and raised toward the chest.

skilled care: medically necessary care given by a skilled nurse or therapist.

special diets: diets for people who have certain illnesses; also called *therapeutic* or *modified diets*.

specimen: a sample that is used for analysis in order to try to make a diagnosis.

sputum: thick mucus coughed up from the lungs.

Standard Precautions: a method of infection prevention in which all blood, body fluids, non-intact skin, and mucous membranes are treated as if they were infected with an infectious disease.

sterilization: a method used to decrease the spread of pathogens and disease by destroying all microorganisms, including those that form spores.

stoma: an artificial opening in the body.

straight catheter: a catheter that does not remain inside the person; it is removed immediately after urine is drained or collected.

stress: the state of being frightened, excited, confused, in danger, or irritated.

stressor: something that causes stress.

subacute care: care given in a hospital or in a long-term care facility for people who need less care than for an acute illness, but more care than for a chronic illness.

subjective information: information that a person cannot or did not observe, but is based on something reported to the person that may or may not be true; also called *symptoms*.

substance abuse: the repeated use of legal or illegal drugs, cigarettes, or alcohol in a way that is harmful to oneself or others.

sundowning: becoming restless and agitated in the late afternoon, evening, or night.

supination: turning upward.

supine: body position in which a person lies flat on his back.

suppository: a medication given rectally to cause a bowel movement.

surgical asepsis: the state of being free of all microorganisms; also called *sterile technique*.

susceptible host: an uninfected person who could get sick.

sympathy: sharing in the feelings and difficulties of others.

systemic infection: an infection that is in the bloodstream and is spread throughout the body, causing general symptoms.

systolic: first measurement of blood pressure; phase when the heart is at work, contracting and pushing the blood from the left ventricle of the heart.

tactful: showing sensitivity and having a sense of what is appropriate when dealing with others.

terminal illness: a disease or condition that will eventually cause death.

therapeutic diets: diets for people who have certain illnesses; also called *special* or *modified diets*.

total parenteral nutrition (TPN): the intravenous infusion of nutrients administered directly into the bloodstream, bypassing the digestive system.

transfer belt: a belt made of canvas or other heavy material that is used to help people who are weak, unsteady, or uncoordinated to stand, sit, or walk; also called *gait belt*.

transient ischemic attack (TIA): a warning sign of a CVA/stroke resulting from a temporary lack of oxygen in the brain; symptoms may last up to 24 hours.

transmission: passage or transfer.

Transmission-Based Precautions: method of infection prevention used when caring for persons who are infected or suspected of being infected with a disease.

tuberculosis (TB): a highly contagious lung disease caused by a bacterium that is carried on mucous droplets suspended in the air.

tumor: a cluster of abnormally-growing cells.

unoccupied bed: a bed made while no person is in the bed.

urinary catheter: a thin tube inserted into the bladder in order to drain or collect urine.

urinary incontinence: the inability to control the bladder, which leads to an involuntary loss of urine.

validating: giving value to or approving.

verbal abuse: the use of spoken or written words, pictures, or gestures that threaten, embarrass, or insult a person.

verbal communication: communication involving the use of spoken or written words or sounds.

vital signs: measurements—temperature, pulse, respirations, blood pressure, pain level—that monitor the functioning of the vital organs of the body.

void: urinate.

VRE (vancomycin-resistant *enterococcus*): bacteria (*enterococci*) that have developed resistance to antibiotics as a result of being exposed to the antibiotic vancomycin.

wandering: walking aimlessly around the facility or facility grounds.

workplace violence: verbal, physical, or sexual abuse of staff by other staff members, residents, or visitors.

Index